Guide to Healing Chronic Pain is not only an absolute must-read for anyone suffering from chronic pain, but also for anyone wanting to stay perfectly healthy for the rest of his or her life. In the book, Dr. Karen Kan has set a new precedent of health care for Western physicians to follow in the 21st century and beyond. Taking the reader on a thorough exploration of drug-free, innovative, and alternative medicine modalities such as infrared nanotechnology patches (acupuncture without needles), grounding, energy healing, nutritional therapy, Qi and nervous system balancing, detoxification, and EMF pollution shielding, Dr. Kan synthesizes ancient Eastern healing techniques with cutting-edge science. A medical doctor, spiritual teacher, energy healer, and law of attraction authority, Dr. Kan's balanced "Spirit-Mind-Body" approach to healing chronic pain is not only revolutionary but is exactly what is needed now in Western medicine. Dr. Karen Kan is indeed a role model for the Next Human physician.

Jason Lincoln Jeffers, Spiritual Teacher,
Author of The Next Human
www.JasonLincolnJeffers.com

Karen Kan is a brilliant M.D. who is also a true healer—an unusual combination! In her new book, "Guide to Healing Chronic Pain," she has brought together decades of study and a practical approach to the relief of suffering. If you're in pain, order this book and read it. You'll learn dozens of techniques to bring about changes in your physical, emotional, mental, and spiritual bodies. Engage in some of the many practices she offers, and you'll experience transformation and healing. Her encyclopedic knowledge of the body and medicine is put into practical, usable terms. She brings in every approach to the problem, so if one doesn't work for you, another one will. This book is a work of genius.

Lion Goodman, Author of Creating on Purpose
and Creator of the BeliefCloset
www.BeliefCloset.com

Not only has Dr. Kan put together a comprehensive, user-friendly resource for a variety of well—proven healing modalities, but she totally honors the journey of illness and pain—something that many holistic practitioners shy away from. She invites you into how to lovingly taking responsibility for your pain, but not from the perspective of guilt and judgment. Rather, she leads you into a beautiful, practical, exploration of what your pain can teach you, and how to remain present and joyful, despite the daily challenges of living with chronic pain. What a gift!

Patricia Lee Jones,
Founder of Healing Adventures and KIA Reiki™
www.HealingAdventures.com

Fabulous! Enlightening! As I read through Dr. Kan's Guide to Healing Chronic Pain—A Holistic Approach, I had so many "Aha's!" pop into my mind. I'm no stranger to chronic pain and I sorely (pun intended) wish I had a comprehensive guide like this one years ago. This book is truly a gift to anyone suffering from pain who doesn't want to take drugs. This is a must-read!

Keith Leon, Book Mentor and Bestselling Author of
Who Do You Think You Are? Discover the Purpose of Your Life
www.BakeYourBook.com

When your health is failing, when you're experiencing chronic pain, or when you learn of a new affliction stealing your wellness away, even if it's just to learn that you must begin to take steps to avoid the loss of your health, it is natural in this day and age to turn to the internet, books and other sources of authority to learn all that you can. Indeed, this is not peculiar behavior for a loved one or caretaker to indulge in. The seeker quickly discovers that there is no dearth of information about wellness, or limit to the advice including contradictory opinions, available. What we all seek in circumstances of this kind is a complete approach from a reliable source whose advice treats us as whole human beings instead of some mechanical assembly of parts knitted together like gears and wheels. Enter Dr. Karen Kan and her ground breaking work, "Guide to Healing Chronic Pain: A Holistic Approach." I cannot recommend this book too strongly to anyone seeking relief from illness and pain! Dr. Kan addresses the subject from beginning to end in straight forward easy-to-understand language, and she offers a number of alternative methods that have been proven effective that may avoid expensive drugs and other interdictions with potentially frightening contraindications. You owe it to yourself to read this book before you need to!

Eldon Taylor, Ph.D.,FAPA,
New York Times Bestselling Author of Choices and Illusions
www.EldonTaylor.com

Wow. What a valuable God-Send resource this is! So full of wisdom and insightful gems!! I personally appreciate Chapter 29: 'Not all psychics are good intuitives . . . A well-trained professional intuitive . . . is someone who reads energy accurately, but also knows how to communicate the information appropriately to best serve the client's highest interest.'—I'll definitely be recommending your work to many of my clients, my friend!

The Corporate Woo-Woo™, Michelle Skaletski-Boyd, C.Ht.,
Named one of the Best Psychic Mediums in the Nation
www.Soul-Felt.com

Guide to Healing Chronic Pain

A Holistic Approach

Karen Kan, MD

BALBOA.
PRESS

A DIVISION OF HAY HOUSE

Balboa Press books may be ordered through booksellers or by contacting:

Balboa Press
A Division of Hay House
1663 Liberty Drive
Bloomington, IN 47403
www.balboapress.com
1-(877) 407-4847

Because of the dynamic nature of the Internet, any web addresses or links contained in this book may have changed since publication and may no longer be valid. The views expressed in this work are solely those of the author and do not necessarily reflect the views of the publisher, and the publisher hereby disclaims any responsibility for them.

The author of this book does not dispense medical advice or prescribe the use of any technique as a form of treatment for physical, emotional, or medical problems without the advice of a physician, either directly or indirectly. The intent of the author is only to offer information of a general nature to help you in your quest for emotional and spiritual well-being. In the event you use any of the information in this book for yourself, which is your constitutional right, the author and the publisher assume no responsibility for your actions.

Any people depicted in stock imagery provided by Thinkstock or Fotolia are models, and such images are being used for illustrative purposes only.

Certain stock imagery © Thinkstock.

ISBN: 978-1-4525-7407-3 (sc)
ISBN: 978-1-4525-7408-0 (hc)
ISBN: 978-1-4525-7409-7 (e)

Library of Congress Control Number: 2013908336

Printed in the United States of America.

Balboa Press rev. date: 06/06/2013

FREE TIPS AND TRAINING . . .

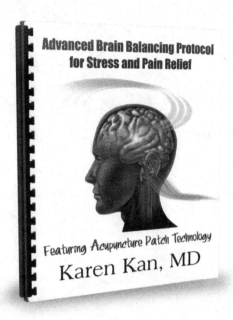

*Please kindly review this book on Amazon
and let me know how it helped you!*

Subscribe to receive additional holistic health tips, instructional videos mentioned in this book, and a free copy of my Advanced Brain Balancing Protocol for Stress and Pain Relief:

www.KarenKan.com/bookbonus

DEDICATION

To my mom, whose health challenges inspired me to become a healer and dedicate my life to helping others. Her belief in me has fueled my dreams.

To my dad, who encouraged me not to give up on science in high school despite my first miserable year. Because of the compassionate way he counseled me, I took another year of science and fell in love with it. If it wasn't for him, I would never have become a doctor.

To my patients, whose lives have touched me in ways that have opened my heart.

Lastly, to my dear partner, James, whose unwavering love and support has made it possible for me to do what I love.

DISCLAIMER

The purpose of this book is to empower people to heal their chronic pain without the use of drugs or surgery. The information in this book represents the personal observations, research, and experiences of Dr. Karen Kan. You, the reader, must take 100% responsibility for your own health, physically, emotionally and mentally.

This book is not intended to be a substitute for the services of a qualified health care professional. Neither the author nor the publisher is responsible for any consequences incurred by those employing the treatments or remedies discussed or taught in this book. Any application of the material set forth in the following pages is at the reader's discretion and is his or her sole responsibility.

The information contained in this book is intended for personal use and should not be considered professional training. No representation contained in these materials is intended as medical advice and should not be used for the diagnosis or medical treatment of diseases. The stories in this book are all true, but the names have been changed in most circumstances to protect privacy.

TABLE OF CONTENTS

FOREWORD

During my neurosurgical residency, I was appalled that the methods of choice for helping patients with chronic pain included cutting the front half of the spinal cord or destroying the frontal lobes (lobotomy). This had been the preferred approach for over 30 years. I discovered that cordotomy, cutting the front half of the spinal cord, had a complication rate of 130%:

- 100% of the patients would never have another sexual orgasm
- 10% would become paralyzed on one side of the body
- 10% would lose bladder and bowel control
- 10% would develop a new pain far worse than their original problem-post-cordotomy syndrome-for which there was no treatment!

And lobotomy destroyed the personality forever! The only other approach, narcotics and tranquilizers, destroyed the personality almost as much as lobotomy.

Shealy, C.N., Borgmeyer, V. and Thomlinson, P. (2004) Reduction of free radicals by electrical stimulation of specific acupuncture points. *Subtle Energies & Energy Medicine*, Vol. 13, No. 3, pp. 251-259

As I finished my residency and joined the faculty at Western Reserve Medical School, I dreamed of finding a non-destructive approach to chronic pain. Over a three year period I proved my theory that we could control pain by stimulating the dorsal columns of the spinal cord (DCS), the back part of the spine, and later by electrically stimulating various areas on the skin—Transcutaneous Electrical Nerve Stimulation, TENS. Both are now used world-wide. Although DCS certainly can be considered in difficult cases, I quickly decided that even though it carries a small surgical risk, it should be undertaken ONLY in extreme circumstances. I knew very early that patients with extreme anxiety and depression, often worsened by narcotics and tranquilizers, were not candidates for another surgical procedure. I ruled out 94% of the 400 patients sent to me each year for DCS!

In 1971, I started a Behavioral Modification program for Pain Rehabilitation. Within a year, I had a 75% success rate in the first 400 patients. I then learned about Autogenic Training and Biofeedback, incorporated them into the program, and soon achieved an 85% success rate in patients who had failed every known conventional approach. This program led me in 1978 to found the American Holistic Medical Association, joined within two years by the American Holistic Nurses Association.

Over the years I treated well over 30,000 chronic pain patients, using the broadest possible holistic approach, with an ongoing success rate of 85%. The major reason for developing Holism was to reincorporate the Spiritual component to healing. Three hundred years ago, "Science" rejected everything spiritual and most things emotional! Fortunately in the 1960's, Humanistic Psychology and Transpersonal Psychology opened the door to reintroduce the critical role of all things Spiritual.

I am delighted to recommend Dr. Karen Kan's Holistic approach to help you achieve pain relief, safely and efficiently! We have come a long way and this book offers you the benefits of our last fifty years of scientific progress, the return of common sense and the role of Spirit in our essential well-being.

C. Norman Shealy, M.D., Ph.D.

President, Holos Institutes of Health
Professor Emeritus of Energy Medicine
President Emeritus Holos University Graduate Seminary
www.normshealy.com
www.holosuniversity.org

PREFACE

Even Smart People Get Sick

It was the summer of 2002. I was teaching at UCLA and my husband was a molecular biologist. Disillusioned with "big city" life and job politics, my husband decided we should move back to a small town to build our eco-friendly passive solar dream home. Being an idealist and dreamer, I had no idea how much energy was required to build a home nor the financial stress involved in funding the project alone.

We moved from a modest three-bedroom house in Los Angeles to a one-bedroom apartment in our neighbor's basement. Our computer and office equipment were crammed into the bedroom and we slept on the floor on a futon. I've never been a morning person so my wake-up partner was a "sunrise" clock, an expensive device whose light mimicked a rising sun. Its large transformer resting on the floor was just inches from my head.

I accepted the first job I was offered in order to fund the "dream" project. It required a two-hour daily commute through slick mountainous roads and carried an enormous responsibility of being the only medical doctor in town. Eventually, I started my own part-time acupuncture practice as well, so I could be closer to home. On weekends, I'd try to help out with the house-building-not my forte, but my idealism fueled the effort. Pride prevented me from admitting that the stress of moving across country, being the main breadwinner, working two jobs, and house-building was taking a toll on my body.

My parents were dead-set against our plans because they knew building this "dream home" was too much for me. Their protective criticism only served to fortify my stubbornness to make this dream come true. In my mind, I was a responsible loving wife who would do whatever it took to make her husband happy. *Bad idea!*

As I juggled the demands of my new life, I wasn't aware my body was falling apart from the inside out. One morning, I woke up and couldn't turn my head. The intense pain in my neck was unyielding and multiple visits to the chiropractor didn't help. Within two months, my condition rapidly deteriorated and I experienced pain in almost every joint. I required twelve to fourteen hours of sleep per night and never felt rested. I dragged myself to work, put on a smiling face for people who "needed me", and then collapsed on the couch as soon as I got home.

My husband, already stressed from building all day and worrying about finances, had to pick up the pieces at home. I couldn't cook, clean or do laundry without intense pain or exhaustion. One day at the Laundromat, while folding a bed sheet, I burst into tears from pain and exhaustion. I wondered, "Where have I gone wrong? I'm trying so hard. I'm a good person. I don't deserve this!"

One of my medical colleagues was kind enough to treat me free of charge. Dorit Gaedtke, M.D. diagnosed me with fibromyalgia, an "incurable" and debilitating pain disorder. Most of my patients with this diagnosis never recovered despite the slew of anti-depressants and pain drugs I prescribed in conventional medicine. Not only did they suffer pain and fatigue, they suffered the side effects of the drugs and remained disabled. Few had the education or financial resources to seek alternative care. Deep down inside, I was terrified I would become another statistic.

My mother struggled with fibromyalgia so I wasn't completely surprised to have the same diagnosis. Nevertheless, I felt defeated and small. My naïve medical mind thought that someone who was as hardworking and smart as I, could never fall prey to such a nebulous pain disorder. But I was wrong.

Even smart people get sick.

Healing is a Journey

Good news! You don't have to suffer any longer. If you are reading this book, it's likely you are tired of being in pain. Maybe now, healing yourself is your top priority. I know it is for me.

Years have passed since that dreaded diagnosis of fibromyalgia. Thanks to my illness, I no longer take my life and health for granted. No longer do I live my life unconsciously, on autopilot, on a diet of stress and to-do lists, in order to achieve success and security in the pursuit of the ultimate goal for all of us-*Happiness.*

My illness was a message to stop pursuing happiness outside of myself and instead make conscious decisions. The first important decision was to get a divorce because I was unhappy in my marriage. Second, was to stop people-pleasing. Third, was to focus on integrative and holistic medicine instead of conventional medicine. Today, I live my life's purpose: *to empower and inspire thousands of people across the globe to manifest the life of their dreams-filled with radiant health, prosperity and loving relationships.* I live my passion of figure skating with my soulmate, and experience the satisfaction of winning multiple gold medals. I have a fun, rewarding life and fabulous relationships with family and friends.

Most of all, I'm happy.

I want you to experience all of your dreams and more. Why? Because it's your birthright! Think of your quest for pain relief as an invitation to a more connected and fulfilling life. Believe everything happens for a reason and you can have fun on your journey to healing chronic pain. Really-I'm serious.

I have treated hundreds of people in pain within my practice as well as teaching thousands of others across the globe. There are few things more heartwarming than witnessing the transformation of someone finally experiencing freedom from pain.

It Doesn't Matter How Bad Your Pain is

Everyone has the capacity to heal. No matter what diagnosis your doctors have given you, how many MRI's and CT scans you have had or how many surgeries you have endured, you can still feel a heck of a lot better than you do right now. I remember a woman, Matilda, who attended one of my pain relief workshops. Matilda had undergone several surgeries and still had intractable back pain. She couldn't play with her grandchild, let alone do any housework. To her surprise, eighty percent of her pain vanished within a few minutes of doing "acupuncture without needles". Soon after, she was able to play with her grandchild and do her housework . . . completely pain-free!

Is This Book For You?

This book is for anyone suffering from chronic pain who wants to learn how to maximize his or her body's natural healing mechanisms. Chronic pain has been defined many ways. Traditionally, acute pain is described as pain lasting less than thirty days. Chronic pain is pain lasting more than six months. Pain that remains between thirty days and six months is considered subacute pain. Personally, I'd rather use the following definition of chronic pain: "pain that extends beyond the expected period of healing". If you're fed up with feeling pain, then this book is for you.

This book is perfect for people struggling with chronic pain who have not been helped by conventional medicine, which usually consists of drugs, surgery and physical therapy. It is also for people who, like me, would rather use holistic or natural approaches to healing rather than cover up symptoms with drugs. Lastly, this book is for people who are ready or are interested in delving into the deeper realms of healing beyond the physical: the mental, emotional and spiritual.

Why I Wrote this Book

I wrote this book because of my own experience in healing chronic pain. There are many wonderful books on natural healing available today. Some of these books focus on the physical modalities and therapies that can be employed to relieve pain. Others focus on harnessing the power of the mind. Few books focus on the role of Spirit in chronic pain. And by Spirit, I don't mean religion. None focused on what I'm attempting to do in this book, which is to integrate Mind, Body, and Spirit in the healing of chronic pain. Notice that I used the word "healing", not "relief", not "management", not "cure".

The word healing denotes much more than the absence of, in this case, pain symptoms. Healing occurs at a much deeper level, and must include the Spirit. My intention in writing this book is to help chronic pain sufferers relieve their physical pain symptoms as well as experience healing on mental, emotional and spiritual levels. A person can experience physical pain relief, but still be in a mental state of anxiety or worry. Another may feel victimized by his/her circumstances. The purpose of my book is to provide a beacon of hope to anyone who has suffered or is suffering from chronic pain. If that's you, I want to let you know that you're not alone. You can become empowered to heal your own pain. If you experience miraculous pain relief like so many of my chronic pain patients, you might even decide that you want to teach others how to become empowered too.

Your experience of pain is not random, back luck, bad genes or co-incidence. Believe it or not, it has a purpose. In addition to helping you find quick relief for your pain symptoms, I'm hoping you'll be willing to go deeper to find the true purpose and meaning your pain provides.

A true holistic approach to healing pain must involve all aspects of our Selves. That being said, not everyone is ready to integrate body, mind and spirit at once. Focus on what resonates with you right now. Be compassionate and patient with your learning. As a recovering perfectionist, I can attest to the value of accepting yourself in this moment. In time, it is my hope you'll be open to perceiving your pain as a gift. It might seem like a big stretch for you right now, but that's okay. Where you are right now is just fine.

What's in this Book?

Much of the book contains my personal research into what has helped my own chronic pain as well as that of my patients. By integrating knowledge from different healing specialties and modalities, my intention is to give you plenty of self-empowerment choices. I will be focusing on empowering tools and strategies you can use at home to heal yourself. Many are based in energy medicine-a subcategory of medicine hardly acknowledged in either natural or conventional Western medicine.

Think of this book as a "do-it-yourself" guide to self-healing. Although I would encourage you to seek support and therapy from natural health care professionals such as holistic physicians, naturopaths, acupuncturists, holistic chiropractors, holistic osteopaths, homeopaths, massage therapists, holistic nutritionists and energy workers, much of the responsibility for your self-care rests with you. For those who don't have access to the holistic support of professionals, not to worry. This guide will ignite the wisdom within to promote self-healing. I've included many patient stories within these pages to illustrate what is possible. I hope these stories will inspire you and let you know you're not alone.

The toughest part of writing a book of this magnitude is that there is always more to learn, more to experience and more to write about. My greatest challenge was probably choosing a stopping point. My patients can confirm the fact that I'm constantly learning new things. As soon as I have found a better, faster, more effective way to treat my patients, I integrate it immediately into my medical practice. If my current "tool chest" of therapies is inadequate to help a patient, I go on a search-and-discovery mission to find a therapy that does. It's just the way I am. As you can imagine, I never get bored.

Financial Disclosure

Please note that I use many of the products recommended in this book, either for my own well-being or in my medical practice. Because of that, I have become an affiliate or distributor for some of them. Please understand that I would never recommend a product just to get paid for selling it. I have been very careful in only recommending high quality products that I would and do use myself. If you are interested in knowing which ones I have financial ties with, you can visit www.karenkan.com/disclosure for details.

Acknowledgments

I'd like to take this opportunity to thank my support group for spurring me on to complete this book. This includes my Patch Training Team consultants; my book mentor, Keith Leon; my Mastermind group members James P. Gann, Marie McMahon, Melissa Gerdes and Greg Gerdes. Thanks to Martha Pickard Palmer for her feedback on the nutrition sections of the book. I'd also like to thank my book writing support team of Marie McMahon, Bronwyn Seal and Linda Sanicola as well as my assistant Jennifer Burns. Lastly I'd like to thank Patricia Lee Jones, my spiritual advisor, and the many coaches, mentors, teachers, and colleagues who have inspired me on this amazing healing journey.

Karen Kan, MD
January 2013

1

How to Use this Book

This book is divided into five sections. The first section involves understanding your pain. Although I was very tempted to skip this chapter and go right to teaching you how to relieve your pain, most people I meet want to understand why they are experiencing pain and discomfort. I don't blame them. As a Western-trained medical doctor, I've spent decades learning the so-called biological basis of why someone gets sick. It's a very left-brain, logical pursuit that most of us in Western civilization still cling to. Understanding why you have pain is helpful, but only to a point. The Achilles heel of being given an official diagnosis is that it can hamper your healing process.

The Mind section will introduce how thoughts influence your recovery and healing. We'll examine currently held beliefs which are often non-supportive to the healing process. Techniques and strategies will be taught to discover more supportive thoughts. I'll also be sharing how our emotions are tied to our well-being and how to use them to your advantage. I'll go over several fun and effective strategies that I've used myself and with my patients to eliminate negative or trapped emotions that might be contributing to your chronic pain.

In the Body section, I'll be covering several topics on healing through nutrition, lifestyle changes, and energy therapy. You'll find nutritional therapies take time to implement and see results from, but they are supportive to your overall health and well-being. Energy-based therapies, however, often work immediately. Whatever you are willing to try will be beneficial.

The Spirit section will provide opportunities to perceive your pain as a conduit through which your soul can grow. By reframing your current experience from one that feels like, "Why me?" to one that is "Wow, this experience is so cool!" you can begin manifesting a consciously-driven life based on spiritual evolution versus physical gratification. It might be hard to conceive how pain relief can be a spiritual practice, but in my experience, it truly is!

Keep in mind that there isn't a division between the Mind, Body and Spirit. The only reason they are divided in this book is so I can present the information in a coherent form. You'll decide how to integrate all these aspects for yourself. Some people may focus only on the Body section because their physical bodies and environment are primary concerns. Others may be drawn to strategies in the Mind section because they know that lingering negative emotions are likely affecting their pain. Yet others will find great solace in reading the Spirit section because they long to understand the meaning behind their pain and illness.

Always remember that it *is* possible to heal. By reading this book, your intention to heal will begin attracting exactly what you need for your journey. Follow your curiosity and start by reading the section that appeals to you the most. You don't need to read the sections in order. The goal is just to begin.

The final section in the book delves into getting appropriate support. Healing chronic pain is a journey that feels easier when you attract the right people to your support team. The last chapter shares other natural healing modalities you may wish to explore. The Resources section lists links to online resources that you can go to for further education and the topics are listed in the order they appear in each chapter.

Let's begin the journey now, shall we?

Section A

Understanding Your Pain

"Man's mind, once stretched by a new idea,
never regains its original dimensions."
-Oliver Wendell Holmes

2

HOW PEOPLE EXPERIENCE PAIN

I would like to describe the various types of chronic pain people experience. A formal diagnosis, such as "herniated disc" can limit one's perspective of the source of pain. The descriptions that follow are fairly detailed. Many people experience a variety of symptoms so if you don't fit into a particular category, don't worry. The point of this chapter is to further your perception about the pain you're experiencing. You'll be pleased to know that there are many natural alternatives to drugs and surgery when it comes to pain relief. But before we delve into those, let's talk about what you might be feeling.

Dull, Achy Pain, Pounding, Throbbing Pain

Achy pain can come from muscles, joints, bones or internal organs (also called viscera). With achy pain in the muscles, people often report that the pain gets better with movement. In Traditional Chinese Medicine (TCM), we would attribute this type of pain to stagnation of Qi, i.e. poor energy flow through the energy channels. Pain relieved by movement means more blood and Qi is flowing through that area of soft tissue. Achy muscles and joints that worsen with damp weather or an impending storm signify "dampness" in TCM which roughly translates to having too much dampness in the tissues. Eating "damp-producing" foods such as milk, cheese, sugar, fried foods, wheat, cold raw foods, and cold drinks may exacerbate this type of pain.

Believe it or not, a common cause of achy low back pain is intestinal problems. Often when my patients have a flare of low back pain, I'll ask them what they've been eating the past few days. Usually they look sheepish because they've been overindulging in sugar, wheat or unhealthy snacks. We'll cover how intestinal issues can cause chronic pain in the Body section.

The last type of achy pain I'd like to describe is literally "tooth-achy" pain. This type of pain is extremely uncomfortable and medications generally do not work well. If you've ever had a toothache, you'll know what this type of pain feels like. It can throb and feel as if it's coming from deep within your bones and muscles. I used to have this type of pain whenever I ate cheese and it would keep me up at night.

Sometimes there is inflammation of a tiny fluid-filled sac acting as a cushion between the bones, tendons and muscles. With repetitive motion and continued inflammation these sacs can fill with fluid and become painful. This condition is referred to as bursitis and it can cause achy, throbbing pain. The major bursae are located adjacent to the tendons near the large joints, such as the shoulders, elbows, hips, and knees.

Sharp, Piercing, Stabbing, Shooting or Knife-like Pain

This type of pain usually occurs with movement. People describe it as a sudden severe pain associated with a specific motion or body position. Occasionally, a sudden loss of strength can occur particularly when two joints are misaligned. The most typical example is the sacroiliac joints. These joints consist of the pelvis bowl and the triangular bone called the sacrum. Stand with your backside to the mirror, see any dimples? Those dimples represent both sides of your sacrum where the sacroiliac joints are located. The pelvis can lose its symmetry in various ways, thereby causing a misalignment of the sacroiliac joints. Bending or twisting movements can exaggerate this pelvic misalignment and cause sudden sharp pain. This sharpness can literally bring a person to his knees, so he cannot walk. Unfortunately SIJ (sacroiliac joint) misalignment is never recognized by conventional radiologists reading X-rays of the spine or pelvis, although it is by most chiropractors.

Sharp pain can also occur when soft tissue is being squeezed or rubbed with movement. An example of this is impingement syndrome whereby a tendon gets trapped in a joint space during movement. In shoulder impingement syndrome, there is often no pain on moving a straight arm out to the side until it gets to about ninety degrees from the torso. As the shoulder joint space narrows past this point, the tendon of the supraspinatus muscle gets trapped and causes a sudden sharp pain in the shoulder.

Burning Pain

This type of pain is a form of neuropathic pain (pain coming from the nerves) and it can be very severe. People with uncontrolled diabetes can experience burning foot pain because their poor circulation has deteriorated the small nerve endings in their feet. This type of nerve damage is a complication of uncontrolled diabetes.

When bigger nerves are trapped, such as the sciatic nerve (a huge nerve that runs from the spine through the buttocks area and down the leg) the same burning pain can occur. When people "slip a disc" in their lumbar spine, the extruded disc can entrap the nerve roots coming out of the spine and cause severe burning pain. Classic "sciatica" is severe burning leg pain.

Cold, Numb, Stiff Pain

Yes, this type of pain sounds weird. I have a lot of experience with this one. It is the feeling that not enough blood or warmth is travelling to an area of your body. In Chinese Medicine, we would say that the energy (Qi) is stagnant in the area. In other words, because the energy is low or nil in the area, it produces this type of "cold" pain. Usually with this type of pain, movement or exercise improves it to a degree, as well as using a heating pad. Prolonged inactivity, such as sitting or sleeping makes the pain worse. The sensations of cold and numb often go together. The sensation of numbness often travels down an acupuncture meridian or a nerve.

Pins and Needles Pain

Also a form of neuropathic pain, pins and needles pain can be a milder form of pain caused by compromised or damaged nerves. Some patients refer to it as feeling "buzzy". One common diagnosis is called meralgia paresthetica. The cause of meralgia paresthetica is compression of the nerve that supplies sensation to the skin surface of your outer thigh and it can be caused by tight clothing, obesity, local trauma or diabetes.

There is another cause of "buzzy" pain which stumps most doctors and some chiropractors, simply due to a lack of understanding and/or training. I was ignorant as well until I experienced it myself. Myofascial pain syndrome (MPS) is a condition involving the connective tissue. Specially trained MPS massage therapists and physical therapists know beneficial treatment techniques proven to ease symptoms.

Myofascial pain occurs when a muscle knots up and stays in constant contraction without the ability to relax. The fascia is the thin layer of connective tissue that envelopes the muscle. The fascia can also be tight or tighter than the muscle itself. These knots are tender when pressed on, but often the pain is temporarily relieved upon release of the pressure. These painful knots are known as trigger points. Janet Travell, M.D. is probably the best known in this field for her work with myofascial pain syndrome.

Have you ever performed a shoulder massage on anyone with tight, painful knots? They often say it hurts but feels good at the same time. Typically myofascial pain is achy; however, I've had many patients with pins and needles or numbness sensations running down a limb because the muscle and fascia were literally strangulating the flow of Qi. In severe cases, blood flow to the skin is affected and the painful limb can even look a different color (usually bluish) from the normal limb. People sometimes worry that the color disturbance is due to a blood clot, but are reassured when the color returns to normal after appropriate treatment. Nerve damage or even a trapped nerve may not be necessary for this symptom to occur. With the release or relaxation of the associated trigger points, often the pins and needles pain diminishes or disappears.

A short time ago, I experienced pins and needles in my left calf when doing a left hamstring stretch. I didn't have damage to any of my nerves yet wondered why the feeling resembled classic "nerve" pain. I realized that the fascia extending from my hip to my foot was tight and was sending electrical signals every time I tried to stretch. I've learned by releasing the tight fascia, the pain sensation melts away. If the fascia is chronically tight, as mine was, it can be an indication that something systemic is causing the fascia to be tight. One of the most common causes I've found in my practice is gluten sensitivity i.e. inflammation from eating wheat products. I'll discuss more about dietary issues related to chronic pain in the Body section.

Electrical Shock Pain

As you can imagine, having this type of pain is horrible. It's not unlike putting your finger into an electrical socket. Most often this pain occurs in the arms and legs where there are long nerves. This is true nerve pain. Carpal tunnel syndrome can cause this kind of pain whereby the median nerve is trapped in the wrist and sends pain signals into the hand. Sciatica can also present as electrical shock pain as a result of compression of the sciatic nerve due to spasm of the piriformis buttock muscle. This condition is called piriformis syndrome. Just by invoking relaxation of the tight muscle, the pain signals go away.

Doctors often recommend a nerve conduction test which determines exactly which nerves are affected and to what degree. A slowing of nerve conduction indicates nerve damage. Many people worry that the only treatment for nerve compression is surgery; however, in my experience, if addressed early, natural non-surgical options can work well.

Cramping, Squeezing Pain

People refer to these as charley-horse pains. The muscle gets locked into spasm and cannot release. Multiple muscle groups can be involved. Occasionally, muscle twitching under the skin may be observed. Recurrent muscle spasms are often caused by nutritional deficiencies, namely minerals like magnesium and potassium. Too much calcium relative to magnesium in our Western diet can cause a mineral imbalance that encourages muscle contraction and spasms. The average American consumes far more calcium in his diet than magnesium, although both may be low. In fact, the soil in which we grow our conventional produce has been depleted of important minerals like magnesium for at least eighty years, so even if you think you eat a healthy diet, you may still be magnesium deficient. Furthermore, common medications such as blood pressure lowering medications often deplete the body of vital minerals such as magnesium and potassium.

Old-fashioned Epsom salts are used to treat muscle cramps because of the magnesium sulfate in Epsom salts. In the Body section, I'll discuss how magnesium chloride works even better, as well as what you can do to improve mineral balance in your diet.

Pressure, Tight, Expanding, Vice-like, Swelling, Heavy Pain

Some people say that certain body parts, such as their head, neck or back, feel as if they are in a vice or are about to explode. Standing upright can compress the spine increasing back or leg pain and causing a heavy feeling in the lower body which causes the person to prefer sitting. The causes of these types of pain are more difficult to determine using traditional Western medicine approaches. In Chinese medicine, we can describe it as blood and Qi being stagnant in one area and not flowing properly.

People with migraine headaches will describe that their head hurts so badly that it feels like it is about to explode. I've had similar experiences when the barometer changes rapidly or when a storm is approaching. In Traditional Chinese Medicine, this is a symptom of "dampness", meaning that there is extra fluid stagnated in the body where it shouldn't be. Examples of internal "dampness" would be diarrhea, nasal congestion or swollen legs.

In my practice I treat several young Nordic ski racers. Whenever they practice with roller skis (skis with wheels), their lower legs can get extremely stressed and swollen. Sometimes the chronic swelling requires surgery to literally cut the fascia that separates the layers of muscle in an attempt to decompress the leg. This condition is called compartment syndrome and can be dangerous as it shuts off the blood supply to the lower leg. Unfortunately, the roller ski manufacturers have yet to design a system of boot and skis that eliminates compartment syndrome in its skiers. By using some of the energy tools I'll mention later, as well as dietary changes, my patients are able to avoid potentially disabling surgery and perform better in their sport.

Dull, Stiff, Cold Pain

Although relatively low on the pain severity scale, morning stiffness or stiffness with inactivity (like sitting for prolonged periods of time) is a common symptom of chronic pain. In Western medicine, we consider morning stiffness that gets better with movement to be caused by inflammation. Yet, as you'll read later, inflammation is related to almost all forms of acute and chronic pain as well as many chronic diseases, so this description isn't terribly helpful.

What I learned recently from Dr. Robert Cass, a naturopathic doctor in Canada, is that stiffness brought on by inactivity (sleeping, sitting in a chair too long etc.) is due to calcium precipitating out of solution into the tissues. In other words, the calcium starts becoming solid and is no longer dissolved in the fluids of your muscles, joints and tendons. This apparently happens in environments of low phosphorus or magnesium. Adequate levels of these minerals are required to keep the calcium in solution. Medications are notorious for depleting minerals such as magnesium and phosphorus. In addition, processed foods containing fructose (high fructose corn syrup for example) seem to promote the loss of phosphorus in the urine.

According to Dr. Carolyn Dean, author of The Magnesium Miracle, you can do your own experiment at home to demonstrate this phenomenon using a calcium tablet and a magnesium tablet. Dissolve a calcium tablet in a little bit of water and notice how there is still some solid left over. Then add a magnesium tablet and watch how the rest of the calcium dissolves into the solution.

"Run over by a truck" Pain

This type of pain is also described as "all over achy" or "flu-like". Typically people diagnosed with fibromyalgia will suffer from this type of debilitating pain. I can tell you first-hand that I wouldn't wish it on anyone! Just imagine the last time you had the flu. It felt awful, didn't it?

People with fibromyalgia and other chronic pain conditions can feel "flu-like" symptoms twenty four hours a day, seven days a week, for months or years on end. The pain literally drains the energy right out of them. They have no life and are often depressed. They are told by their doctors to get exercise, but if they overdo it, they suffer worse pain. Usually this type of pain gets worse with too little or too much exercise, as well as too little or too much sleep. If you suffer from this type of pain, even just once-in-a-while, know that holistic treatments offer hope. The underlying cause may take time to resolve, but the pain relief doesn't have to.

"Mixed Bag" of Symptoms

The grand majority of chronic pain sufferers experience two or more of the various pain symptoms I've discussed so far. The mixture of pain symptomatology can be confusing for both patients and doctors. As a young doctor, I remember that occasionally a new patient would present with inexplicable and weird symptoms that I could not explain using traditional biology and physiology. My professors would sometimes dismiss this type of patient as a hypochondriac or would assume it was all psychogenic (created by psychological disturbances). It wasn't until I became very sick myself that I understood what some of these patients were actually feeling. I'll give you an example of a patient complaint that would typically drive a doctor insane:

> *"Doctor, I'm getting these annoying eye twitches every day and they are getting worse. And I just began having a buzzy electrical feeling in my body, but it's only on the right side of my body, including my head. I get it mostly at night and I can't sleep. I can see little muscle twitches in my arms and legs sometimes and I can see my veins poking out for no reason, even if it isn't hot or cold out . . . and I'm bumping into walls. Why is that? Can you test me for multiple sclerosis? Then there is this heavy feeling behind my eyes. No, it's not a headache exactly, just a heavy feeling . . . and my memory is getting worse. I get to the top of the stairs and can't remember what I went upstairs to get! I know I'm only 30, but I think I'm getting Alzheimer's. Can you test me for that? Oh, yeah, I almost forgot, I have a weird metallic taste in my mouth and my stool smells like metal too. What is that from?"*

Imagine how overwhelmed a doctor might feel hearing a litany of seemingly unrelated symptoms like that? Most doctors label patients like these "extra sensitive" and a few actually think they are crazy. Western trained doctors get trapped into ordering a multitude of tests on these patients, partly because they ask for them, and partly just to placate them. Little time, however, is spent actually on healing. Why? Because neither doctor nor patient really know what to do in order to heal.

I had to learn how to heal myself. I didn't know that many of the symptoms in the above example were symptoms of magnesium deficiency!

Sadly, most doctors are not trained adequately in nutrition. We are not taught to treat patients with nutritional therapy, only with drugs. Who do you think funds a lot of medical school education programs such as hospital Grand Rounds? The pharmaceutical industry does, spending the majority of their money on marketing to both doctors and consumers.

Are You Extra Sensitive?

A friend of mine, Andrea, is sometimes able to see the outside world in pixels, just like on a computer or television screen. If you've seen the movie, "The Matrix" with Keanu Reeves, you'll understand what I'm talking about. According to quantum physicists and spiritual teachers from ancient traditions, our "real" world is no more real than the pictures in our mind. In other words, we apparently "project" our environment from within. In traditional Buddhist teaching, everything is an illusion. Of course, you may argue that if you stub your toe, as the resulting bruise and pain feel real! Whether you believe in quantum physics or spiritual traditions, it is still important for you to be able to function in everyday life.

Andrea searched for years for the cause of her "condition" and went through many scans, eye exams, blood tests and x-rays. Her doctors couldn't find a single thing to explain her symptoms. My intuition told me that Andrea had extraordinary abilities to sense things the rest of us could not, like auras (colorful energetic fields) around living things, so I told her she was gifted. At first she didn't believe me. It wasn't until she met with famous energy healer, Eric Pearl, D.C., that she began respecting her divine healing gifts. After being trained by Dr. Pearl, she is now a certified Reconnective Healer and is able to harness her sensitivity into a healing skill to help others like her. This is what Andrea says about her visions:

> *I want you to know that I do not see in pixels all the time. It is not*
> *something that is continuous that I move through. It is more like seeing*
> *very fast moving tiny lights in objects, for example, the television . . . but*
> *I can look out the window and see them too in the whole sky. The time I*
> *saw an entire dresser turn into pixels, it looked like fast moving black dots,*

but still held the shape of the dresser. It is hard to explain. What I see is wavy-like energy, almost what you see with a mirage or when heat is rising off the road. Things can and do become illuminated and golden especially when I am experiencing my higher states and feeling love intensely; then they get wavy, not solid. Wish you could borrow my eyes when this occurs, to better help explain this. I really enjoy it now and like to go there often. Sometimes I will cry spontaneously. Tears will just begin and it feels like bliss, ecstatic joy and can be overwhelming, but in a good way!

Sometimes "sensitive" individuals like Andrea can initially suffer from their sensitivity until they learn that it is both a gift and a curse. Once "sensitives" are taught how to harness and protect their energy, they can turn that talent inwards to not only heal themselves, but also others if they choose to do so.

Please understand that your pain can manifest as anything, but you are not alone. Allow the frustration with the lack of improvement within traditional medicine fuel your efforts to explore alternative or energetic treatments. In fact, if you're reading this book, you are likely to be the perfect candidate to take advantage of what holistic medicine has to offer.

Chapter Summary

- People experience pain in all sorts of ways so you are not alone.
- Myofascial pain is a common source of chronic pain and most traditional doctors are not taught to diagnose or manage it.
- Mineral deficiencies such as magnesium, potassium and phosphorus can contribute to or cause chronic pain.
- Traditional Western medical doctors may not be adequately educated to treat chronic pain without drugs or surgery.
- Sensitive people may suffer more from their symptoms until they learn how to harness and protect their energy field in order to self-heal.

3

CAUSES OF PAIN—
EASTERN PERSPECTIVE

In Energy Medicine, there are only two main causes of chronic illness of any type. That's it! Just two! The first is energy depletion in the body and the second cause is energy imbalance. Every health problem *originates* from one or the other. It is that simple. And to think, I spent seven years in medical school and never learned this until I went to acupuncture school. All physical illnesses first manifest as energetic imbalances, often years before the first overt symptom.

According to Traditional Chinese Medicine, the symptom of pain often arises from a blockage of energy flow in the body. Often the blockage of flow is preceded by a decline in energy reserves. This energy is referred to as Qi, Chi, Ka, Ki or Prana. In modern terms we can refer to it as Life Force, Vital Force, Subtle Energy, Life Energy, or Bio-Energy. Even if you don't understand the concept of Qi, just think about how you actually perceive it in other people.

For example, do you know anyone who exudes vibrant energy and health? This person likely has a good reserve of Qi. On the other hand, I'm sure you can think of at least one person you've met that makes you feel tired just being in the same room with her. That person has a low reserve of Qi. The more Qi or vital force you have, the healthier you are. The more balanced and free-flowing the Qi, the healthier you feel and the better your body functions.

Energy Depletion

Think of life force as the energy that makes all the processes in your body work-the feeling of being alive. As an analogy, think of your body as a laptop computer for a moment. If the energy in the battery wears out, the laptop stops working until you can plug it into the wall outlet right?

14

If your body's energy battery is low, you'll start manifesting symptoms of illness, including pain, because the body doesn't have enough "juice" to heal itself. Even infectious diseases can be traced to a weakened immune system that has resulted from energy depletion. In fact, when your energy is low, the body turns on its survival mechanism and any process that the body considers extraneous isn't tended to. In order to heal, you need to "charge" your battery. In later chapters, I'll be showing you just how to do that through energy tools and lifestyle changes.

So why does your energy battery get low? Namely, it's stress. I bet you could have guessed that! Generally, it is stress that has occurred over a prolonged period of time, often decades, that manifests in a low energy battery.

Stress can be viewed as endogenous, stemming from within the body, or exogenous, stemming from outside the body. Exogenous stressors are things that we experience from our environment that drain our energy. I'll wait until I share the Western perspective to name exactly what those things are in more detail.

Endogenous stress comes from our *response* to the outside world. Do you notice how some people just thrive on stress? Before I became ill, I was one of them. Whenever I had a deadline to meet or a competition to win, I'd savor the rush of adrenaline. I'd feel alive. Feeling stressed made me feel important, like I was contributing to the world. If I became too relaxed, I was afraid someone might think I was lazy. My self-esteem was so fragile that I couldn't bear that label. Thus I did everything in my power to keep myself stressed.

The stress response is a protection response built into our survival genetics. When our bodies feel threatened, a whole cascade of reactions turns on to preserve our lives. You may know it as the *fight or flight response*. The fight or flight response is an important part of our evolution as humans because we wouldn't have survived saber-toothed tigers, plagues and wars without it. This response however wasn't meant to be a daily event.

Imagine yourself as part of an ancient tribe. Most of the time you'd be playing, eating and having fun . . . until the food supply became low and it would be time to kill a beast to feed the clan. As a hunter, your fight or flight response enabled the chase-and-kill to be executed safely and successfully. Once the hunt was over, you'd settle back down into a relaxed state for many days or weeks before you were called upon to hunt again.

Now picture our modern lives. The minute we wake up, we down half a pot of coffee; a stimulant, and the stress response begins. Kids have to be dressed and fed for school while they are still half-asleep and whining. We get stuck in traffic and pray we're not late for work. During lunch we catch up on email while eating. We rush home to make dinner and help our kids with their homework so we don't miss the debut of the new "Transformers" movie. While we are enjoying the movie, our pulse rises and our hearts race because of the exciting images we see on the screen. Back at home, right before bed, we watch the evening news and hear about devastating floods, earthquakes and civil unrest. Is there any wonder why our energy batteries are low? Without an adequate and renewable source of Qi, the self-healing mechanisms of our body grind to a halt.

I've witnessed in my medical practice a certain minimum level of Qi, or energy, that one must have in order for the body to keep repairing itself. If the Qi levels drop below that crucial threshold, symptoms ensue. Here is the key: if you start out with a full battery charge of energy but only get symptoms when it's down to thirty percent capacity, how long do you think it took you to lose the seventy percent? Honestly, it might have taken you decades. The loss in energy charge can be slow enough to be almost imperceptible if you're not paying attention. If year after year, your batteries continue leaking without replenishment, your energy levels will diminish until you *do* pay attention.

Energy Blockage

All pain symptoms are due to the blockage of energy flow in the body, which is why ancient therapies like acupuncture and modern energy therapies work so well in treating it. By increasing the flow of Qi in the area of pain, the body begins to heal the painful area on its own, thus reducing the pain symptoms. I'll be sharing with you various ways of promoting healthy energy flow in the chapters ahead. Once you find the best tools for your body, you no longer have to suffer from chronic pain.

Energy Imbalance

It is well known in Traditional Chinese Medicine that energy imbalances can occur in the body and, if not corrected, can produce pain and illness. Every single chronic disease has an antecedent energetic depletion and/or imbalance associated with it. Often, the imbalances have been present for decades before a person manifests symptoms.

Acupuncture training taught me that it was vitally important to improve the energetic balance in all the acupuncture meridians in order for my patients to heal; yet something was missing that I couldn't put my finger on until recently. In the past, even when using acupuncture and other holistic therapies, I was very successful in treating most people for pain and other issues that Western medicine couldn't improve. Yet, there were always a few patients, usually with the diagnosis of fibromyalgia, whose improvements were short-lasting. These patients never seemed to "hold" their improvements long term. It was frustrating for them and for me.

Finally years later . . . the answer! This discovery has literally revolutionized how I evaluate and treat every new patient who walks into my office.

The patients who could not heal had one thing in common: they weren't *brain balanced*. In Chinese medicine terms, brain balance is the balance of Yin and Yang energy in the nervous system. The energy in the nervous system is responsible for communication to other organs and systems in the body. If every one of the twelve principle acupuncture meridians were balanced, it also means that the nervous system is balanced. A balanced nervous system makes healing possible. In fact it is critical.

I use the term "brain balance" to mean nervous system balance. It is a state whereby the right and left hemispheres of our brains are balanced and communicating with each other, neither side being "dominant" in function. Brain balance is also a state where the stress and relaxation responses of the body are appropriately regulated and balanced.

This is probably the most important point I'm going to share with you in this book: *in order to heal chronic pain, restoring brain balance is absolutely the single most important thing we need to do.* Healing cannot, and I repeat, cannot occur when the brain balance is short-circuited! If you don't remember anything else from this book, please remember this one thing. I don't care how many acupuncture treatments people receive, how many chiropractors they see, or how many herbal remedies they take. If they are not brain balanced, they will find that treatments will rarely work long term. They might feel better temporarily, but they won't heal. Guaranteed.

I know that is pretty strong language, but I can't emphasize enough the importance of this one pre-requisite to healing. Now, are *you* brain balanced? If nothing you've tried to relieve your pain has worked thus far, you probably aren't. In Chapter 6, I'll be teaching you how to recognize brain imbalance and how to rectify it in yourself once discovered. Correcting the imbalance is relatively simple and straight-forward when minimizing the controllable risk factors.

The reason that ancient techniques like acupuncture have not been as effective at rebalancing the nervous system as in the past is because of our modern lifestyle. Acupuncture was "invented" long before mercury-laden vaccinations, computers, cellular phones and food additives ever existed. It is no wonder why we need to use complementary energy tools to counter the negative effects of our modern lifestyle.

The bottom line is this: energy depletion and energy imbalance (including brain imbalance) is responsible for the development of chronic illnesses including chronic pain. By managing and rebalancing your energy, you'll be well on your way to healing your pain!

Chapter Summary

- Energy depletion, imbalance and/or blockages are the causes of chronic pain and illness from an Eastern perspective.
- Energy depletion is common and is caused by long-term stress.
- Brain balance whereby the right and left sides of the brain are communicating well with each other is crucial for healing.
- Brain imbalance blocks the healing response of the body and could be why you are still experiencing pain.
- Even acupuncture cannot rebalance severe brain imbalance that is caused by modern living which is why we require complementary energy therapies.

4

CAUSES OF PAIN—
WESTERN PERSPECTIVE

As compared with the Eastern perspective on the causes of pain, the Western perspective is much more complex. Here in the West, we're not satisfied with just knowing that energy depletion, blockages and imbalances cause all pain and all illness. If you are new to Eastern medicine, you'll probably want "more". So the rest of this chapter will piece together a holistic, yet Westernized, view of why you're still in pain. Interestingly enough, the Western perspective has summarized the causes of chronic pain under two major umbrella categories which are separate but interrelated. The categories are stress and inflammation. Since we covered the topic of stress earlier, let's move on to inflammation.

Acute inflammation is a natural and appropriate immune response to an infection, an irritation, or an injury. Immune cells are called to the site through the blood stream. The blood vessels near the site become permeable and the site becomes warm and red due to the increased blood flow. The inflamed site also becomes swollen which is supposed to protect the area from further injury. Inflammation is the body's way of repairing itself, but it isn't meant to be a permanent state.

Chronic inflammation, unlike acute inflammation, is pathological. Soon, modern medicine will link chronic inflammation (as a root cause) of all chronic diseases including heart attacks, diabetes and cancer. Acute inflammation during infection is easy to understand because you can see the swelling and redness, along with feeling the pain. Chronic inflammation, however, is more insidious and harder to appreciate. Chronic inflammation probably underlies all types of chronic pain, but the reasons aren't so obvious. It's as if the healing mechanism of the body is hung up and can't complete its cycle. Many of the physical and non-physical causes of chronic pain induce an inflammatory response in the body. Even nutritional deficiencies of anti-oxidants, for example, can prevent the scavenging of free radicals and promote chronic inflammation.

Free radicals are atoms or groups of atoms with an odd (unpaired) number of electrons and can be formed when oxygen interacts with certain type of molecules. Once formed these highly reactive free radicals can start a negative chain reaction, like dominoes. When they come into contact with important components of the cell like DNA or the cellular membrane, they can cause significant damage. Cells may then function poorly, age or die. To prevent free radical damage, the body has a defense system of antioxidants. Some, we make on our own, like glutathione, and others we get from our food, like Vitamin C. Drugs or toxins that interfere with antioxidant activity can thus contribute to chronic inflammation and that is why we want to be conscious of what we expose our bodies to on a daily basis.

Almost every other physical "cause" of pain I've listed below is linked to inflammation. The underlying causes of inflammation are the real story behind why your pain is hanging around. In the Body section, I'll be sharing strategies to lower your inflammation regardless of the cause.

Trauma

As a family practitioner trained initially in Western medicine, I'm well aware of the tomes written about the causes and conventional treatment of pain conditions. Some of the causes are fairly easy to understand such as physical trauma. When someone sprains an ankle, the ligaments either stretch or tear and microscopic shearing of the blood vessels creates the fluid accumulation. The body begins the healing process by creating an inflammatory response to clean up the area and rebuild the structures that were damaged. Swelling protects the area, but often is a source of pain in addition to the pain caused by torn ligaments. Pain signals travel along nerves to the spine and up to the brain where the brain sends the message to the body to "protect" the joint by discouraging excessive movement.

Western medicine is unable to explain why some people heal completely from trauma and why others don't. Nothing is more frustrating to a patient than hearing that every single test her doctor has done has come back "normal" and no cause for the pain has been found. In today's hurried medical climate where insurance companies are paying less for medical visits, doctors often rely on laboratory tests, x-rays and scans much more than on their clinical diagnostic skills to evaluate pain. In America, doctors often practice "defensive medicine" which translates into ordering as many diagnostic tests to avoid a malpractice suit for missing something crucial, like a tumor. To make matters worse, patients often request diagnostics because of a belief that these tests will accurately diagnose the cause of their pain.

Obviously trauma will cause pain, stress and inflammation to the body. What isn't obvious is why some people seem to get better quickly and others don't. Occasionally the trauma is repetitive and the area never rests enough to heal completely. For example, people who lift heavy things or play tennis with bad form may develop inflammation on a bony prominence on their elbow called the lateral epicondyle. This can become chronic and known as tennis elbow or lateral epicondylitis. These types of injuries are also called repetitive strain injuries.

As I'll explain in the Body section, people who suffered head injuries, such as concussions, neck injuries, and whiplash are at higher risk of not being able to heal their chronic pain. If you've experienced a head injury at any time in your life, even as a child, it could have caused brain imbalance and it may explain why your pain lingers. Car accidents, rough sports like hockey or football, can predispose you to experiencing chronic problems that show up later in life.

Toxins

In order for the body to heal, it must be able to efficiently get nutrients into the cells and get toxins out of the cells. If the toxic load on the body is too heavy, then the toxins will affect the functioning of the cells in the body. Toxins come in two forms, endogenous (coming from within us) and exogenous (coming from outside of us).

Endogenous toxins are normal waste products the body creates during the process of normal cellular function. If the body does not eliminate them adequately, they will remain in the body. Uric acid, a by-product of protein metabolism is a fine example. Exogenous toxins come from outside our bodies and can take the form of many things we are exposed to on a daily basis, including:

   ×   Volatile organic chemicals (paint, exhaust, new carpet)
   ×   Pesticides/Herbicides
   ×   Smog
   ×   Heavy metals such as mercury and lead
   ×   Synthetic food additives and preservatives
   ×   Synthetic chemicals in skin care products
   ×   Household cleaners
   ×   Cigarette smoke
   ×   Viruses, bacteria and parasites
   ×   Fluoride and chlorine in tap water
   ×   Bromine in baked goods and home furnishings
   ×   Plastic containers leaching chemicals into our food
   ×   Microwaved food
   ×   Low frequency electromagnetic radiation (EMF) from appliances, computers and lights
   ×   High frequency electromagnetic radiation (EMF) from wireless devices such as cordless phones, cellular phones and Wi-Fi
   ×   Genetically modified food (most commonly corn, soy, cotton, sugar beets and canola)
   ×   Processed food (food that comes in boxes, bags, cans or bottles)
   ×   Foods you are allergic or intolerant to

Even watching the nightly news on television can be viewed as a potential toxin depending on how your mind and emotions are processing the information. You'll learn in the Mind section just how powerful your thoughts and beliefs are when it comes to healing chronic pain.

Toxins will gum up the energy flow in your body and stress your detoxifications organs such as the colon, liver, kidneys, lymph, lung and skin. If toxins back up because the detoxification organs are overburdened, then they can leach into your muscle and joints and cause pain. Gluten, a protein component derived primarily from wheat, used to cause stiffness and pain in my muscles and joints whenever I ate it, as did dairy foods. Although I have desensitized myself to many foods that used to cause me pain, I don't often get the urge to eat wheat or dairy because they don't taste good to me anymore.

Living in the modern world, you deal with a plethora of toxins in your daily life, even if you eat organic and use only vinegar to wash windows.

Since it's impossible to avoid every single toxin, it is important to be at least aware of the role toxins play in your ability to heal.

In an ideal world, toxins, either exogenous or endogenous, are harmlessly transformed and excreted by healthy organs in the body. The primary organs of detoxification are the colon, liver, gallbladder, kidneys, lungs, lymph and skin. Some detoxification experts will include the nasal passages, blood and reproductive organs as secondary detoxification systems. When these organ systems are functioning optimally, we can theoretically get rid of toxins as fast as we accumulate them. Unfortunately, no matter how healthy your detoxification organs start out, if you are living in North America, your daily toxic burden heavily outweighs your body's ability to process them. The colon is responsible for ridding our bodies of most of the toxic burden through bowel movements. If the colon can't function optimally because of stress or inflammation, then toxins are handed over to the liver and kidneys, neither of which was designed to handle large amounts of toxins on a daily basis. Toxins can then literally "back up" so that the lymph, lung, and skin literally overflow. The toxic load can jam up the flow of lymph through the lymph channels. Thus, instead of the toxins dumping efficiently from the lymph channels into the kidneys for excretion through the urine, they can leak out into the muscles, joints, tendons and skin.

Remember the "achy" muscle and joint pain I described in an earlier chapter? I've discovered people who suffer from this type of pain often have sluggish lymphatic flow. I was one of them. Over the last year or so, I noticed with constipation or abdominal pain, I also experienced achy muscles or joint pain. Once I'd clear out the constipation, the pain improved considerably. I also noticed that when I ate an intolerant food such as popcorn or raw nuts, the pain would return. I went to see a massage therapist who specialized in lymphatic flow and she confirmed my suspicion that every time my abdomen was upset, my lymph flow would grind to a halt and I'd experience pain.

If the toxin-processing organs cannot rid toxins efficiently, the toxins will be stored away in "safer" places away from the bloodstream. Unfortunately these "safer" places may be safer in the short-term, but not-so-safe in the long term. Toxins often get stored in fat cells. Fat cells are metabolically slow and aren't very demanding, so storing the toxins there, especially the fat-soluble ones, require enough fat cells to be available.

Thus one of the symptoms of chronic toxicity is fat accumulation in the abdomen and the formation of cellulite. I look like a slim person compared with most Americans, but yet after succumbing to fibromyalgia, I developed significant cellulite and gained two inches around my waistline.

Aside from pain, problems in the lungs, nasal passages and skin are indications of toxicity. All skin rashes can be traced to an inefficient or sluggish detoxification system. Thus, when I treat someone for a chronic rash that has stumped other medical professionals, I always start by supporting the health of the detoxification organs, especially the colon. Many strange and severe rashes have been "cured", not by cortisone creams and pills, but by increasing the health of the bowels and liver. Other symptoms like chronic sinus infections, nasal congestion due to allergies, are other signs that your detoxification system is backed up and not working properly. In the Body section that follows, I'll show you how you can eliminate these toxins more effectively.

Kerri came to my office with a diagnosis of fibromyalgia. She was extremely negative and complained bitterly about how poorly she was being treated by "the system". She was on government assistance and every word out of her mouth was about how other people owed her. She had terrible body odor. I didn't know too much about body detoxification at that point in my career, so I gently asked Kerri if she would mind showering before her next appointment with me. Well! The venom that came from her mouth was sharp and to the point! *"I've showered twice already today and I still reek like this! I can't get rid of it! I'm so toxic!"* I only saw Kerri in the office for a single visit and she never returned to pay her bill, but I learned something really valuable that day.

When someone is *that* toxic, the sweat glands will bear some of the burden of detoxifying and it won't smell very pleasant to be around them! Not only did Kerri have physical toxins burdening her battered body, the emotional toxins were adding fuel to the fire. She was in a downward spiral of "poor me" and was so physically ill that the only true option for her was healing on a spiritual level. In other words, people like Kerri have to hit rock bottom and totally surrender themselves to spirit before change can happen. That degree of surrender happens when you are too sick and tired to fight anymore.

I know rock bottom. I know the feeling of suicidal thoughts because the pain and fatigue are unbearable. In the Spirit section we'll discuss the empowerment of choice versus victimhood. This change in perspective made all the difference in my healing and in the healing of others I have worked with.

Nutritional Deficiencies

In order for the body to heal, it requires the right nutrients, and not just protein, fats and carbohydrates. Many of our natural sources of minerals have diminished because of food processing and the poor soil conditions in conventional farming. Minerals are essential for almost every job a cell has to do and the lack of minerals may well be one of the major contributors to chronic pain and chronic diseases in North America.

Plants are able to synthesize vitamins from sun and water, but they cannot synthesize minerals. If the soil is mineral deficient, the plant will be too, no matter how big and lovely synthetic fertilizers make them look. I was at a potluck party recently and brought my own food. One couple brought a raw vegetable plate, so I was excited to have something else to eat. Unfortunately, when I took my first bite, I wanted to spit it out. Every single vegetable I tried tasted bland and some even tasted like chemicals. My taste buds, being used to local and organically farmed produce, could no longer tolerate the taste of conventionally grown vegetables! No wonder children these days would rather eat sugar. It tastes better.

Food processing basically strips the nutrition right out of the fruit, vegetable or grain it's made from. Magnesium is the mineral that is most affected by food processing according to Carolyn Dean, MD, who wrote, The Magnesium Miracle. It never ceases to amaze me how some of my new patients don't make the connection between what they eat and why their bodies can't heal. "Garbage in, garbage out" is a term used by computer programmers to describe why computers sometimes don't work-if you program the software incorrectly. I think that this saying applies to nutrition and health as well.

Intestinal Problems

Many people with persistent low back pain have intestinal issues. Think about it for a minute. Your intestines sit all curled up in your belly cozily next to your other abdominal organs: the liver, kidneys, bladder, gallbladder, pancreas, spleen, uterus (if you're a woman), major blood vessels etc. Next to your organs, the spine, spinal nerves, and sacrum are all connected together through thin layers of fascia. Everything is touching everything.

When there are problems in the bowel and the bowel walls become inflamed, they end up being overly porous. In medical terms, we call this porosity "permeability". When the bowel walls become too permeable, then there will be leakage of bowel contents into the pelvis. This relatively "toxic" fluid then leaks through the various fascial tissues and can inflame the nerves of the spine, the pelvic joints and even track down into the hip joints and knee joints. Integrative manual therapists, like my friend Melissa, told me that she has witnessed patients requiring hip and knee replacements due to long term bowel leakage into the joints!

Food Sensitivities

Recently, I've been diagnosing more and more people with gluten-sensitivity. Gluten is type of protein found mainly in wheat, rye, spelt and barley. Severe gluten-intolerance, such as found in Celiac disease, can cause serious health problems including malnutrition, chronic severe abdominal pain, weight loss, weight gain, chronic diarrhea or constipation, chronic fatigue, depression, skin problems, arthritis, and even neurologic disease.

You might not have full blown Celiac disease, but you might have gluten intolerance or sensitivity. In other words, the body has an immune response and creates inflammation. The inflammation can manifest as almost anything, but the most common symptoms I see are intestinal symptoms and chronic pain in the muscles or joints.

My partner, James, found out not long ago that he is gluten-intolerant. Having been a "sugar and wheat addict" all his life, it was a sobering realization. It took us a while to diagnose him because I was gluten-intolerant, so we didn't have a lot of wheat products at home. Over time, I began to notice that James would get annoying little "injuries" when we skated together or would suffer from bouts of recurrent, severe low back pain for no reason. Finally I put two and two together and realized that these bouts of pain only occurred after he had splurge at the deli eating wraps or sandwiches.

James resisted the possibility of being gluten-intolerant because he really craved wheat and needed "proof". One day, I consulted with a retired certified colon hydrotherapist about what bowel cleanse she recommended. James was so intrigued with her stories of parasites and tape worms that he decided to do the cleanse with me. So we did an eight day cleanse using the supplements the colon hydrotherapist recommended and James did not consume wheat, processed food, sugar or coffee for the entire time. To his amazement, he felt absolutely great! He experienced an increase of energy and not a stitch of pain anywhere in his body. We skated wonderfully that whole week and although we didn't push ourselves too hard, we were able to do lifts without any injuries. In fact, James was particularly strong.

Within a week after finishing the bowel cleanse, James re-introduced wheat into his diet. His buddies at work offered him a donut and by the next morning, his back was "killing him". Weeks of experimenting with and without eating wheat continued until, undeniably, he pinpointed wheat ingestion as the cause of his pain. His initial reluctance has now transformed into solid resolve. He's stronger, happier and pain-free when gluten-free. James still loves his junk food, but at least he opts for organic and gluten-free options. Occasionally he makes an honest mistake, such as eating organic granola, not realizing that oats are not necessarily gluten-free, or French fries, where the fryer oil was used to fry breaded chicken fingers. As for me, I'm happy to have a healthier partner!

Although wheat and gluten are the major culprits in causing food-sensitive pain, other foods like dairy can do the same. In fact, in Chinese Medicine, cheese and other dairy foods, sweets, alcohol and cold raw foods are considered too "damp" for people predisposed to arthritic conditions. No doubt you've heard someone with arthritic pain remark that a storm is approaching. I also used to feel pain before a storm even though I don't have arthritis. Whenever I ate cheese, my muscles and joints would ache, and worsen during rainy or damp weather.

The Elimination Diet is the most cost-effective way to determine whether you have a food sensitivity contributing to the pain. In this diet, you abstain from eating the most common allergens such as egg, dairy, seafood, shellfish, tree nuts, soy, wheat and peanuts for at least two to four weeks and see if your symptoms improve. If they do not, then it is unlikely that you are intolerant to these foods. The longer you do the elimination diet, the better. If your symptoms improve, then reintroduce each allergen one at a time every three to seven days, gradually increasing the "dose" until you are sure you don't react to it. Alternatively, you can get a blood test called the ALCAT test to check for food intolerance. I'll share more on this later.

Lifestyle Contributions

Research the causes of chronic pain online and you might read about postural strain, repetitive movements, overuse, and prolonged immobilization. Poor posture and poor body mechanics forces other body parts to compensate for the imbalance. There is no question that how you treat your body daily has an impact on the development and perpetuation of chronic pain. Several male patients in my practice have physically demanding lifestyles. They cut down trees, lift sheetrock, haul wood, etc. They were invincible in their twenties doing heavy manual work and unfortunately they hold the same expectation in their fifties. Heavy manual work is tough on the body and chances are that at some point in time, injury will occur.

Natural healthy aging doesn't mean stopping the activities that you truly love just because you are older. My patients don't understand that they must support the body in other ways that keeps it nurtured and in balance. The harder you are on your body, the more support it needs.

Think of your body as an expensive sports car. If you're just driving around town showing off your car, there isn't much wear and tear on it, but if you are competing in the World Rally Championships racing in gravel, snow and ice, the performance of the car depends on its upkeep. At times I've joked: some people take better care of their cars than of their bodies!

Many people would acknowledge that exercise is good for the body. Conditioning the body means putting "good" stress on the skeleton, muscles, joints, ligaments, heart, lungs, skin and fascia so that they remain robust and flexible. With today's modern lifestyle, we often find ourselves sitting in front of our computers (as I am right now) or television sets, or driving in cars. The lack of regular exercise prevents the flow of energy in the body and can lead to or contribute to chronic pain. Unfortunately, experiencing chronic pain actually prevents people from exercising so it's a never-ending cycle of pain and de-conditioning.

The elite athletes I work with put huge demands on their bodies. To make matters worse, specific sports often cause muscle imbalances because certain muscles are "recruited" more heavily than others. One of my friends is a former luge athlete. He can still bend forward and flatten himself like a pancake, just as he did years ago while training. The only problem is, his back and hamstring muscles are overly flexible as compared to his hip flexors and abdominal muscles, so when I asked him to try a back bend, he just chuckled because he knew he couldn't do it.

The quality of sleep every night has a lot to do with how well your body heals itself. Physical rejuvenation is said to occur during deep sleep. Important hormones and neurotransmitters (chemical messengers) are released during sleep. Caffeine and alcohol can negatively impact sleep. Stimulating activities such as being on the computer or watching television can also negatively impact sleep. Chronic pain can exacerbate sleep issues and can cause multiple awakenings if the pain is moderately severe. We'll discuss in the Body chapter how to get your sleep back on track so that your body can heal.

What you ingest can contribute extensively to your body's ability to self-heal. Low nutrient, low energy food, like processed conventionally made food can harm rather than heal the body. Hippocrates said, *"Let medicine be thy food and thy food be thy medicine"* and he was right. Without the energy from proper nutrient dense foods, our body's cells literally starve and cannot function well. Over time, we can succumb to disease and illness. If you're not ready to cook all of your own food and go totally organic, that's okay. Any little bit helps. My goal is to help you feel better faster because inevitably you'll start making healthier lifestyle choices. How exciting is that?

Lastly, a discussion on lifestyle would not be complete if I didn't include the mental, emotional and spiritual factors of lifestyle. How often do you have "down" time? And I don't mean sitting in front of the TV watching movies. Few people in the modern world give themselves the opportunity to be truly conscious of their thoughts and feelings on a daily basis. Spiritual teachers call this being a "witness" to yourself. Most of us are just too busy getting our "To-Do" list done, myself included. How often do you just sit still, not doing anything, but witnessing your breath? Unless you have been practicing meditation, probably never.

How often do you read non-fiction books? How many per month? Expanding your awareness is part of growing yourself and an integral part of the self-healing journey. My guess is that if you are reading this book, you are already way ahead of the average American who spends nearly four hours a day watching television shows and slick marketing ads from big corporations.

How connected do you feel to your life's purpose? Or are you one of many who feel as if they are just surviving day to day, trying to get out of debt and get out of pain? Have you ever thought that maybe your experience of pain is actually part of your life's purpose? Part of your life journey to share your gifts with others? I can't say for sure. Only you can answer that. Consciously evolving your spirituality as a part of your healing (which I sometimes consider the fast-track route) will help make your journey a joyous one. It certainly has been joyous for me.

Thankfully, small changes in your lifestyle can dramatically improve your health and wellness. In the upcoming chapters you'll get to choose what resonates with you most.

Iatrogenic Pain

Iatrogenic pain means that pain is being caused as a complication or by-product of medical treatment. Unfortunately, most people don't realize that taking medications for other non-pain related conditions can actually cause or perpetuate chronic pain.

For example, drugs for heartburn, or gastroesophageal reflux disease (GERD), diminish or eliminate the ability of the stomach to produce stomach acid. They are categorized as H2 blockers and proton pump inhibitors. Proton pump inhibitors such as omeprazole (brand name Prilosec®) and esomeprazole (brand name Nexium®) are extremely effective stomach acid reducers and there are millions of people taking them on a daily basis. The supposed cause of GERD is that the stomach acid is back-washing (refluxing) into the esophagus and causing pain. Therefore, GERD is not being caused by excessive amounts of acid in the stomach. Can you see a problem with the long term use of stomach acid reducers?

Think for a moment why our stomachs were designed to produce acid. Could it be that we need it to properly digest our food into smaller components so that the nutrients can be absorbed? Could it be that the acid kills harmful bacteria, parasites and viruses in the food and beverages we invariably ingest? What would happen if we stop producing stomach acid? If you're following my train of thought, you'll conclude that we'll eventually become nutrient deficient and be at higher risk of succumbing to infections.

Studies have reported that acid reducing medications can deplete Vitamin B12, folic acid, Vitamin D, and these minerals: calcium, iron, and zinc. If you become nutrient deficient, then the body's self-healing processes slow down or stop functioning all together. Pain could be one of the signals that your body is crying for adequate nourishment.

Let's take another example. Drugs to treat high cholesterol are some of the best-selling drugs worldwide, especially statins. Pravastatin, lovastatin, simvastatin and fluvastatin sales have been greatly dwarfed by the newer more powerful statin, atorvastatin commonly known as Lipitor®. Unbeknownst to the majority of patients taking these statins, the muscle pain these drugs can cause is not just inconvenient, it can be downright dangerous. Cerivastatin (also known as Baycol® in America) was pulled off the market because of severe muscle disease causing deaths.

As well as lowering your cholesterol, statins lower your ability to make coenzyme Q-10 which is a fat soluble antioxidant that is found in virtually all cell membranes, possibly as much as forty percent. CoQ-10 acts as an antioxidant independently, protecting against DNA damage and other forms of oxidative damage. Coenzyme Q-10 is also an essential component of the mitochondria (the "power-house" of the cell), playing a critical role in the formation of ATP, the body's fundamental energy unit, from carbohydrate and fatty acid metabolism. Without adequate coenzyme Q-10, your cells can't repair as well nor can they produce the molecules of energy. Thus many people not only feel muscle pain, but also their muscles can't actually repair themselves after the normal wear and tear of daily living.

Before I became more holistic, I had always wondered why my patients on cholesterol lowering diets and medication still ended up with heart failure. Now I know the heart needed coenzyme Q-10 to stay healthy. So what I was giving them to control their high cholesterol and hopefully prevent heart disease might have actually been causing it! If your doctor has encouraged you to take a statin, please read The Great Cholesterol Myth by Jonny Bowden and Stephen Sinatra, M.D. before you make a decision on whether to take it.

Here is a brief list of common medications that can cause nutrient deficiencies that may be related to the development or the perpetuation of your chronic pain:

- Oral contraceptives (birth control pills)
- Synthetic estrogen replacement therapy
- Anticonvulsants
- Anti-diabetics
- Anti-hypertensives (blood pressure lowering)
- Anti-inflammatories (ibuprofen, aspirin)
- Anti-ulcer and heartburn drugs (H2 blockers)
- Cholesterol-lowering drugs
- Beta-blockers
- Phenothiazines
- Tricyclic antidepressants
- Benzodiazepines
- Antibiotics

If you are taking medications right now and are concerned about their causing or contributing to your pain, don't just stop them suddenly. Stopping certain medications suddenly can cause a rebound effect and can be dangerous to do without consulting a medical professional. Instead, consult with a holistic physician or naturopath who can assess how to gradually replace your medications with natural remedies that work with your body and not against it.

A great resource to have in your library is a book by Dr. Hyla Cass called Supplement Your Prescription. In it, she outlines how psychiatric patients coming to her for depression and anxiety were often nutrient deficient from other medications they were taking. Instead of giving them yet another prescription such as an anti-depressant, she gave them nutritional therapy based on knowing the patterns of drug-induced nutrient deficiency. The results were spectacular-these patients recovered their mental health without drugs. In her book, simply find the medications you are currently taking and which nutritional supplements would be helpful to offset nutritional deficiencies.

In addition to iatrogenic pain caused by drugs, surgical procedures can also contribute to the development of chronic pain. I've had many patients who have had back surgery for a herniated disc and who later complain of recurrent, unremitting back and hip pain even though MRI's do not show a new cause of their pain. In many of these patients, the scar tissue from the original surgery is now impinging on the proper functioning of the soft tissue around the area causing muscle spasm and nerve entrapment. And in Traditional Chinese Medicine or energy medicine terms, the scar tissue has created a significant block to the proper flow of energy, thus creating a cycle of chronic pain.

Brenda suffered from chronic neck pain and dizziness after being in a car accident. No matter how many doctors and therapists she saw, her neck pain and dizziness remained. When she finally saw me, we corrected her brain balance and her pain markedly improved. Her dizziness, however, was more difficult to treat so I sought out the expertise of Marie McMahon, L.M.T., a good friend of mine, who is a craniosacral therapist. After speaking with Brenda for only five minutes, Marie knew exactly why she was still experiencing dizziness.

Marie has discovered that many women who have undergone a hysterectomy often have head and neck issues including dizziness. This was the case with Brenda. Not only did Brenda have a hysterectomy, she also had a C-section earlier with the birth of one of her sons. The scar tissue arising from the surgeries pre-disposed her to having tight fascia internally, and Marie could literally feel Brenda's sacrum pulling on the structures above whenever she moved her head. I found this fascinating since I never knew how delicate the fascial balance can be between the brain and the sacrum. I certainly didn't learn this in medical school!

Although seemingly benign, I've seen debilitating pain arise in one area of the body after a patient has been given a brace to wear to support another injured area of the body. Walking casts for broken legs tend to elevate one leg higher off the ground compared to the other non-casted leg. The resulting imbalance creates strain on the hips, spine and ligaments and can contribute to the development of chronic pain. Even a thick supportive knee brace can cause an unusual walking pattern that then throws the hips out of alignment. Alas, most doctors who prescribe casts and braces don't consider their negative effects on body mechanics.

What about Aging?

The one belief that no longer resonates with me is that our bodies fall apart with age. How many times have you heard *"Oh, it's arthritis. I'm getting old, so what should I expect?"* You'll learn in the Mind section that we manifest in our reality what we believe. Thus it is vitally important to question our beliefs. For example, I used to think cancer was incurable until I saw a provoking video called The Science of Miracles by Greg Braden in which a bladder tumor completely disappears (as documented by live ultrasound) with Qi Gong healing within minutes! Then I saw several documentaries and read several books about how cancer is curable and my mind blew wide open. I no longer believe that cancer is incurable. If you'd like to know more, check out the annual Healing Cancer Summit at www.healingcancersummit.com.

I highly recommend that you remove the belief from your psyche that your body falls apart as you age. It doesn't have to be true. If you look for more so-called "exceptions to the rule," you will find that there are many older folks who live vibrant active lives without having to take medications. There are few things as "cool" as witnessing an eighty year old doing a perfect back bend or a head stand. One of my heroes is adult skating legend Barbara Kelly of Lake Placid. She's over eighty five years old and still skates during our Coffee Club sessions. I plan to still be skating in my nineties. How about you?

There is a big difference between graceful aging and pathological aging. Graceful aging occurs when the body is still strong, healthy and flexible and the mind is sharp. Pathological aging occurs when our bodies seem to "fall apart". Many anti-aging experts feel that the aging process can be delayed through various natural means including toxin removal, stress and inflammation management, nutritional therapy, stem cells and bio-identical hormone therapy, to name a few.

Getting old is not synonymous with getting sick. There are plenty of ways to reverse your chronic pain and even the aging process if you learn how to take care of your body. It's never too late to start. By involving all the physical, mental, emotional and spiritual aspects of yourself in your healing plan, you'll have the opportunity to grow old gracefully.

Unfortunately, most of the skills I use today were never part of my medical school curriculum. They still aren't part of the curriculum in most schools today. Despite my being in the top ten percent of my medical school graduating class, the most important hands-on skills I have learned are not those I learned in school. In fact, I learned them almost exclusively from non-physicians such as massage therapists, physical therapists, holistic osteopaths, acupuncturists and holistic chiropractors.

In Western medicine, x-ray will show us that someone has an aging degenerative joint whereby the cartilage has eroded away. We never expect anyone to be able to "grow back" his cartilage. But people do!

Modern medicine has made great strides. New diagnostic equipment continues to be developed. Surgical equipment and less invasive surgical techniques are constantly being created. Our ability to save someone's life after an acute trauma such as a car accident has never been better. Yet, despite the advances in modern medicine, we have a growing number of people experiencing chronic disease, cancer or chronic pain. Something is missing.

Traditional Western medications only affect one chemical reaction among an extremely large network of chemical reactions in the body. In doing so, they can put the rest of the body out of balance. For example, a common medication used for pain is acetaminophen, also called paracetamol. Even the makers of acetaminophen (brand name Tylenol ®) can't explain how Tylenol relieves pain, but we know there is a risk of liver damage even at proper doses.

Other pain medications under the class of NSAIDs (non-steroidal anti-inflammatory drugs) include common over-the-counter drugs such as ibuprofen (brand names Motrin®, Advil®, Nuprin®), naproxen (brand name Aleve®), ketoprofen (brand names Actron®, Orudis®) and aspirin (brand name Bufferin®, Bayer®, Exedrin®). All carry warnings of an increased risk of gastrointestinal bleeding, i.e. ulcers, and kidney damage. The prescription NSAIDs, although more expensive, are not necessarily safer and have been implicated in increasing the risk of heart attacks and strokes in regular users.

Narcotics are usually the drugs of last resort for most doctors because of their potentially addictive nature. Narcotics such as codeine, hydrocodone, propoxyphene, meperidine, hydromorphone and morphine can also cause vomiting, confusion and shortness of breath. Most commonly, they cause constipation, and you'll learn in the Body section why you never want to become constipated if you're trying to heal your chronic pain.

Personally I feel that taking pain relievers for acute pain for short periods of time isn't necessarily dangerous; however, the growing trend of long term use of these medications is worrisome. There are not adequate studies showing long term safety and there is an ever-increasing incidence of deaths due to adverse reactions documented by the American Food and Drug Administration.

Chapter Summary

- The underlying cause of chronic pain from the Western perspective is stress and inflammation.
- There are a multitude of contributors to stress and inflammation in our daily lives, many of which are not commonly recognized by traditional Western medicine.
- Medications can contribute to or even cause chronic pain due to their toxicity or nutritionally-depleting nature.
- Lifestyle is a major contributor to health and wellness.
- There is a major difference between pathological and graceful aging.

5

CAUSES OF PAIN—
SPIRITUAL PERSPECTIVE

The Mystery of Life

I used to believe that if I did everything "right", I could think myself well, and my body would heal to perfection. If someone's cancer can disappear within minutes through Qi Gong healing, surely I'd be able to heal myself to physical perfection, right? Even James' mother, who developed liver cancer, went into spontaneous remission, after almost dying of pneumonia after toxic chemotherapy weakened her immune system. So I thought to myself, why do I still get pain? What was I doing wrong?

I've since made marvelous discoveries about how experiencing pain serves me as well as others. Being inspired to write this book to help people in chronic pain is just one example. Although we have great influence over our personal lives, there is much we still don't understand about the mystery of life and how our experiences evolve the human species. Asking "why me?" is often not a valuable question to ask if you are wondering what you did wrong. Asking in this way puts you in judgment-an energy that is anti-healing. Instead, ask "why me?" in the context of wanting to know how your experience is supposed to evolve you or humankind - that's the key!

Your Unique Journey

Everyone's experience is truly unique. Chronic pain has a way of forcing us to stay more present in our bodies, rather than up in our heads. As my parents will tell you, I'm quite a dreamer, so I love spending lots of time dreaming, imagining and thinking. During those times, I forget I even have a body! When that happens, sometimes I don't even eat or drink because I'm not "in" my body . . . I'm in my head. Pain has a way of reminding me that I *have* a body and if I want to feel good, I need to pay attention to it and treat it well.

From a spiritual perspective, your chronic pain serves a purpose. It isn't just an inconvenience to "fix" as quickly as possible so you can get back to normal life. Only your higher guidance can reveal the purpose of your chronic pain. Through self-inquiry, you can transform from feeling victimized to feeling empowered and peaceful. This is possible at any stage of physical healing. In the Spirit section, I'll be taking you through an inquiry process and giving you real life examples of how chronic pain can be a doorway to your personal evolution. In the meantime, here is one example of how a patient discovered that for herself.

Frannie worked as secretary for a State institution. She was the perfect secretary, always knowing what her boss needed her to do before he even asked. Everyone loved Frannie because she was the "go to" person and generously offered assistance to her co-workers. Yet, despite her popularity and feeling useful at work, Frannie was not feeling well. She'd wake up feeling as if she had been run over by a truck. She felt slight relief from an anti-seizure medication prescribed by her doctor. Unfortunately this medicine caused extreme brain fog and Frannie referred to it as her "stupid pills". When Frannie came to see me for acupuncture, she was lovely and intelligent. Under her calm demeanor, however, Frannie was desperate. She didn't understand why she had such pain and why prescribed medication wasn't offering complete relief. Discouraged, she was even taking anti-depressants because her doctor said that some of her pain might be "in her head".

It was obvious that Frannie was everything to everybody. She loved being adored by family, friends and co-workers and rarely said "no" to anyone, even if she was too tired or achy. Frankly she was so busy helping others that she didn't have a clue how to help herself. She was hoping that I would just magically "fix" her, but that's not how healing works in the real world.

Frannie's healing began with the realization that she was trading her health to be liked by others. Her self-sacrificing habits had been imprinted as a young child from parents who couldn't differentiate between selfishness and self-care. Frannie learned that taking care of herself meant that she was selfish and "bad". Her self-esteem was fragile and dependent on pleasing people. When people liked her, Frannie felt great, and when people didn't, she felt horrible. Frannie exhausted her energy stores doing whatever she could to guarantee that people would like her. Of course, this strategy proved only to feed into the pain/illness cycle.

While working with me for over two years, Frannie finally took responsibility for her own healing by setting healthy boundaries with family, friends and co-workers. She practiced saying "no", and with my support and encouragement, applied for a promotion enabling her to direct others. Once she experienced true empowerment with healthy boundaries and accepted that she might be disliked by someone, her pain literally vanished. Not surprisingly, so did everyone whose needs were not met by Frannie. You see, Frannie's pain had a purpose. It was there to say "no" when others encroached on her boundaries. Once she created healthier boundaries, the pain no longer had a purpose so it dissolved.

Frannie's experience is witness to how pain can be a helpful guide and blessing. Her soul was directing her to a state of higher awareness, to take action out of choice rather than out of habit. Hopefully when you read the Spirit section, you'll experience an "Ah ha!" like Frannie did, as to how your pain is currently serving you.

I believe that through what Rupert Sheldrake refers to as Morphic fields, those of us who can successfully navigate through our painful experiences transforming them into empowering journeys, evolve the entire human race.

Chapter Summary

- Pain has a way of forcing us to become more present and in our bodies instead of being up in our minds.
- From a spiritual perspective, the symptom of pain serves a higher purpose.
- Pain is a way for your body to say "no" when you aren't empowered enough to say "no" aloud.
- Pain is an avenue through which you grow your Soul and help evolve the human race.

Section B

Your Mind—Harness Your Internal Healer

"There is no medicine like hope, no incentive so great, and no tonic so powerful, as expectation of something better tomorrow."
-Orison Swett Marden

6

BALANCE YOUR BRAIN

Without brain balance, life will feel like a struggle. You won't stick to your goals and you won't follow through on your own intentions. Without it, other therapies just don't work well, even natural ones, like acupuncture or chiropractic. Once I am able to restore brain balance in a patient, the trick is to maintain it, so that he continues to self-heal. The problem lies in the malleability of our nervous systems in response to negative or harmful energy. Just like we can initiate and support healing through exposure to positive energy (such as music therapy); we can destroy it through exposure to negative energy.

Brain *imbalance* can be viewed as a "short-circuit" in the brain. Here's the bad news. Approximately 95% of people (even so-called healthy people) are not brain balanced according to John Diamond, MD, innovator of Behavioral Kinesiology and the author of the book, Your Body Doesn't Lie. Before I tell you why we are all at risk of being out of balance, here is an analogy that might help you understand in simpler terms. Imagine old-fashioned circuit boards with wires coming out of one spot and plugging into another. Your brain and nervous system are similar to this circuit board but with thousands of wires. What would happen if a circuit board was shaken so hard that some of the wires got loose? The circuit board wouldn't work as well, would it? No matter how much electricity, or Qi, you deliver to the circuit board, communication would still be "lost" in some areas. Right?

Every single one of my patients who couldn't heal had, in a sense, short-circuited their nervous systems in *two* ways: their right-left hemispheric balance and their ability to regulate the stress response. Right-left brain imbalance occurs when under repeated stress; the brain hemispheres become desynchronized. Most often, the left, logical side of the brain becomes dominant and the right, intuitive side of the brain becomes passive.

The other type of short circuit occurs when the nervous system gets locked into a stress (fight or flight) response and can't manage to get back

42

42

into the relaxation response. This imbalance can manifest if someone has been under severe stress for a significant period of time. Both short-circuits can also occur with any repeated or significant stress to the brain such as trauma, toxins or radiation.

The stress-relaxation responses in the body are governed by what's called the *autonomic nervous system*. The autonomic nervous system regulates all the non-voluntary functions of the body like breathing, circulation, sweating, intestinal function and salivation. You don't have to think about breathing. It's automatic. You also don't have to tell your stomach to digest your food. It is also automatic. The autonomic nervous system is of vital importance and when not regulating properly, can prevent the body from going into "healing" mode.

There are two parts to the autonomic nervous system: the sympathetic and the parasympathetic. The sympathetic nervous system, when turned "on" is best known for the stress response, also known as the fight or flight response. The parasympathetic nervous system promotes the relaxation response. In my patients with the most severe symptoms of chronic pain, insomnia, anxiety and stress, the autonomic nervous system is no longer regulating properly and in fact, is stuck on "stress mode". My patient Kate, who had this condition, explained it best: *"It's like being in a car and you've got the accelerator to the floor, but the gear is in neutral, so you're expending a lot of energy but not going anywhere!"*

The nervous system uses electronic signals and messenger chemicals to communicate with the rest of the body and thus is susceptible to particular stressors. In addition, some of the cells in our brain contain magnetite, which are crystals that can be affected by magnetic energy, which explains why some people (myself included) can feel when a severe storm or an earthquake is imminent. So, in my humble opinion, the brain's energetic imbalances seem to be the crux of all the other energetic imbalances in the body.

In this chapter, I'll be teaching you how to treat brain imbalances using energy tools. Most people associate the mind with brain functioning, which is mostly what we're going to be talking about in this chapter. The remainder of the Mind section, however, will focus on shifting your thoughts, beliefs, and emotions from negative to positive. By the way, when I refer to the word "negative", I really mean non-supportive, rather than bad. Same goes for the word "positive". Positive means supportive, rather than good. I prefer, whenever I can, to refrain from making judgments such as good or bad. Judgments themselves can thwart the healing process.

The reason I'm providing you with energy tools to balance your brain is because I have found that without balancing the brain first, people can't easily change their thoughts, beliefs, and emotions! If you cannot shift your thoughts, beliefs and emotions, you will not take actions toward your goals. As I mentioned in Section A, there is not a single thing that is more important in your healing than balancing your nervous system.

Opening up the communication between both hemispheres of the brain gives you the ability to creatively solve problems. This is called brain synchronization. In life, it is the feeling when you get a wonderful "Ah-ha!" about something. It is also the feeling of being in the "zone" as you do what you love with grace and ease. When I won my first Adult National gold medal in figure skating, I felt like I was in the zone.

Restoring a healthy autonomic nervous system is foundational to all holistic healing strategies. Without first attaining brain balance, other holistic therapies won't "stick". In other words, the improvements, if any, will not hold no matter how much work you do to help yourself.

How to Know if You're Brain Balanced

Sadly, most people aren't. To determine brain balance, I do a simple muscle test in my office on every new patient that comes to see me. Approximately 95% percent of new patients fail this test. You can learn this simple test too, but you'll need to practice it on quite a few people to become consistent at it. I have videos on my YouTube channel that will show you how to check your own brain balance as well as that of others. See Resources for links.

Don't worry if you aren't comfortable with self-testing brain balance. By examining the list below, you'll have a pretty good idea if you are brain balanced or not. If you have all or most of the symptoms, it is likely that you need to balance your brain:

☐ You can't sleep through the night without waking
☐ You trip or bump into things by accident

☐ You have dyslexia or right/left disorientation etc.

☐ You have ADD/ADHD (attention deficit disorder)

☐ You are addicted to drugs, sugar, alcohol, caffeine, or wheat

☐ You don't remember your dreams

☐ You feel stressed or panicky all the time

☐ You can't relieve chronic pain

☐ You have tried all sorts of therapies but nothing seems to work

☐ You feel better with treatment but the results don't last

☐ You experience chronic tiredness or brain fog

☐ You tend to be edgy, irritable, quick to anger, or sad

☐ You can't easily let go of negative thoughts

☐ You have mood swings or symptoms of depression

☐ You have difficulty with decision making and remembering things

☐ You feel chaotic and disorganized much of the time

☐ You feel overwhelmed, lost or unmotivated

☐ You get migraines easily, especially when the weather changes

☐ You feel sick whenever there are significant shifts in earth energy such as electromagnetic storms, earthquakes, hurricanes etc.

Causes of Brain Imbalance

There are many things that can cause brain imbalances. The most common include head injuries and exposure to electromagnetic radiation including those emanating from popular wireless devices (microwaves). The greatest threat to health in this millennium is electropollution from wireless technology according to Dr. Stephen Sinatra of the HeartMD Institute. Many experts and scientists now understand that the outer membrane of our cells (cellular membrane) is the location where chemical and energetic signals are processed to establish important cellular functions.

Communication via receptors on the cellular membrane tells the genetic code of our cells, the DNA in the nucleus, what proteins to make to accomplish each important task of keeping the body alive and healthy. According to Dr. Sinatra, these receptor sites on the outer membrane of our cells are responsible for keeping bacteria, viruses and microwaves out. When the microwaves start coming into the cells, the receptor sites shut down. Because we are exposed to microwaves via wireless devices on a constant basis, cellular function can also shut down. The cell membranes block microwaves from entering the cell, but also block the assimilation of vitamins, minerals and hormones! Furthermore, waste products produced by the cell cannot escape. The cell then rapidly ages, the cell voltage diminishes, and the cells become sick.

Food additives such as monosodium glutamate (MSG), artificial sweeteners such as aspartame, can cause cell death in the brain and predispose you to brain imbalances as well. Mercury and lead are heavy metals that are extremely toxic, particularly to the nervous system. Heavy metal toxicity causes chronic inflammation in the body which can lead to hardening of the arteries and heart disease in addition to contributing to pain. Most holistic experts agree that the number one risk of heavy metal toxicity is having mercury fillings in your teeth (often called "silver" fillings).

The American Dental Association has yet to admit that using mercury for fillings is toxic despite ample evidence that mercury volatilizes easily from the tooth when it is exposed to heat or pressure, and can then lodge in other areas of the body. Instead, they blame eating fish for the majority of mercury exposure. Go to the International Academy of Oral Medicine & Toxicology for more information on this topic. See Resources for the link.

I remember vividly years ago at a holistic health conference seeing slides of mercury vapor escaping from a mercury-filled tooth. Most disturbing was seeing sequential photographs of radioactive-labeled mercury fillings in a sheep. Within thirty days of inserting the amalgam, the mercury had volatilized (became gaseous) and lodged in the jaw, stomach, liver and kidney. A similar experiment with monkeys found mercury lodged in their jaw, kidneys, liver, intestines and heart. After that conference I tested myself for mercury toxicity and found that I had excessive levels of mercury in my body, even though I only had two small fillings in my mouth! Today, you can easily view videos online and watch mercury gas escaping from dental amalgam.

However, if you have mercury fillings don't run out and get them removed right away. It can be more dangerous to have them removed by a regular dentist. Instead, you need to consult with a holistic dentist. There are special precautions dentists need to take when removing mercury fillings. Only holistic dentists routinely use *all* of these necessary precautions to protect the patient as well as the staff from mercury exposure. Regular dental offices do not have elaborate venting systems for preventing the mercury from vaporizing and contaminating patients and staff. Just working in a dental office can be dangerous.

Jacob, a dentist, had a good diet and swam competitively. His cholesterol wasn't high and neither was his blood pressure. Despite having no family history for early heart attacks, he suffered two. "It's not fair!" exclaimed his sister-in-law. "Jacob's lifestyle is so healthy. He shouldn't have had a heart attack". But I think I deduced what the cause was. His regular exposure to mercury most likely set him up for having chronic inflammation, the real cause of heart disease.

Aside from electropollution, food toxins and mercury, there are natural causes of brain imbalance in the form of geomagnetic disturbances. Examples in this category include severe storms, earthquakes, typhoons, solar activity, eclipses and hurricanes. Here is a checklist you can use to evaluate your brain balance risk factors:

- ☐ I or someone living in my home uses a cell phone or Bluetooth device
- ☐ I use a baby monitor, or walkie talkie
- ☐ I talk on my cell phone/Bluetooth while driving in my car
- ☐ I or someone living in my home uses a cordless phone
- ☐ I have a cordless phone next to my bed while I sleep
- ☐ I use a laptop or desktop computer on a regular basis
- ☐ I have a clock radio or transformer beside my bed
- ☐ I use a wireless-enabled tablet device such as an iPad
- ☐ I carry a wireless device on my body such as a cell phone
- ☐ I use or am exposed to wireless internet (Wi-Fi)
- ☐ I am exposed to fumes or volatile organic chemicals
- ☐ I use artificial sweeteners such as sucralose or aspartame (diet soda)
- ☐ I eat a lot of processed salty snack food (that might have MSG or flavor enhancers like autolyzed yeast extract or yeast extract)
- ☐ I have had a concussion, whiplash, or a severe fall at some point in my life
- ☐ I have been in a car accident
- ☐ I live in an urban area (where there are many cell towers)

☐ I eat a lot of large fish like tuna or swordfish (mercury risk)
☐ I have or have had "silver" amalgam fillings (mercury risk)
☐ My mother had amalgam fillings before I was born
☐ I work in a dental office or a salon (toxin risk)
☐ I am extremely stressed or have a very stressful life
☐ I drink fluoridated water
☐ I do not get enough quality sleep
☐ I have a neurological diagnosis such as multiple sclerosis, stroke, epilepsy

I don't know about you, but I've had a few concussions in my life. I wasn't very athletic until I became a figure skater. But before that, I experienced several episodes of head trauma while downhill skiing, cross-country skiing, bicycling and even playing tennis! The latter was caused by my former husband hitting the tennis ball into the back of my head by mistake. In 1995 I also had a head-on motor vehicle collision and lost consciousness. Stubbornly, I didn't take any time off work to rest. After a CT scan of my head and a night's stay in the hospital, I promptly went back to work. I now realize that I suffered from post-concussion syndrome that could have been avoided if I had taken some time off to rest.

One Christmas, I made the mistake of accompanying my partner and my brother, to an electronics store. It was during Canadian Boxing Day, so the place was jam packed with customers, all carrying cell phones, of course! The store was alive with wireless devices, security systems, computers and televisions. Within ten minutes of entering the store, I developed a severe migraine headache. I rarely get migraine headaches, but that day, I felt as if my head was going to explode. I had not yet discovered the importance of brain balancing at that point, but now it all makes sense to me.

Needless to say, given my traumatic history, my nervous system is rather sensitive to "bad" energy. I don't like handling a cell phone without a protective device on it, because within minutes I'll start feeling tired and headachy. I also wear a necklace that helps protect me from harmful electromagnetic frequencies when I'm away from home. Sleeping in a hotel with wireless internet is a recipe for morning stiffness and achy joints, so I make sure I use every single energy tool at my disposal to protect myself. I'll be sharing many of my tools with you in the Body section of this book.

Maybe you aren't as sensitive to electropollution as I am, or maybe you are, but just don't realize it. Maybe your chronic pain or fatigue stems from chronic brain imbalances due to exposure to electropollution. An unfortunate myth exists in our society: people erroneously believe that any product that is available for sale must be safe. Nothing could be further from the truth. The United States government does not require independent safety testing of cellular phones or other wireless devices. In Switzerland, on the other hand, the government was so concerned about the negative effects of wireless technology on children that they banned wireless use in schools. Instead, SwissCom, inventors of the World Wide Web, opted to install fiber optic internet cable free of charge in all Swiss schools. Here in America, the opposite is true. More schools than ever are incorporating wireless computing into their classrooms. It is no co-incidence that the incidence of attention deficit hyperactivity disorder (ADD/ADHD) is on a sharp rise and that wireless technology may be partially to blame.

Achieving Brain Balance

There are several methods that I know of and have used to achieve brain balance. By far, the fastest and easiest to use is an energy tool called the LifeWave Y-Age Aeon anti-stress patch. I'll call it the Aeon patch for short. This patch was released on the market in January 2011 and has fast become LifeWave's biggest seller. Not only does this patch balance and calm the nervous system of the body, it has a dual action of also decreasing inflammation. Thus I've used this patch, as well as the LifeWave IceWave pain patches (which I'll show you how to use in an upcoming chapter) to reduce or eliminate pain in over ninety percent of people who are willing to try them. Allow me to give you a little background on LifeWave patches, which I consider one of the greatest breakthroughs in the history of energy therapies.

LifeWave patches are the brainchild of inventor, David Schmidt, who was working on natural ways to safely enhance the energy of Navy SEAL soldiers who were confined in mini-submarines for months at a time. Because these ships were so small, storing caffeinated energy drinks were not an option. Schmidt developed a prototype acupuncture energy patch, which finally came onto the market as the Energy Enhancer patches in 2004.

In 2005, I was introduced to these patches by a chiropractor. At first I was skeptical that a patch could work as well as acupuncture, but after doing some research I was willing to try them. The only patch LifeWave had available at the time was the Energy Enhancer patches, so I used them for my figure skating. I wore them on my Stomach 36 acupuncture point during my first-ever Adult International Figure Skating Championship in Oberstdorf, Germany, and won a gold medal for the United States! After that experience, I was hooked. Recovering from the fatigue of having fibromyalgia took months rather than years, thanks to these patches, and today I'm as productive as ever. Then with the advent of the IceWave pain relief patches, and the Aeon anti-stress patches, I am now able to return to doing things I couldn't do when I was sick-like back bends.

LifeWave patches contain nano-sized organic crystals in a homeopathic solution that reflect a specific spectrum of infra-red light frequencies in our bodies. Because the patches communicate to our bodies via light, nothing transfers through the skin into the body. In fact, they are just as effective when taped onto clothing. The organic crystals inside the patches are activated by your body's warm electromagnetic field. Once the patches come within close proximity to your body, they "turn on". If they are removed from the body, they "turn off". Each patch stays active approximately 12 hours. The patches can become ineffective if exposed to heat, so make sure you don't leave the package on the dash of a car in the middle of the summer or wear them in a hot tub!

Brain Balance Protocol Using Acupuncture Patches

Just a quick disclaimer before I teach you my Brain Balancing protocol: this patching protocol is not officially endorsed by LifeWave because it has not been researched by the company. Thus you will not find this protocol in any company literature. Rather, I developed it from my own clinical research and experience.

To balance the brain, you will need to purchase a package of LifeWave Y-Age Aeon patches from a LifeWave distributor. By the way, I highly discourage you from purchasing these patches from just any online discount reseller for three reasons. Firstly, LifeWave does not honor the 30-day money back guarantee if the patches were bought from an online discount reseller such as Amazon or eBay. Secondly, LifeWave distributors are strictly prohibited from reselling patches on a separate website and are thus breaking the rules of ethical conduct if they do. Thirdly, the whole point of selling the patches through distributors is so that you, the customer, can get personalized training and support. If you take the risk of purchasing LifeWave patches from online discount stores, do not expect help, training or support from a LifeWave distributor. See Resources for the customer service link to find a distributor you can work with.

Please feel free to download a free PDF version of the protocol below from my LifeWave Patch Training team's website: www.patchtrainingteam. com.

General Guidelines:

- ✓ Use one patch per day, maximum 12 hours a day, daytime or nighttime, whichever feels better to you.
- ✓ Hydrate with plenty of water, about ½ oz. per lb. of body weight per day or approximately 2 Liters.
- ✓ Choose any one of the acupuncture points below to use daily or rotate through the points to see which feels the best to you.
- ✓ You may wear the patch stuck to a hat, headband or scarf to hide it if you like. It doesn't have to be stuck onto your head in order for it to work.
- ✓ When not in use, keep patches away from heat and your body.
- ✓ Keep in mind that you do not have to place the patch exactly over the acupuncture point.
- ✓ Approximate location will work just fine.
- ✓ Do not reuse patches once the adhesive backing is removed.

What to Expect:

- • You may feel more relaxed, calmer, happier, or have less "brain fog".

- You may feel you have more energy. But if your life has been stuck in "stress-mode" for a long time, you may actually feel overly relaxed or sleepy.
- With continued use, you may experience deeper sleep, less awakenings, more vivid dreams.
- You may feel more refreshed on awakening in the morning.
- The patches are powerful activators of acupuncture points. If you feel unwell, headachy, flu-like, it means your body is detoxifying (healing response). If it is mild, drinking more water or taking some Vitamin C may ease the symptoms. If it is moderate or severe, simply remove the patch and try again the next day for a shorter period of time.

Four Options for Placing the Aeon Patch

Option 1: You can place the patch on the hairless area of the skull behind the right ear. The approximate acupuncture point is Triple Burner 17 (see Figure 1). This area is close to the brainstem of the nervous system, the part of the brain controlling many automatic nervous system functions such as breathing. People who have a lot of fear or anxiety tend to like using this acupuncture point.

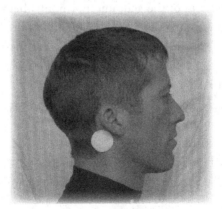

Figure 1: Triple Burner 17

Option 2: You can place the patch over the "third eye" which is just above and between the eyebrows. This acupuncture point, Governing Vessel 24.5 (see Figure 2), stimulates the pineal and pituitary glands. Many women in my practice like to sleep with the patch activating this acupuncture point to encourage deep sleep and hormonal balance.

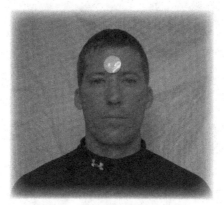

Figure 2: Governing Vessel 24.5

Option 3: You can place the patch on top of the head at Governing Vessel 20 (see Figure 3). This point can be found by drawing an imaginary line from the tips of your ears intersecting the midpoint of the top of your head. This acupuncture point is used to lift the energy into the head and is good for people with foggy thinking or low mood.

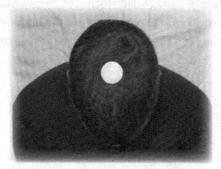

Figure 3: Governing Vessel 20

Option 4: You can place the patch over the thymus area (see Figure 4), which is on the breast bone, about one third of the way down from the notch in the front of the neck. Although the image is shown with the patch on top of clothing, you may place it directly on the skin for optimal effect.

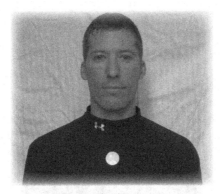

Figure 4: Thymus

It's a good idea to rotate through the points daily or every couple of days to see which points make you feel the best. Continue patching with Aeon patches on a daily basis for at least two weeks. Then you can graduate to patching your head four days a week while patching other acupuncture points listed in the company's brochure on the other three days of the week. Alternatively, you can patch nightly to help you sleep. If you hear about severe weather, geomagnetic storms or big earthquakes above 6.0 somewhere in the world, you may wish to use the brain balancing protocol for a few days in a row to prevent the stress from affecting your nervous system.

Brain Balancing Using Affirmations

Dr. John Diamond found that when the thymus gland was balanced, both hemispheres of the brain were also balanced. You'll notice that one of the brain balance points is on the upper chest. That point is right over the thymus gland. He discovered that if any one of the acupuncture meridians were imbalanced, the thymus would test "weak" on his kinesiology testing, and the brain would test imbalanced. Each of the meridians is connected to a different emotional response. Dr. Diamond found that by saying a specific positive affirmation for each meridian, a person could rebalance his brain. Once the brain was rebalanced, the thymus would then test "strong". You can view my brain balance test videos at www.YouTube.com/karenkanmd.

Meridian imbalances caused by negative emotions can be corrected with verbalizing specific affirmations as verified by applied kinesiology testing. I have tested my patients in the office and found that brain balance can be achieved easily within three to five repetitions of the affirmation(s). Unlike Aeon patches, however, which last twelve hours on the body, you may need to repeat the affirmations regularly throughout the day to maintain your brain balance. The nice thing about the affirmations is that they are free. I'd recommend repeating these affirmations as often as you can during the day. Say them out loud, quietly and authentically, to reinforce your brain balance. The more you can "feel" the words, the better your results. Here is the list of daily affirmations listed in Life Energy (reproduced with the permission of Dr. Diamond):

I have love, faith, trust, gratitude and courage. (Thymus)
I am humble. I am tolerant. I am modest. (Lung meridian)
I am happy. I have good fortune. I am cheerful. (Liver meridian)
I reach out with love. (Gallbladder meridian)
I am basically clean and good. I am worthy of being loved. (Large Intestine meridian)
I have faith and confidence in my future. I am secure. (Spleen meridian)
My sexual energies are balanced. (Kidney meridian)
I renounce the past. I am generous. I am relaxed. (Pericardium)
I have forgiveness in my heart. (Heart meridian)
I am content. I am tranquil. (Stomach meridian)
I am buoyed up with hope. I am light and buoyant. (Triple Burner/ Thyroid meridian)
I am jumping with joy. (Small Intestine meridian)
I am in harmony. I am at peace. (Bladder meridian)
I have faith, love, trust, hope, gratitude and courage (Thymus)
Close with: *My life energy is high. I am in the state of love.*

Brain Balancing Music

Dr. Jeffrey Thompson, a chiropractor and musician, has pioneered the best brain balancing music I've ever listened to. Used ideally with headphones, his music balances both hemispheres of the brain and encourages a balanced nervous system. His technology uses three coordinated methods for bringing the mind-body into a state of deep relaxation and balance: "Primordial Sounds," "Brainwave Entrainment" and "multi-layered music" recorded in 3D. The body responds positively to primordial sounds that include womb, nature and space sounds.

Dr. Thompson's healing music can train the brain to establish coordinated brain waves of beta, alpha, theta, delta, gamma and epsilon. This process is called brainwave entrainment. Delta waves are required for deep sleep and physical rejuvenation, so if you are not sleeping well, you can't truly heal the body. Dr. Thompson's delta wave music, when used for at least twenty days in a row, entrains the brain to produce relaxing delta waves. Some people feel results from their first listening.

Unlike other brainwave entrainment music, Dr. Thompson doesn't try to entrain the brain by introducing audible repetitive beats to the music, which I find rather stressful and annoying. He has a special technique that he uses that entrains the brain without any audible beats. I find his music particularly effective for myself and my patients. In the office I have one of his patented Neuroacoustic Sound Tables, a massage table specially equipped with a patented speaker technology that vibrates your body as you relax while listening to his brainwave music. Almost all of my patients experience profound relaxation on the Sound Table and it enhances their healing.

In order to maintain your brain balance, you will want to listen to Dr. Thompson's music on a daily basis. Remember not to listen to the relaxation ones in the car in case you fall asleep! Children and adults with attention deficit disorder (ADD/ADHD) should avoid theta wave music and may wish to play beta wave music instead during the day to enhance their focus. The Brainwave Massage 2.0 audio CD is for beta wave enhancement. Some of my patients who are teachers play this CD in the background for their classes to enhance their children's relaxation and focus.

Alpha wave music is for general relaxation and meditation, whereas theta wave music enhances the dream state (which is why it isn't recommended for ADD). Delta wave music is good for everyone and I highly recommend that you listen to Delta wave music before going to bed each night. Some people prefer listening to it all night long to enhance sleep.

Epsilon and Gamma brainwaves are advanced brainwave states found in advanced meditators, some of whom are known to have the ability to leave their physical bodies and travel in the astral plane. I particularly enjoy Dr. Thompson's gamma brainwave music because I notice that it enhances my intuition and insight.

To achieve and maintain brain balance using brainwave entrainment music, it is very important to listen to it daily for at least an hour. Dr. Thompson's brainwave entrainment music can be found listed on my website at www.KarenKan.com/products.

Alternate Nostril Breathing

As we breathe normally throughout the day, one nostril demonstrates more airflow than the other and this alternates approximately every ninety minutes. According to Dr. Leonard Laskow in his book Healing with Love, the hypothalamus, a glandular part of the brain, is responsible for regulating the switch in nostril dominance. The hypothalamus controls many activities including activities of the autonomic nervous system. Blood vessels that supply the mucous membrane of the nasal passages are under the control of the autonomic nervous system which is composed of the sympathetic (fight or flight) and parasympathetic (relaxation). Through alternate sympathetic constriction and parasympathetic dilation of these small blood vessels, the nasal passages either allow more or less air flow.

When air flows in through the right nostril, the left hemisphere of the brain is stimulated. When air flows in through the left nostril, the right hemisphere of the brain is stimulated. D. A. Werntz, a researcher conducting a study at the University of California at San Diego School of Medicine, demonstrated that breathing through one nostril generated EEG activity in the opposite brain hemisphere.

While doing research at a biofeedback lab, Dr. Laskow decided to practice the ancient yogic breathing science of pranayama, in particular, alternate nostril breathing, in order to see what would happen to his brain EEG patterns. As taught in yogic traditions, as you breathe in through the left nostril, you occlude the right nostril with your right thumb. At the peak of inhalation, you switch nasal passages and there is a slight pause in breathing at this point. As you slowly breathe out through the right nostril, you then occlude the left nostril with your right ring finger. Then to balance the brain hemispheres, you are supposed to continue occluding the left nostril with your right ring finger as you proceed to breathe in through the right nostril. On the out-breath, release the occlusion and breathe out of the left nostril while occluding the right again with your right thumb.

Dr. Laskow discovered that when he used one of his hands (as in the above traditional instructions) to practice alternate nostril breathing, he surprisingly imbalanced his brain hemispheres. Instead he decided not to use his hands at all and imagined the air flowing just through one nostril or the other. This had the intended effect of balancing his brain hemispheres as evidenced on EEG testing. It would be interesting to see if you used the same finger of each hand to do the alternate nostril occlusion whether or not you would get a more balanced effect than by using the traditional one-handed approach.

Alternate nostril breathing can be changed to single nostril breathing to calm the brain. You can breathe in through the left nostril and breath out through the right nostril over and over again, activating the right side of the brain. This has a relaxing effect on the nervous system. Alternatively, if you're feeling a bit sleepy and want to wake up, try breathing in through the right nostril and out through the left repeatedly in order to activate the left side of the brain. Translated into Chinese medicine, the right side of the brain would be Yin (feminine) and the left would be Yang (masculine). Balancing the brain would then translate into balancing the Yin and Yang in your nervous system.

Although I don't know if there is any research about how long the brain stays balanced after doing several minutes of alternate nostril breathing, it is safe to say that frequent daily practice will be necessary.

Subtle Energy Therapeutics

Dr. Yuri Kronn, a Russian radio-physicist, invented Vital Force Technology. Utilizing a plasma-based generator to generate sophisticated frequency patterns of low intensity alternating magnetic fields, he infuses them into "substance-carriers" that dramatically enhance and intensify nutritional and therapeutic effects on the body. Both Energy Tools International's Vital Force formulas as well as Nutrilink Energy's formulas utilize this advanced technology.

Energy Tools International's Vital Force formulas are only available through practitioners like me. They have several formulas that help with re-establishing brain balance including Clear Mind, Master Brain Formula, and Meta-Stress. Nutrilink Energy's Dr. D's Master Brain and ANS Support are potent subtle energy formulas that are available to consumers online.

I use muscle testing to determine the correct dose for each patient (see later chapters on how to do this yourself), but you can start at a low dose of 5 drops per day and work up to a maximum of 30 drops a day. If you are currently taking conventional medication, it may be wise to start at a very low dose, such as 2 drops a day diluted into a large water bottle. I usually recommend spreading out the dose throughout the day so that you are slowly trickling in the energy. Dr. Steven Davis, co-creator of the Nutrilink Energy formulas, calls this process "trickle charging".

The subtle energy formulas help your body reestablish the correct energetic pattern which has been lost through stress and illness. They also increase the overall energy available to the cells. The LifeWave patches do something very similar. All cells function according to underlying energetic patterns. Through stress and toxins, these patterns become distorted over time and re-create "sick" cell functions. Think of the underlying energetic pattern as a blueprint. If you were building a house with a distorted blueprint, it wouldn't matter what materials you used; it would not stay standing for very long. Same goes for your body. If your blueprint is wrong, then it doesn't matter what food or supplements you take in, your cells won't know how to properly absorb or assimilate them.

The above formulas contain vibrational frequencies that are enhanced and preserved in trace minerals. Don't be surprised if the ingredient list only lists "trace minerals". Here in the United States, it is not required to label "energy" ingredients per se, and even if they did, there wouldn't be enough space on the bottle to list them. Unlike homeopathic medication, these formulas are not simple dilutions of known organic and inorganic substances. They are much more powerful. I often use a combination of LifeWave Y-Age Aeon patches and subtle energy formulas to help my patients heal faster.

How Soon You Will See Results

Your brain will begin balancing right away with these energy tools. The challenge is *maintaining* and deepening the balance. The more hydrated you are and the healthier your diet and lifestyle, the easier it will be to maintain your brain balance. I've noticed that people who patch their heads daily with Aeon not only become brain balanced very quickly, but also experience profound shifts in their mood, awareness and pain levels within two weeks of consistent use.

If you're using Dr. Thompson's brainwave entrainment music, you need to listen to it daily for at least twenty one days in a row for optimal results. Similarly, consistent daily practice is important if you are using Dr. Diamond's affirmations or yogic breathing techniques for brain balancing. Subtle energy therapeutics take about two to three weeks at most before you begin feeling results. A combination of the methods would be, of course, the most powerful, as each technique uses different technologies and can thus influence the brain's circuitry in synergistic ways.

Preventing Brain Imbalances

Get protective devices for your electronic equipment and phones. As a result of testing in my office, I've noticed that the new generation iPhones are notorious for causing brain imbalance, more so than any other brand. I suspect, however, that as cellular and smartphone technology increases, we will have even more radiation to contend with across the board. For mobile phones, there are three microwave radiation-protection devices that I currently recommend: the Quantum Cell (EarthCalm), the Matrix

2 (LifeWave) and the EMF Transformer (Energy Tools International). For cordless phones I recommend a single Quantum Cell device on the base station. For tablets, such as iPads and other wireless-enabled portable devices, I recommend the EarthCalm Torus. EarthCalm devices have circuitry that grounds harmful microwave radiation, rendering it harmless even if the device is on your body. I'm grateful for the EarthCalm protective devices because without them, I wouldn't be able to tolerate having cell phones or Wi-Fi in my home because I'm so electrically-sensitive.

If you're unwilling to purchase a protective device for your phone, there are other, albeit less effective, ways to minimize the radiation harm to your nervous system and brain. We discuss these ways in a later chapter.

Dr. Diamond feels that the thymus gland is the first gland that "takes a hit" when you are stressed. It can literally shrink with stress! According to Dr. Diamond, people who have a weak thymus can easily lose their brain balance due to other causes (in addition to what I have already outlined). For example, he has noted in his experiments that hats made of synthetic material can affect the brain balance.

Poor posture, such as slouching, can cause a slowing of the energy system and brain imbalances. Metal in necklaces, eye glasses and belts can sometimes contribute to weakening the energy system in susceptible people. Not surprisingly, certain types of music, particularly rock and heavy metal, can cause brain imbalances in many folks whereas classical music and classical rock-and-roll do not. You may wish to experiment with changing what you wear and what you listen to in order to see if you have more energy and feel better.

Avoiding brain toxins such as aspartame, food additives, MSG, as well as toxic fumes (from paint and household cleaners) may also prevent you from losing your brain balance. I have found that avoiding excessive ingestion of sugar can also be helpful in most cases.

Listening to Dr. Thompson's brain balancing brainwave music on a regular basis, even without headphones, can help you maintain your brain balance. I have speakers in my bedroom so I can listen to healing music throughout the night when my system is most receptive to energetic input.

After someone has achieved brain balance using the Aeon patches, I will often recommend that they maintain their balance by patching "their heads" at least three times or four times a week. On the other days of the week, the Aeon patch can be used on other acupuncture points found in the LifeWave brochure to help ease stress and inflammation.

Beware of Self-Sabotage

The number one mistake that all my patients make is assuming that once they feel better, they don't have to continue paying attention to and maintaining their brain balance. Here's a typical scenario:

Jean sought acupuncture to treat her insomnia and back pain. I tested her brain balance and it was abnormal. I brain balanced her using daily Aeon head patching and within a week she was sleeping better than she had for the prior eleven years and her back pain was history. A couple weeks later, she showed up again with insomnia and back pain. On questioning her, I found out that she discontinued using the Aeon patches that I had given to her to maintain her brain balance. Moreover, she had been talking quite a bit on her cordless telephone. She sheepishly admitted that after the first week when she felt so much better, she didn't follow through on my suggestion that she replace her cordless phones with landline phones or purchase a protective device for the cordless base station.

Once you are feeling better and having less pain, you too will forget all the wonderful new habits and the skills you have learned to get your body to heal itself. We literally sabotage our success! When the symptoms go away, we forget that there is often a lot more healing that needs to take place to reverse the damage. By the time you experience symptoms, your body has been out of balance for a very long time, often decades. You can't expect *everything* to heal in an instant, so it is important to maintain your improvement with good habits and effective energy tools. Ok, maybe you are just interested in symptom control, but even so, wouldn't it be great to build up some resilience so that your body doesn't "fall apart" when life gets too busy or overwhelming?

Even the best of us sabotage ourselves, although I'm getting much better at catching myself in the act of self-sabotage. Part of the self-sabotaging habit is a self-esteem issue. Deep down, many of us don't really feel like we deserve love or deserve "the good life", especially when there are so many other people who are miserable. We feel guilty if we feel too good, as if there wasn't enough "good" to go around. This unconscious line of thinking is labeled as scarcity thinking as opposed to abundance thinking. A key mantra in scarcity thinking is "there is not enough".

Did you ever notice that it is human nature to notice when we are feeling bad rather than notice when we are feeling good? When we feel good, we become unconscious of our healthy habits. It is only when we feel bad (again) that we "wake up" to the fact that we're not feeling good anymore! Let me give you an example. Steven came to my office complaining of brain fog and joint pain. Every two weeks, I noticed a pattern whenever I asked him how he was feeling. He would hand me a detailed one or two page diary of all of his symptoms over the last two weeks. I began noticing that some of the older symptoms were no longer mentioned, but that new ones had sprung up. Basically Steven was getting better, but he only mentioned what was still wrong in his life rather than what was now right. When I pointed this fact out to him, he was really shocked that he hadn't noticed this habit. I gently encouraged him to give equal billing to both what was going well in his life as well as what wasn't going well. He really liked this suggestion and it's not co-incidental that his healing sped up.

Chapter Summary

- Brain balance is vital to health and healing. Without it, you cannot heal your chronic pain.
- Brain balance improves your ability to shift your thoughts and beliefs from negative to positive.
- Trauma, electropollution, mercury and food additives are common causes of brain imbalance.
- One of the most effective ways to balance the brain is using LifeWave Y-Age Aeon anti-stress patches on specific points on the head or thymus.
- Brainwave entrainment music, Dr. Diamond's affirmations, alternate nostril breathing, and subtle energy therapeutics are alternative ways to balance the brain hemispheres.
- You can protect yourself from electromagnetic radiation which can cause recurrent brain imbalances.
- Be prepared for self-sabotage so you can get back on track quickly.

7

CHANGE YOUR MIND

How Your Thoughts Shape Your Health

Dr. Bruce Lipton's pivotal book, The Biology of Belief, proved to me beyond a shadow of a doubt, that our thoughts and emotions can affect the health of our cells. As a former biochemist and molecular biology student working in the lab, I can attest to the indoctrination that I received in school. We were taught that our genes are responsible for everything; that our DNA could predict our future health, and that "outside" factors didn't matter. Throughout my early years in biochemistry and medical school, the belief that our genes predicted our health was ingrained into my consciousness.

Have you ever been told that you are at high risk for a disease because it's in your genes? I certainly have. According to my family genetic history, I am apparently at risk for diabetes, heart disease, stroke, depression, colon cancer, high cholesterol, osteoporosis, osteoarthritis, and dementia to name a few. With those genetics, most people would feel depressed, as if they've been handed a death sentence. Not me though. I know that I can change my genes and so can you. One of those ways is by changing your mind.

Epigenetics is an emerging science that teaches us that our environment is more important than our genetic code (DNA) when it comes to health and wellness. The DNA is like a blueprint, just waiting for signals from outside the cell to tell it what to do. Our genetics may predispose us to various diseases, but it doesn't mean that we have to succumb to these diseases. In fact, you can turn on the "good" genes and shut off the "bad" genes in your cells by living a healthier lifestyle.

In the book, The Genie in Your Genes, author Dawson Church, writes about a 92 year old woman, Josephine, who is vibrantly healthy, living independently and working part-time in a hospital gift shop. She participates in four bridge groups and has outlived many of her friends and three of her six brothers. Josephine has one sister who has had a hip replacement, is incontinent and is essentially blind. In addition she has dementia. So what's so special about Josephine and her sister?

They have identical genes. *They are identical twins.*

How could two people with the same genes, growing up in the same family and living all their lives in the same place, as these two did, age so differently? Many epigenetic experts would answer: lifestyle. Lifestyle would include preventive health strategies like good nutrition, regular exercise, good sleep habits, healthy living environment etc. Thanks to Dr. Bruce Lipton's work and the work of other incredible scientists interviewed in Lynne McTaggart's book, The Intention Experiment, we now know that even our beliefs and attitudes can shape our health by turning on and off genes within our cells.

Dr. Robert O. Young, author of The pH Miracle, has done research that has found that negative thoughts can create acidity in the body two to three times worse than eating acid-forming foods, such as dairy. A body that is too acidic can create all sorts of health problems according to Dr. Young. Isn't it amazing how powerful our thoughts can be?

What Have You Been Telling Yourself?

I'm going to share something really personal with you right now. Like every other person on the planet, I can't stop having negative thoughts. I'd prefer not to have them, but they just happen. Isn't that true for you too? The only difference between how I experience negative thoughts now versus five years ago is that I don't take them all that seriously anymore. But that wasn't always the case. Like many people, I used to believe my negative thoughts. I used to believe that every single one of them was true. And if I happened to have a positive thought once in a while, I wouldn't believe it! How silly! Now I know that a thought is a thought. They are just photons of energy with different frequencies. None are better than another, but they can affect you positively or *infect* you negatively depending on which you choose to focus on.

When I was crying in the middle of the night during the worst of my fibromyalgia symptoms, hurting from every pore of my body and exhausted beyond belief, I had a lot of negative thoughts. They kind of sounded like these:

What did I do to deserve this?

God must hate me.

I'm a bad person; otherwise this wouldn't happen to me.

I'm weak.

I hate myself.

Just kill me already!

Why do I have to suffer?

What's the point in living?

This is what it must feel like to be ninety years old.

I can't be sick. My patients need me.

I'm not trying hard enough. I need to be better than this.

I am not good enough.

I wonder how I could kill myself without it looking like suicide.

I don't deserve to be happy. I'm a bad person.

I have to stay in this marriage. That is what God wants.

I can't divorce or my parents will have a heart attack.

My family will hate me for leaving my marriage.

My husband will hate me for leaving the marriage.

I will ruin my husband's life if I end the marriage.

My job is to make my husband happy.

I'm a bad wife.

I'm a bad daughter.

I'm a bad sister.

I'm a bad niece.

I'm a bad granddaughter

I suck as a human being.

I'm a phony. What if my patients find out?

I can't live with myself anymore.

I don't want to live if I can't do what I love.

Why couldn't I be a strong mountain woman like my husband wanted?

I'm going to be all alone. No one really cares.

My friends will judge me and I deserve it.

I have to stay strong for my patients. I'm their rock.

I could go on, but I think you get the picture. I was miserable. I was depressed. The pain and fatigue were unbearable and I just wanted them gone. Do you resonate with any of this? Have you thought negative things about yourself and believed them? Many people know that the more negative thoughts they have, the worse they feel but most people can't help it. When you feel bad, isn't it natural to have negative thoughts?

Since we can't shut down our negative-thought factory, we have to develop practical strategies to deal with this negativity. Otherwise, we'll just dive into a deep black hole that is hard to crawl out from. I hope you are not feeling suicidal because of your pain, but if you are, please reach out to a professional for some immediate support. You might not need it for long after you learn the emotional freedom techniques discussed in an upcoming chapter, but having an empathetic relationship in your life is important.

Don't just rely solely on your spouse, parents or children for emotional support. They aren't trained professionals and because they have a vested interest in your feeling happy, they may say or do inappropriate things that can have the opposite effect. At least a trained professional counselor can be objective as well as empathetic.

The Power of Belief

Beliefs can be considered thoughts that you hold to be true. Unlike random negative thoughts that come and go, beliefs are rather steadfast in their nature. Therein lies the problem. If we believe something to be true, we will actually subconsciously manifest our reality to prove that we are right! For example, if a woman believed that all men are untrustworthy, then the *only* men she'd attract into her reality would all be untrustworthy. I've seen it happen time and time again. So let's pause so you can take a quick quiz on what you believe right now about yourself and your ability to heal. Read the following set of non-supportive beliefs and see if any ring true for you. Be as honest as you can. There is no one to judge you.

> *My diagnosis is incurable, so there is a limit to what extent I can get better.*
> *I've got severe "bone-on-bone" arthritis so of course I'm in pain.*
> *The doctor said I can't do anything about my herniated discs.*
> *I'm getting old and I'm falling apart.*
> *It's just part of getting old. Having aches and pains is normal at my age.*

I've got too much scar tissue to heal.

I've had three surgeries already, so there is no way I can get out of pain easily.

It's going to take a lot of work to get out of pain.

I've tried everything for my pain and it hasn't worked yet, so why try more?

You just don't understand the kind of pain I'm in. It's worse than most.

I've been to twenty doctors and they couldn't help me. How can you?

If strong drugs can't touch this pain, how is anything you are offering going to help?

I'm too far gone to heal.

I'm too old to heal.

The doctor said I'll stay in pain until I lose some weight.

I've just been rough on my body over the years so I've got a lot of wear and tear.

I've tried acupuncture and it hasn't worked. I don't think you can really help me.

I've tried chiropractic care and it hasn't worked. It doesn't work.

I've taken a bunch of herbs and supplements and it didn't really help, so why try more?

It just wasn't meant to be.

I think I'm supposed to suffer.

No one can help me.

Somehow I brought this on myself.

My case is too complex.

You just don't understand what I'm going through, do you?

Just notice your internal reaction as you read those statements. Did a few of them resonate with you? Can you think up some more for yourself in your situation? If so, you're not alone. Many of us have been conditioned to believe certain things because other people close to us have believed in them as well. I know a ton of people who believe that they'll eventually get old and decrepit and that there is nothing they can do about it. They've seen their parents go through it, so they believe they will too.

I recently saw What If? The Movie in which Dan Brule, breath coach, went to visit a prison inmate in order to interview him. Apparently the inmate had been in several fights where his teeth had been knocked out, but to everyone else's astonishment, his teeth always grew back! He told

Brule that as a child, no one had ever told him that he was only supposed to get two sets of teeth in his lifetime! Such is the power of belief.

I am finding in my own life that as each week passes, an old belief is dissolved and another one has taken its place. The reason for this is that I am continually expanding my knowledge through books, documentaries, courses and workshops. I was shocked, for example, when I learned that there are people out there who have chosen not to eat food, but instead diligently train to get all their sustenance from solar energy. They are called sun gazers. After seeing interviews with these interesting people, and proof of their existence, a hard-held believe that we need food to survive was wiped away from my belief system. Now, don't get me wrong, I love food and I'm not willing to give it up, at least not yet, but it is interesting to know that it isn't absolutely necessary for our survival.

Just so you know, there aren't "good" beliefs and "bad" beliefs, just supportive beliefs and non-supportive beliefs. Supportive beliefs are ones that help you and non-supportive beliefs are ones that hinder you. The belief that "life is awesome!" is probably going to serve you better than a belief that "life sucks!" It is a great idea to question your own beliefs on a regular basis and decide whether they are helping or potentially harming your health and happiness. Optimistic beliefs, like positive thoughts, can support your healing. Even just being open to new possibilities is better than not being open.

Positive thoughts hold a higher vibrational frequency than do negative thoughts. The same goes for emotions. The higher your vibration, the healthier your biochemistry will be. But how do we shift from negative to positive? How do we shift from lower vibration to higher vibration without forcing ourselves? Since waving a magic wand isn't an option, I'm going to share with you some fantastic strategies that you can implement today.

We've already covered one method in this section that can already produce profound changes in your attitude: patching your head with LifeWave Y-Age Aeon patches. In my clinical observation, brain balancing with this acupuncture patch tends to elevate one's vibration to a higher, more positive state. I've seen extremely negative people shift dramatically in just a day or two from this single intervention. The next holistic healing method I'm going to introduce to you is the concept of changing your thoughts and beliefs through subliminal programming.

Subliminal Programming

Subliminal programming is a way of changing how you talk to yourself from within. The subconscious mind is the part of your mind that actually manifests your reality, according to John Kehoe, author of Mind Power into the 21st Century. If we could effectively program the subconscious mind with what we want versus what we don't want, we would be able to manifest anything we wanted. Unfortunately, our subconscious mind is constantly listening to all of our thoughts, both positive *and* negative. From birth onwards, our subconscious mind also absorbs the negative and positive programming from others such as our parents and teachers.

Subliminal programming involves inserting specific messages in visual or audio material so subtle that only the subconscious mind picks it up. The conscious mind doesn't notice the messages at all and thus there is no resistance to the messages. An example of a subliminal message would be a brief flash of the words, "buy me", during a commercial on television. Your conscious mind doesn't see these words but your subconscious mind does.

Dr. Eldon Taylor, bestselling author of Choices and Illusions, and Mind Programming, has created a unique subliminal technology that may help support you in healing your chronic pain. Dr. Taylor used to be a criminalist, specializing in lie detector testing. Twenty to twenty-five percent of lie detector tests showed inconclusive results and Dr. Taylor heard a rumor about a subliminal program used by the Los Angeles police department that was so successful that they had to terminate the program for safety reasons. He was intrigued to find out whether using subliminal technology could reduce the rate of inconclusive lie detector test results.

While researching subliminal audio programs on the market, he was dismayed to find that none had any decent scientific backing despite their claims. Shockingly, after buying every single subliminal audio program on the market, he had them tested by an audio professional and was told that "there was nothing on them". Undaunted, he delved more deeply into researching how the brain works and created his own patented subliminal audio technology to help people reprogram their subconscious mind for good purposes.

What I love about Dr. Taylor's technology is that it is the only subliminal technology that has been validated through independent research. Given the power of subliminal technology to either help or harm a person, it was important to me that I only recommend safe and effective technology. That is why I recommend Dr. Taylor's InnerTalk technology. His technology has worked with lowering aggression in incarcerated inmates as well with increasing performance in Olympic athletes. How it works is that the left hemisphere of your brain is receiving passive positive messages like, "It's okay to be healthy. It's okay to be happy." whereas the right hemisphere of your brain is receiving more assertive affirmations like, "I am healthy. I am accepted. I enjoy my life". The major difference is that the right brain gets an audio message that is played backwards and is undecipherable by the conscious mind, yet is still understood by the subconscious mind!

The reason that the assertive affirmations are not played for your conscious mind to hear is that many people will rebel against positive affirmations with an automatic negative response. When they are played backwards, your "guard" is down and you won't reject the affirmations. Amazingly, the right brain can understand these backward messages. The audio programs record a man's voice, a woman's voice and a child's voice, knowing that your subconscious mind will respond to at least one of them. You don't have to play the music loudly nor are you supposed to pay attention to the positive statements. So, just go about your day normally with the subliminal music playing in the background. That makes this form of therapy very appealing because the only effort on your part is pressing play on your CD or MP3 player.

One of the most important studies I want to share with you is the one involving terminally ill cancer patients. Seventeen terminal cancer patients were given Dr. Taylor's subliminal Cancer Remission CD audio program to listen to over forty-two months. Questionnaires were given to both participants and their doctors and they were asked to rate to what degree the mind had an impact on physical health. Of the fourteen remaining subjects terminally ill with cancer, 43% went into remission. That is an astounding percentage even if you take into account the small number of subjects in this study. Remember, these people were sent home to die. They weren't supposed to survive. I'm telling you this story, though, not because I want you to be impressed about the survival rate but because of this next piece of vital information.

When both the patient and the physician agreed strongly to the statement, "I believe that the mind or attitude of the patient is relevant to his/her health and/or health care", one hundred percent of these patients survived! If the physician believed, but the patient didn't, some survived but some died. However, if the physician responded neutrally or negatively to the statement, *one hundred percent of the patients died*, even if the patients believed that their mind or attitude was important.

This suggests that a negative physician attitude could harm a patient regardless of the patient's attitude. Scary. Since reading about this study in Dr. Taylor's book, "Choices and Illusions", I've made a conscious effort to believe in my patients' ability to heal, even if they don't. I now realize that as a physician, an authority figure, my attitude has a lot of clout. If your doctor has clearly demonstrated that she does not believe that you can get better, then you might want to fire her! You need to be around people who believe in you and who support you. Surrounding yourself with positive life-affirming people can be part of your healing. Likewise, severing your ties with negative people as much as you can is equally important.

How You Use InnerTalk

InnerTalk technology comes in audio CD format and some MP3 and you can choose from a large selection of titles. Each InnerTalk title comes in two styles, one with music and one with ocean waves in the background. If you are planning on sleeping with it on, then I'd suggest you purchase the latter. Please note that the Cancer Remission audio CD is free to any patient with cancer who produces a note from his doctor. There are several free downloadable MP3 programs available as well. Just scroll down the left hand navigation on the InnerTalk website and you'll find them.

In addition to purchasing the Natural Pain Relief InnerTalk CD, I highly recommend that you also purchase some of his other CDs that deal with emotions, relationships and self-esteem. A holistic approach to using the subliminal technology will not only support you as you become free of your chronic pain, but also help you to effortlessly develop healthier boundaries, relationships and self-esteem. Here are some of my personal recommendations:

- Soaring Self-Esteem
- Freedom from Back Pain

- Pain Management and Relief
- Accelerated Healing and Well Being (one of my favorites!)
- Ending Self-destructive Patterns
- End Co-dependency
- Healing Emotional Pain
- Sleep Soundly
- Freedom from Arthritis
- Be Well, Stay Happy
- Serenity

Listen to an InnerTalk CD for an hour or more per day seven days a week. The more you listen to it, the more effective it becomes. In one study on depression, participants who successfully went from depressed to non-depressed had logged at least seventeen hours of InnerTalk listening time. Sometimes I will play the CDs on my home stereo on the repeat setting, so that as I putter about my house or work at my computer, I'm passively letting the technology act on my subconscious mind. Often I sleep with one playing all night long because I know that night time is when my subconscious mind is wide open and receptive. That's the reason why you shouldn't fall asleep while watching television and worst yet, watching the news. Why would you want negative or marketing messages programming your subconscious mind as you sleep? Remember, it is your subconscious mind that manifests your reality. Read Dr. Taylor's Mind Programming book and you'll understand why I don't watch television and I almost never watch the news.

With all the negative programming out there in the world, it takes conscious effort to continually shift your thoughts from negative to positive. At first, it seems very difficult and that is why I've provided you with a few strategies that I've found to work well. Balancing the brain and using positive subliminal technology are two of the fastest ways I've found that can positively change your mind.

Self-Hypnosis

Self-hypnosis is a skill in which you put yourself in a state of trance in order for your subconscious mind to be open to healing suggestions.

By tapping into your subconscious mind and bypassing the conscious mind, self-hypnosis can be a powerful tool to help you heal at many levels. Although there are many self-hypnosis books out on the market, I recommend that if you are interested in learning how to do it, you should get a copy of Eldon Taylor's book, Self-Hypnosis and Subliminal Technology: A How-to Guide for Personal-Empowerment Tools You Can Use Anywhere! Extensive research backs the power and efficacy of self-hypnosis and Dr. Taylor shares this information in a simple way while teaching you step-by-step how to create your own subliminal CD program as well as how to induce self-hypnosis.

The BeliefCloset Process®

My friend and colleague, Lion Goodman, created a coaching process that eliminates-permanently-deep-seated beliefs once and for all. According to Goodman, our deepest beliefs about ourselves became programmed into our subconscious in the first two years of life, before we had language. These beliefs are associated with feelings and experiences rather than words, which is why saying positive affirmations doesn't change much for most people. Although there are many good belief-changing processes taught by many wonderful teachers, the BeliefCloset Process works consistently, even when others fail.

The BeliefCloset Process uses a unique guided visualization that invokes physical sensations and images associated with the belief you wish to change. After honoring the belief for the way it has served you in the past, you can then delete the belief from the subconscious mind. Utilizing the power of the Imaginal Realm, the subconscious is invited to participate fully in the process, and since that is where beliefs are stored, they can be cleaned out completely. Using the analogy of clothing to represent our beliefs, the process is not only effective, but entertaining and fun. Your mind literally conjures up an outfit of clothing that represents the belief, the feeling, and how the belief has impacted your life.

In my first BeliefCloset session with Goodman, I experienced the following: my long-standing and interfering belief appeared as a Big Bird costume from Sesame Street. It was gangly, large and uncomfortable, with feathery tentacles reaching out in all directions. Goodman guided me through the process of honoring the belief, choosing to let it go, and incinerating it in my BeliefCloset incinerator. After it was gone, I felt open, free, and light. The shift was palpable. Then, with his guidance, I chose a new, empowering, and more supportive belief. This one felt like an angelic white gown with big wings that carried me gracefully up into the air. I was amazed at how much better my body felt when I planted this new belief in the open space that was created. This feeling has stayed with me since the process, giving credence to Goodman's claim that his method produces a permanent change in the deep core of the psyche.

I highly recommend that you experience the BeliefCloset Process for yourself. Change the beliefs that are interfering with your healing and that are preventing you from enjoying vibrant health. There are many BeliefCloset Practitioners around the country. You can find them at www.BeliefCloset.com/Practitioners. Lion has offered his beautiful multimedia eBook on beliefs and the BeliefCloset Process to my readers. Register at www.TransformYourBeliefs.com and you'll get immediate access to the book, which contains a guided journey to give you a sample of the process.

Chapter Summary

- Thoughts and beliefs can change your biology and your health.
- Negative thoughts happen naturally especially when you don't feel well, but knowing how to handle them makes all the difference in the world.
- In addition to using LifeWave Y-Age Aeon anti-stress patches, you can use subliminal technology to naturally and painlessly shift your thoughts from negative to positive.
- Subliminal programming and self-hypnosis are powerful self-healing tools you can take advantage of.
- The BeliefCloset process is a way of permanently ridding yourself of negative or non-supportive beliefs.

8

HARNESS THE LAW
OF ATTRACTION

Start with the End in Mind

Imagine yourself taking a trip in your car. You have your GPS device installed and maps at your disposal. You get into your car, buckle your seatbelt, start the engine and press on the gas pedal. There's only one problem. You have no destination, so you drive along and just avoid obstacles that get in your way. This seems like a silly scenario doesn't it, but most of us never learn the power of intention and so we live our lives on autopilot hoping that no obstacles get in our way . . . until one does! So what would you do if you were planning a real trip? You would first decide on a destination, wouldn't you? Once you decide on a destination, then you would plug in that address into the GPS device so that it could guide you on your way. In order for you to heal your chronic pain, you must "plan" the journey as well. Your destination, in this case, is your health and your ideal vision of it.

In the book, The Intention Experiment, Lynne McTaggart, an investigative journalist by trade, shares the results of scientific research from all over the world about how powerful our thoughts can be in shifting reality. In some of these experiments, thoughts could change the pH of water, skew the results of a random event generator (sort of like an electronic version of a coin flipper), or make plants grow faster.

What is most clear from these experiments is that in order to create a particular result, the intention, also known as the outcome, had to be very specific and clear. One of my favorite wealth trainers, T. Harv Eker, is known for saying that *"People don't often get what they want because they don't know what they want"*. The same is true for healing your chronic pain. It may seem obvious that your intention is to get rid of your pain. That's fine and dandy. But believe it or not, that might not be specific enough. In this chapter, I'm going to stretch your imagination so that you can use your mental abilities to dream up your ideal outcome.

The law of attraction is a law you may or may not have heard of. It has been popularized by the movie, The Secret, and if you haven't already seen this movie, I highly recommend it. Another great movie to watch is The Cure Is, which shows us the power of our minds to heal ourselves. The law of attraction states that what you think about you bring about into your existence. Another movie, What the Bleep Do We Know, is also a great resource to learn about the law of attraction. The attraction is literally on the level of the quantum field, so it doesn't refer to magnetic attraction, yet it is just as real as the law of gravity. The law of attraction uses your thoughts and feelings as fuel for the attraction. The Universe (called The Field in Lynne McTaggart's books) responds to your thoughts by giving you more of what you are focusing on.

So if you are focusing on wellness in your thought processes and with your emotions, you'll get more "wellness". Unfortunately, most of us are focused on the opposite when we're feeling bad. The good news is that as we go through the exercises in this chapter, you'll begin to neutralize the negative thoughts that may be contributing to your experience of chronic pain. Before we do that, however, let me give you a couple of concrete examples of how the law of attraction works if we focus mainly on what we don't want, rather than on what we do want.

Trish has rheumatoid arthritis. She is terrified of becoming permanently disabled. Much of her time is spent fighting with insurance companies and researching all the side effects of drugs and complications of her arthritis. She focuses solely on what's going wrong with her body. The more she focuses on the negative, the more negative circumstances she seems to attract into her life. Now the good news to this story is that once we balanced her brain with LifeWave Y-Age Aeon patches, her whole attitude turned right around, and now she is a woman who sees possibilities where she used to only see limitation. If you've had trouble with recurrent negative thoughts and emotions (evidence of intense stress), I'd highly recommend patching your head acupuncture points with the Aeon patch. I've seen miraculous results just using this simple energy tool.

Here's another example of negative manifesting. Dave thinks he has a lot of debt. He worries about the debt and about how he might not be able to pay his bills. He works hard at his job and tries to save as much money as he can, but no matter what he does, he piles up more debt. Approximately ninety percent of his worries are about debt. He thinks about it day in and day out. He talks about it. He complains to his friends and family about it. He blames the government and corporate America. The more he thinks about debt, the more debt comes knocking on his door. Just as he pays off one credit card, a disaster happens to his house and he has to go into debt again just to repair it. Success coach, Bob Proctor, one of the stars of the movie, The Secret, would say to Dave, *"Set up an automatic debt repayment plan and the focus on prosperity!"*

How to Set Intentions

One of the best ways to get the law of attraction working in your favor is to create a clear intention. The way I teach people to do this is to first pretend that you have a fairy Godmother and she can grant you whatever your heart desires. Make a big list of what your healing will look like. Writing one sentence like, "I want to be out of pain" isn't good enough. Ask yourself what you would be doing and enjoying in your life if you weren't in pain? What new things would you try? What would you pursue if pain weren't limiting you at all? What passions do you have that you have put on hold because of your health?

Write as many things down as you can in a journal or on a piece of paper. One of the secrets to harnessing the law of attraction is to understand that if you don't have a big enough "why", then you won't attract the resources to you that you'll need to get better. In other words, if you are just going to sit around all day and watch television, it isn't a good enough reason to ask for vibrant health. Does that make some sense to you? Compare someone wishing to become a millionaire. If the only thing on her wish list is to buy all her favorite clothes from Macy's department store and nothing else, she isn't going need a million dollars. Clothing doesn't cost that much. On the other hand, if she listed reasons like wanting to enjoy a second home in Vail, Colorado where she loves to ski during the winter, being financially free so that she can travel to Europe and learn eleven languages, learn surfing in Hawaii, and set up a foundation for needy children in Haiti, then maybe becoming a millionaire makes sense.

After you have made your list, then what I want you to do is write everything in the positive sense. In other words, if you wrote, "I don't have pain", then re-write it as "My body is flexible and comfortable", for example. Because I want you to focus on the positive and because the Universe doesn't register the words "don't" and "not", this step is rather important. Secondly, rewrite your sentences as happening now or has having happened already instead of writing them in the future tense. In order to practice this, I want you to re-write the following intentions in the positive sense and the present tense:

1. I don't have cancer.
2. My arthritis will disappear.
3. I will be out of debt.
4. I become pain-free.
5. I'm not being criticized any longer.
6. I'm not depressed.
7. I will lose weight.
8. I'm not working for minimum wage any more.
9. I'm no longer addicted to diet soda.
10. I don't have diarrhea and stomach cramps.
11. I'm out of this horrible relationship.
12. I am married to a non-alcoholic.

So how did you do? It's not as easy as you think. I've done this exercise in workshops with groups of people and much of the time, people can't help but insert negative terms into their intentions. It's not the end of the world if you do, but words have significant power, especially if you say them out loud as a declaration. It is this power that you are purposefully taking advantage of to help you manifest your good health. It takes practice shifting your perceptions, so be patient with yourself. Here are some of my answers for the above. Yours may be very different, but that's okay. That's what makes us unique. I'm hoping that some of my answers will inspire you to stretch your imagination and "upgrade" your intentions list.

1. I have vibrant health.
2. My joints feel strong and flexible.
3. I am financially free.
4. My body is comfortable and strong.
5. I am being appreciated and loved.

6. I am joyful.
7. I am slim and healthy.
8. I'm earning $500 an hour coaching self-development clients 20 hours a month.
9. I crave healthy food.
10. My intestines are working perfectly.
11. I am enjoying my life with my soul mate.
12. I am married to a happy, health-conscious man.

Imagine Your Ideal Life

The second exercise in this chapter is super fun, or at least I think it is. Most of my coaching clients love doing this exercise. Don't worry, it isn't hard at all. You're going to be using your imagination to write the story of your future life. The only catch is that you have to use your imagination and you have to write it in the present tense. The paragraph should read like a short story and it should feel fun. Use your list of intentions from the first exercise as material for this one. Remember to make things as specific as possible and to keep the wording positive and in the present tense. First I'm going to give you an example of a story that is not very specific; then I'm going to give you an example of a story that is.

> *Story #1: I am enjoying vibrant health. I am enjoying exercising. I have a great job and am earning lots of money doing what I love. I've found the love of my life and we live in a big house in the woods. I have great neighbors and my kids are happy and well-adjusted.*

Now there is nothing wrong with Story #1 and if your story reads like that, it's still good! Notice that everything was written as being positive and there were no negative phrases. For some people being less specific feels more relaxed for them and so if you're one of them, you can stick to more general intentions and let the Universe fill in the gaps.

I, for one, like writing stories that are more specific, based on Lynne McTaggart's findings, but if you try writing one and you get more anxious than you get excited, then maybe you'll want to stick to generalities until you get your "intention" muscles trained. Here's another story for you to compare with Story #1.

> *Story #2: I am enjoying vibrant health. I wake up each morning with lots of energy and spend the morning meditating and doing yoga after which I eat a scrumptious breakfast prepared for me by James. James and I train at least five hours a week at the rink and we win a gold medal at the next Adult National Figure Skating Championships. We also win a gold medal at the Adult International Figure Skating Championships in Oberstdorf, where we have our best performance ever. We get a standing ovation! We inspire other adult skaters to take up pairs skating. I'm thoroughly enjoying directing my brand new eco-designed wellness center that has a nice big dance studio/workshop space. I see patients a few days a week, while my book reaches number one on the bestseller list. I'm the "go-to" expert on healing chronic pain in my profession and I have a blast on the Dr. Oz show where I brain balance people and get them out of pain with the LifeWave patches. My business expands exponentially and requests for interviews and television appearances flood my email. I'm helping thousands upon thousands of people heal their lives through my books and workshops. I am enjoying financial freedom—I work because I choose to, not because I have to. I take a week off from work to unwind every six weeks or so and am thrilled to be enjoying vacations visiting the most beautiful ice rinks and eco-vacations spots in the world with James and spending quality time with my family!*

So what do you think? How did you feel when you read my story? Did you judge it as being "over the top" or fantastic? Did the thought, "She's too greedy" enter your mind? Or did it inspire you to stretch your imagination more? Whatever your reaction, it will give you a clue about whether you have any mental blocks that might be holding you back from healing your body and your life. Your reactions are a mirror to your subconscious, so if you judged my story harshly as being too extravagant or outrageous, then you have a subconscious story that runs your life in a way that tells you that you can't really have what you want. On the other hand, if you read my story and got as excited as I did writing it (and yes I got very excited!), then your subconscious is biting at the bit to be reprogrammed to help you manifest your dreams.

Just in case you're wondering, my expertise in harnessing the law of attraction first came from practicing how to manifest my ideal love partner. After my divorce, my number one wish was to manifest the perfect skating partner. Details about how I did this (using the method I am teaching you) can be found on my law of attraction website: www.LawofAttractioninLove.com. I can't say that I'm an expert in manifesting abundance in *all* areas of my life yet. However, as I practice on a daily basis, I witness dramatic shifts that are like signs showing me that I'm on the right path.

Take some time to write out your ideal story. Normally, mine take about five revisions until I can read them out loud without stumbling and with full unadulterated enthusiasm. If you have read your own story and you are not one bit inspired, then try again. The energy or inspiration is vital to harness the law of attraction to do your bidding. And if you are having trouble, balance your brain first, then try again after a few days. If you are brave enough, read your story out loud to a couple of trusted friends and get their honest feedback about whether this story rings true for you. Let them know that this story is supposed to inspire you, and ask them whether it inspired them to hear it.

Your Story as a Meditation

The last exercise in this chapter uses your energy field to create a pattern by which the Universe can bring you what you have intended. The law of attraction states that *like attracts like*. When your energy field is vibrating at the level of having already been healed, you will attract similar vibrations to create that reality for you. This stuff isn't rocket science, but it takes discipline and openness to becoming more conscious.

One of the most powerful mental exercises you can do is meditation. In this case, it isn't just mental because you're going to use your entire body to feel the reality of the story you wrote in the last exercise. If you like music, you might want to play inspiring music as you do this meditation. Here's what you do. Sit quietly in a comfortable chair or on a cushion so that your spine is upright and your posture is good. Alternatively, you can do this lying on your back if you are comfortable this way. Or, if you are like me, you will dance around the room. Close your eyes and start to imagine your story coming to life. Use all of your common senses: sight, smell, sound, touch, and taste to imagine what you would experience if your story were happening right now in the present moment. Feel the entire experience in your whole body.

Often people report that they feel waves of energy permeating their bodies as they do this mediation. My intuition teacher, Laura Day, author of The Circle, calls this exercise *Embodying Your Reality* and she instructs you to feel your new reality extending out from your core, out through your pores into the Universe.

If you aren't feeling anything in your body, don't worry. For many people, being energetically "in" their bodies is very foreign since they live in their heads most of the time. People who bump into walls or who have a lot of accidents are people like that. Be compassionate with yourself. You will get better at sensing your body with more practice. Practice this mediation daily. It may take you five minutes or twenty minutes. You can just take a piece of your story and use that for meditation if you don't have much time and if you have a detailed story like mine. The point is to really enjoy your meditation. You should feel exhilarated.

I remember that when I used this technique to imagine winning my first Adult National Figure Skating Championships, it was so real that tears were streaming down my face during one meditation session. After the meditation, I felt as if I had already won and didn't need to skate the following week! It was *that* real to me. If you can convince your subconscious that the pictures it sees in your mind (and feels in your body) are real, then you can harness its abilities to manifest the realities you want rather than the ones you don't want. I've used this meditation to win several gold medals since.

Chapter Summary

- To heal yourself, you first have to create your desired outcome through intention-setting.
- The law of attraction responds to your predominant thoughts and emotions and brings similar vibrations and experiences into your reality.

- Be creative in imagining your ideal healthy life because enthusiasm helps to fuel the manifesting process.
- Keep your story positive and in the present tense as if it is already happening right now.
- Use a daily meditation practice whereby you experience your ideal reality with your entire body and make it feel as real as possible.
- If you're having trouble with these exercises, use the brain balancing techniques in Chapter 6 for a few days before attempting them again.

9

CLEAR EMOTIONAL BAGGAGE

If you read the title of this chapter and thought to yourself, "Hmmm, I don't have any emotional baggage", then you are mistaken. *Everyone* has some degree of emotional baggage and it is easy to appreciate this after I share with you what emotional baggage is and what happens to it when we don't clear it.

What Constitutes Emotional Baggage?

Emotional baggage can be any reaction you still have to any events or situations that have happened in the past and are not happening in the present . . . as in right at this moment! Think back to a situation where someone really embarrassed or betrayed you. It could be a spouse, parent, co-worker or friend. Do you know of anyone in your life whom you are afraid to call or confront? Anyone you'd rather not be around because he or she is critical or negative? In every single example from your past where you had an emotionally charged situation, unless you can recall the story and feel completely neutral or even grateful for it, it is likely that you have emotional baggage.

One of the most important concepts presented in this book is this: *in order to heal your physical body, you need to have most of your energy in present time.* Any traumatic experiences from your past which you have not yet let go of, forgiven, or become thankful for, siphon your energy from the present into the past. If a lot of your energy is going to your "past" via emotions that have not yet cleared from past experiences, then you will not have enough energy, Qi, in the present to heal your body.

For example, almost everyone can recount at least one incident in childhood where they were humiliated or embarrassed. If you can't, then think of a more recent incident. I remember several from childhood that made a big impact on me, but since have cleared. I remember walking home from school and having two neighboring boys making fun of me and trying to choke me with my winter scarf. More memories resurface as I go deeper into my own personal healing. Although some of the stories don't seem to be a big a deal on the grand scale of things, any little bit of emotional "charge" that remains in the past is an energy loss.

I remember that in fourth grade, my teacher asked all the students to raise their hands if they felt happy with their bodies. As I began to raise my hand, I noticed that *none* of the other students raised their hands. Because I didn't want to be singled out as "different", I quickly dropped my hand. The silence was unbearable. My teacher was shocked and so was I. I couldn't understand why the class jock or the class beauty didn't raise their hands. From that moment, the belief that was etched into my subconscious was that I didn't deserve to feel good about my body if no one else did. Wow! An incident as innocent as a simple question from a teacher could have set up a life-long belief system that may have contributed to my chronic pain.

Here's another story. In the sixth grade, students were forced to recite speeches in front of their fellow students. Most of us were terrified including me, not only because we had to speak in front of our fellow students, but also because they would be grading us. After each speech, the teacher would ask the classroom students to raise their hands to a corresponding grade. If the student didn't like the speech, they could grade it a "1" or if they loved it, they could grade it a "10". Well, I had a terrible time figuring out what to speak about because I absolutely hated speaking. I wasn't exactly the most popular kid in class. I was the smart nerd. My parents, being Asian, had no personal experience with this type of assignment. I was on my own. I decided to do my speech on the subject of "kindness", and my mother helped me the best she could.

After the speech, during which my heart pounded so hard I felt like everyone could see it popping out of my chest, my class had to vote. In typical fashion, the "popular" kids gave my speech low marks and the "outcasts" of the class gave me high marks. It was degrading to see exactly who hated my speech because in my mind, it translated into hating me. I was so angry at my teacher for forcing us to endure this type of humiliation, but I just swallowed my pride and said nothing. I probably went home and cried to my mother. Being a straight-A student at the time, anything less than an "A" was horrible in my mind.

Incidents like these from our childhoods can leave emotional scars that need to be healed. Otherwise these scars can have a profound impact on our happiness and healing. If you can't remember most of your childhood, that's a sign that you probably experienced enough trauma in childhood that your mind decided it was safer to forget it than to remember it. Emotional baggage does not always have to come from things in the distant past. Even things that happened yesterday that you are still reacting to will affect your energy in the present moment. If you recently found out that your co-worker has terminal cancer and you have been feeling upset for days, you have developed emotional baggage associated with this event.

Experiencing emotions are a natural and healthy part of our humanity, but re-experiencing emotions from past events over and over again is not. Think of a young child playing on her own. Maybe the child falls and starts to cry, but then looks around and realizes that no one is there to comfort her, so she just carries on playing, completely letting go of her emotional reaction. If we could all let go as easily as young children, we would all be healed! Unfortunately, we learn to catalogue and hang on to our emotional reactions for future reference. Certainly my own school experiences testify to this "hanging on" factor!

Why do we often hang on to our emotional reactions when they can't possibly help us heal in the present? The most common unconscious reason is that we want to prove our victimhood. On some level, we really don't want to be fully 100% responsible for our current experiences, so we look to the past to explain why we are what we are. Consider someone who has suffered childhood abuse. Abuse should never be condoned or tolerated, yet it is undeniably rampant in many countries and in many societies including our own. Victims of abuse can suffer immeasurable psychological and physical damage. The physical damage, however, fades with time, but the psychological damage often lingers on.

I know several abused patients who have never been able to forgive their abusers and continue to suffer emotionally and physically (because they are now chronically ill) because they don't appreciate the link between their current state of health and their energy currents. Instead of blaming the abuser for their psychological impairments years after the abuse ended, the most courageous "victims" step out from the victim role and instead learn self-empowerment by letting go of the past and moving forward.

So many great spiritual teachers, such as Louise Hay, author of bestseller, Heal Your Body, have gone through horrible abuse in their past, yet have let go of their victim mentality and emotional baggage, so that they are free to share from their heart and empower others to do the same.

Take an Emotional Inventory

So-called negative emotions, such as anger, fear, and sadness are not "bad" for you. They are only "bad" for you when they stick around indefinitely. It is completely human to react with anger, fear and sadness to life events. Life throws us curve balls and that's how it has always been. In the ideal world, we would feel our feelings completely and fully in our bodies, and then in a short time, when we are ready to move on, we let them go. The time span could be as short as a few seconds or as long as a few days. Aside from the benefit of having more of your energy currents in present time so your body can heal, there are side benefits as well.

I'll give you an example as an illustration. I decided one day to do an "anger" experiment. There was an online store that I was using to market some fun T-shirts with cool Law of Attraction slogans. I had uploaded a logo from a company who had given me special permission to use their logo. Unfortunately, the store wasn't able to contact me to verify that I had this special permission, so they shut down my account. After multiple unsuccessful attempts to get my account reinstated, I decided that I was going to consciously stay angry at the store for a while. I could feel "big" energy running throughout my body and it gave me a false sense of power. Further attempts at communication were futile. Nothing I did managed to reinstate my online store.

Finally after three weeks (yes, a whole three weeks!), I decided that I'd better do an exercise to let go of my anger. So I did. I used TAT, one of the energy tools I'm going to share with you in this book, during which I forgave "them" for their "incompetence" while at the same time asking for forgiveness. In this exercise, neither they nor I needed to communicate further. This exercise was completely private and silent and no one knew that I was doing it. After performing this letting go exercise, I knew that by the next morning I would receive an email from the online store owners. Sure enough I was right! The owners had reinstated my account overnight! The moment I let go of my anger was the moment when things started going my way.

The side benefit of letting go of emotions that no longer serve you is that you attract more positive circumstances into your life. Now it's your turn. I want you to take your emotional inventory, which means doing some honest work to determine where your energy has been going these days. If we all had our energy circuits in present time, none of us would need any "healing", so don't feel guilty for having held onto emotional reactions. We all do it unconsciously, but now you get the opportunity to bring them into consciousness for final resolution.

Review the questions below and use a journal or notepad to answer them. Consider yourself an emotional baggage "detective" and note down every single negative reaction you still have to events in the past as well as in the present, without self-judgment or guilt.

1. Is there anyone in my past with whom I am still angry for what he/she did or said to me or my loved one?
2. Whom or what do I resent?
3. When I think back to stressful or traumatic situations in the past, do I still have an emotional reaction? And if so, what is that reaction?
4. Whom do I blame for things going sour in my past or in my current reality?
5. Who didn't support me when I was growing up when I felt they should have?
6. How do I feel about being chronically in pain? Are there feelings of frustration, anger, sadness, fear? What do they represent?
7. Aside from experiencing chronic pain, what else is bothering me emotionally right now? Finances? Spouse? Children? Job? And how do I feel about each of these?
8. Write down all the people who hurt you in the past and what they did to you and rate on a scale of 1 to 10 how much charge you still feel about it.

To make things easier, ask yourself what bothers you, if anything, about:

- The environment
- The news on television
- The government
- The Internal Revenue Service (IRS)
- Religion
- Your relatives
- Your career or job
- Your co-workers
- Your hired-help
- Your income
- Your savings
- Your future

Everything we judge negatively, such as government irresponsibility, contains seeds of emotional reactions that may not be serving us. Even if we are a staunch environmentalist and do not condone the toxins spewing out into our environment, we don't have to hang on to our anger and resentment. Instead, we can take that energy and put it into action through our mission to create a better future for everyone.

Anger as Your Ally

Just in case you get the notion that there are "good" emotions and "bad" emotions, I want to set the record straight. Different emotions are just different qualities of energy frequencies. They only become "bad" to us when they get stuck in our system or prevent us from moving on to a healthier place.

Anger has gotten a bad rap. I don't know about you, but I got the distinct impression that when I was angry as a child, it was completely unacceptable. In fact, my parents had a nickname for me. In our Cantonese dialect, my name is pronounced as Gun Ga Mun, or "Kan, Karen". The surname goes first. Because of my bouts of irritability as a toddler, I was nicknamed, Gun Ga Mung, which translates into "Karen the Grumpy". When I was young, my parents were struggling new Canadian immigrants and my mother was in poor health. She was needy and depressed at the time, so no wonder I was grumpy. It's taken me years to finally feel self-compassion for my childhood "grumpiness".

So think for a moment about when you were a child? When did you get angry? When you didn't get what you wanted or needed? Or when you felt something was unfair or unjust? Or when you were hurt? Given this context, our anger is a useful part of our survival instinct. Thus anger can be a useful tool to uncover the areas of our lives where we haven't treated ourselves as well as we should or have let others mistreat us.

Instead of judging anger as "bad", let it be your guide to develop ways in which you can feel more nurtured, respected and loved. Commonly, angry people need to develop and hold healthier boundaries so that other people don't mistreat them or deplete their energy. In our society, it is not polite to rant and rave when we're angry. We might seriously injure someone, either physically or emotionally. What's great, however, is that we can use energy psychology tools to turn down the volume (intensity) of the anger as we move through it. Notice that I didn't say "get rid of it" in this instance. Many times, especially with perfectionists, anger isn't even properly felt in the physical body! Some of us stay mostly in our heads and don't feel any emotion at all. That's a problem.

Stuck emotions live in our tissues and cause physical pain. I know that someone is really healing when she finally is able to feel, acknowledge and honor her anger and its place in her life. Anger can be your soul calling out to you and letting you know that you deserve better! Feelings of anger can be scary to most people, but they don't have to be. With the energy techniques that I will share you with in this chapter, you will be able to move through intense emotions in order to release them, but more importantly, transmute them so that you can be in the space of receiving guidance from your Higher Self.

Letting Go of the Baggage

Here's the fun part where we take pieces of our emotional baggage that we determine are no longer serving us and consciously choose to let them go. Even intense emotions of anger and resentment related to abuse, for example, can clear surprisingly fast when you know energy psychology. Energy psychology is a fairly new field of expertise, whereby negative emotions and the energy that they take up are cleared from your energy body. The resultant energy is free to then return to present time where we need it to be if we're going to heal and manifest what we truly desire in our lives.

There are several different types of energy psychology techniques. I'll share with you the ones I know the best: EFT, also known as Tapping, TAT, Tapas Acupressure Technique and the Emotion Code. They have a basis in acupuncture/acupressure, yet are very different in execution. Other techniques such as TFT (thought field therapy), Sedona Method, and PSTEC are equally as powerful, so you may wish to explore these on your own as well. Links are provided in the Resources chapter.

Tapping

Tapping or Emotional Freedom Technique (EFT) requires that you tap specific acupressure points on the head, torso (and sometimes hands) in order to clear energy blocks caused by negative emotions. The most popular tapping form involves two stages. In the first stage you are tapping while expressing the negative emotion. This stage will last as long as you still have an emotional "charge" and repeated tapping will bring that charge down to a minimal level.

The second stage involves reframing the situation positively where you choose a positive thought or emotion to replace the negative ones. Here's what's cool: you can't do tapping incorrectly! Your intention is enough to make it work. Even if you don't think that you are tapping the right acupressure points, you will still release the negative energy.

One of the things I've noticed is that when people are brain balanced, especially with the LifeWave Y-Age Aeon patch, the energy psychology techniques work even better and faster. If you are using the patches I highly recommend that you place an Aeon patch on the top of your head, on acupuncture point GV20 while you are doing the these exercises. Here is a step-by-step protocol on how to do EFT using the basic method. There is a more free-form method I now use. If you've signed up for your bonuses, you'll be getting access to some videos I created just to illustrate the creative ways you can use EFT.

Basic EFT Instructions:

1. Choose an emotion you wish to clear based on a situation that's bothering you. For example, you might be angry at your neighbor Bob for letting his cat poop in your yard.

2. Rate the emotional charge out of ten; ten being the highest and zero meaning none.

3. Fill out the following starting sentence with the emotional situation you're dealing with:

    "Even though I am _____ (angry) at _____ (Bob) for _____ (letting his cat poop in my yard), I deeply and completely love and accept myself and my feelings"

4. While saying this sentence three times, tap the karate chop point on one hand with the finger tips of the other hand (see image).

5. Then, tap the other acupressure points in the picture, one after another.

    a) Inside eyebrow
    b) Outside eye
    c) Under the eye
    d) Under the nose
    e) Under the lip
    f) Collarbone
    g) Under the arm
    h) Top of the head

    Tap each point five to eight times with the fingers of one hand (or both), starting at the inner eyebrow point and ending at the top of your head while you repeat out loud your negative emotion e.g. *"this anger"*. Feel free to alternate hands, if you like, or keep tapping just on one side. It doesn't matter because both will be effective.

6. After one or two rounds, rate your emotional charge again out of ten. If it has dropped to under two out of ten, then you can choose to move onto the positive round or remain tapping until

the charge is a zero. Don't be in a rush to proceed to the positive round if you still feel a charge after the negative round. It may take several rounds. Doing the freeform style that I show you in my videos may help you become more creative in your own Tapping practice.

7. When your emotional charge has diminished significantly and when you wish to do a positive round, then you can tap all of the acupressure points again and state what you'd rather be feeling. For example, as you tap, you might say, *"even though I have every right to be angry at Bob, I choose to forgive him and the cat for pooping in my yard"*, or simply, *"I choose forgiveness"*, *"I choose to be open"*, *"I choose to let go"* etc.

8. To close the EFT session, just close your eyes and take a deep breath to integrate the new energy.

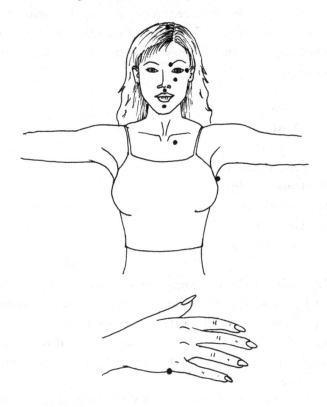

Tips for Success:

Don't worry about doing it "right". Tapping is very forgiving. Your intention is what matters most. I purposefully did not write down the exact acupuncture points because approximating these points work just as well. Some people have had excellent results just tapping in the middle of their chests! Try different techniques and see what works best for you.

TAT—Tapas Acupressure Technique

Tapas Fleming, the creator of TAT, is an acupuncturist who specialized in allergy desensitizing using a complex series of acupuncture treatments. One day, she had the inspiration to try special points on the head instead of the usual series of acupuncture treatments and to her surprise they worked. Not only did they work as well as the other acupuncture treatments, but also she found that she often only needed only one session to cure her patients! She then decided to teach people a specific acupressure hand position to be placed on the head since this method was just as successful.

During one of her early sessions in which she cleared a patient of a salt allergy, the patient shared with her that the emotional baggage from childhood sexual abuse had also cleared at the same time. This was incredibly surprising since this patient had already been in therapy for a long time without being able to let go of the emotional trauma. Apparently as a child, she was given a bag of salty potato chips after the abuse and somehow the body wired the entire experience as "bad". Tapas realized after this experience that her technique, named TAT, could effectively release all types of emotional trauma. The beauty about this technique is that the person doesn't have to re-experience the trauma in order to let it go.

What I like about TAT is that you can neutralize a whole situation all at once without having to specify one emotion at a time. In addition, generational traumas may also be healed without needing to know the exact traumas that have transpired. You don't need to "know" the cause of why you feel the way you do, only that you wish to heal it. The nine step procedure is easy and gentle and can readily be learned. Only do TAT for approximately 20 minutes a day as it is very powerful therapy.

For a free copy of Tapas Fleming's How to do TAT booklet, go to www.KarenKan.com/TAT and click on the banner image.

TAT pose with the hands is as follows. With one hand, place the thumb and fourth fingertips just above the inner corner of each eye (Bladder 1) and the third finger on the third eye point (GV 24.5) and with the other hand, cup the base of the skull. Check out the Resources chapter for a link to a video which shows you the TAT position.

Tapping and TAT may seem very foreign to you if you've never been exposed to energy psychology. When I went through medical school, I loved doing psychotherapy with my patients. Perhaps I was natural at it because as a child I learned to be a good listener while consoling my depressed mother. People need to feel heard and validated to some extent, so counseling and psychotherapy are of value. The difference between doing psychotherapy and using energy psychology tools is that the former may not actually resolve any of the negative feelings, and in some cases, serves to perpetuate them.

Energy psychology, on the other hand, is about releasing old stored negative emotions or trauma that have been stuck in your energy field and are preventing you from moving forward and healing. From what I've experienced in my practice, it only takes minutes to take someone's traumatic emotions from an intensity level of "10" to a "1", even if these emotions have been present for decades. Counseling alone, in my experience, was never that efficient.

Both Tapping and TAT are very effective. Try them both and see which one resonates with you more. With tapping, it works best if you can be very specific about what you are tapping about, but I find that it is very quick and I can do it even while I'm in the middle of something else like driving. I prefer doing TAT just before bed, when I have some quiet time, because it takes me a little longer.

The Emotion Code

So far we've focused on the emotional baggage you have become aware of, but what about emotional baggage that lies deep in your subconscious and that you are not aware of? According to Dr. Bradley Nelson, author of The Emotion Code, healthy emotional processing occurs when we can feel emotions come and go. However, some emotions get trapped when our ability to process them is inadequate or overwhelmed. Dr. Nelson discovered that trapped emotional energies become lodged in the body during intense emotional events. These energies or "trapped emotions" end up distorting the normal energy field of the body and thus result in physical pain, congestion of the acupuncture system, and disease, as well as leading to other common conditions such as depression, anxiety, panic attacks, phobias, self sabotage and so on.

Trapped emotions are not necessarily the sole cause of your body pain, but they may be. In the very least, if they are trapped, they can contribute to your chronic pain. The Emotion Code is a process by which you can determine what trapped emotions you may have and quickly neutralize them. The Eastern-based process uses the body's intuitive system via muscle testing. Muscle testing is a procedure first taught by holistic chiropractors, but is now used by many healthcare professionals and lay people alike to utilize the body's intuitive guidance system to make health choices.

I have found that in cases of chronic pain, trapped emotions are invariably involved even if they are not the initial cause of the pain condition. Sometimes weak or susceptible areas of your body become reservoirs for trapped emotions that wouldn't otherwise be trapped in healthy tissue. Even if doing the Emotion Code procedure does not release the pain, at least you can increase your chances of healing chronic pain by removing an energetic block to healing.

Tim came into the office with pain in his rib. It began mysteriously right after his father died. He used LifeWave patches and acupuncture and with each treatment the pain subsided only to return again between treatments. Confused, Tim sought another cause of his non-healing pain. I decided to use the Emotion Code on Tim after he revealed to me that this pain only began when his father died. Using the Emotion Code, we asked his body whether there were trapped emotions contributing to his rib pain. The answer was "yes". He had apparently absorbed two negative emotions from his mother when he was a baby.

When I released Tim's first trapped emotion, I asked if he could feel anything. He said, "Yes", then turned and sat down with his head in his hands. I was worried that he was going to vomit, but instead his body shuddered in a flow of sobs. Allowing this release for a few minutes, Tim sat up and was ready to release the next emotion. The experience was interesting for both of us since I was still fairly new at using the Emotion Code at the time. Almost immediately after releasing the first emotion, the pain in his rib practically vanished. Even though the emotions trapped in Tim's rib related to his mother, not to his father, it was clear that releasing these trapped emotions helped ease the pain.

When we use the Emotion Code, we assess and release trapped emotions one at a time. For whatever reason, Dr. Nelson has determined that the subconscious mind will release emotions in this pattern. You can ask your subconscious whether there is a trapped emotion related to your chronic painful body part that can be released now. If the answer is no, that either means that you do not have a trapped emotion in that painful body part or that your subconscious is not ready to release one. If the answer is yes, you can then follow Dr. Nelson's emotion code chart (see Figure 5) to ascertain the exact trapped emotion via muscle testing. Once you determine the emotion, then you can release it easily using an energetic or magnetic device such as a magnet, by sweeping it over the Governing Vessel acupuncture meridian.

Dr. Nelson's book and video course has clear instructions about how to use muscle testing on yourself and on others to determine trapped emotions as well as how to release them. In addition to releasing trapped emotions in chronic pain areas, you may wish to search for trapped emotions in your heart wall. A heart wall is an energetic protection that our subconscious builds around our heart. Heart walls start being built when we are extremely young or even before we are born. Children easily absorb emotions from their parents. That is why it is so important for parents to cleanse their own trapped emotions so that they do not inadvertently pass along generational trapped emotions to their children.

Heart walls are made up of trapped emotions and can be made of any material that your subconscious deems strong and impermeable. Although they were made to protect your vulnerable heart, their presence may cost you the ability to truly enjoy your life to the fullest according to Dr. Nelson. Trapped emotions in your heart wall may prevent you from experiencing happy and fulfilling relationships because your perceptions will be tainted by trapped emotions. To learn Dr. Nelson's Emotion Code, go to www.KarenKan.com/Emotion.

The Emotion Code™ Chart

	Column A	Column B
Row 1 Heart or Small Intestine	Abandonment Betrayal Forlorn Lost Love Unreceived	Effort Unreceived Heartache Insecurity Overjoy Vulnerability
Row 2 Spleen or Stomach	Anxiety Despair Disgust Nervousness Worry	Failure Helplessness Hopelessness Lack of Control Low Self-Esteem
Row 3 Lung or Colon	Crying Discouragement Rejection Sadness Sorrow	Confusion Defensiveness Grief Self-Abuse Stubborness
Row 4 Liver or Gall Bladder	Anger Bitterness Guilt Hatred Resentment	Depression Frustration Indecisiveness Panic Taken for Granted
Row 5 Kidneys or Bladder	Blaming Dread Fear Horror Peeved	Conflict Creative Insecurity Terror Unsupported Wishy Washy
Row 6 Glands & Sexual Organs	Humiliation Jealousy Longing Lust Overwhelm	Pride Shame Shock Unworthy Worthless

Image figure 5: Emotion Code chart

How to Super-charge Emotional Balance

I'll share with you a little secret of mine. Despite the fact that Tapping and TAT are incredibly effective in their own right, I've found a way to make them work even better and faster! That goes for the Emotion Code as well. What I've noticed is that the patients for whom these techniques work the best are the ones who are brain balanced while we perform them. Remember, brain balance refers to a healthy nervous system whereby the right and left hemispheres of the brain are synchronizing with each other and the autonomic nervous system is balanced or regulating (and not stuck in "stress" mode).

Quickly reducing the "charge" of negative or traumatic memories or emotions is a desirable process. When you do EFT, TAT or Emotion Code, consider putting a LifeWave Y-Age Aeon patch on your head during the procedure. You can use any of the brain balancing points and can even use an extra Aeon patch on your belly button for when you are clearing extremely traumatic events. If convenient, I like to put the Aeon patch at GV20 on the top of my head since it is out of the way and this point, GV 20, specifically activates the seventh energy center (our seventh chakra) responsible for our connection to our higher power also known as our God-self.

Just as Tapas Fleming described how the emotional baggage associated with allergies was neutralized along with the allergies, I've noticed that the Aeon patches can sometimes do the same if placed on specific points of the body. During one of my office sessions with a patient, she was lamenting the fact that she would always come down with the flu in March every year. She didn't know why she would get so sick but I suspected some sort of traumatic childhood event was involved. We used muscle testing to determine that she would weaken when exposed to a piece of paper with the written statement, *"Frequencies causing annual flu in March"*. We then did the Uhe Method and acupuncture.

Afterwards, not only did my patient test "strong" to the statement, she remembered a painful incident from childhood that caused her extreme embarrassment. The words "SHAME" written in capital letters scrolled across her visual field as she recounted the incident while lying on the acupuncture treatment table. She had forgotten all about that event until the day we did the treatment with the intention of clearing whatever it was that brought on the annual flu. One year later, the patient reported that she remained healthy throughout the month of March. Not only did she not get her annual "flu", she didn't get sick all winter. Simply amazing!

Sometimes the words, emotional baggage, seem so heavy that people deny having any. Please believe me when I say that we *all* have some degree of emotional baggage. If we were all fully present in the "now", none of us would need any self-help books. Being emotional is part of being human. Even slight feelings of frustration, multiplied over days or months, can siphon energy away from healing your body and your chronic pain. So I encourage you to try these techniques and to "clear" your emotional field daily. Compare it to doing the dishes every day. If you only dirtied a couple of dishes per day, it wouldn't seem worthwhile to wash them daily, but if you let the dishes pile up over three weeks, you probably wouldn't have any space left in your kitchen to cook!

Chapter Summary

- Negative emotions from past events and trauma can sabotage your healing by diverting the energy away from the present, the only "place" you can really heal.
- Anger is an ally in your healing and should be honored for its role in guiding you to a more deserving place.
- Clearing emotional baggage can be quick and painless and years of psychotherapy are not required.
- Energy psychology techniques such as Tapping, TAT, and Emotion Code can help clear negative emotional blocks through the acupressure meridian system.
- Energy psychology techniques are enhanced by brain balancing with LifeWave Y-Age Aeon patches placed on specific acupuncture points.
- Daily clearing is recommended so that past emotions are not hampering your present healing abilities.

10

MEDITATION AND MINDFULNESS

The practice of mindfulness and meditation has been growing in popularity since the seventies. Pioneers such as Jon Kabat-Zinn, creator of the Mindfulness Based Stress Reduction program at the University of Massachusetts Medical School have proven that mindfulness based programs can have a positive impact on chronic pain as well as many chronic diseases. Dr. Peter A. Levine and Dr. Maggie Phillips, authors of Freedom from Pain: Discover Your Body's Power to Overcome Physical Pain, have found that people can shift their experience of pain through mindfulness-based practices.

Your Relationship with Pain

Many people understand the term "relationship" when it involves another person, but not when it involves different aspects of our body and life. Believe it or not, you have a relationship with your pain. The most common relationship pattern is one of avoidance. Think about it for a minute. When you feel pain in your body, isn't it kind of instinctual to try to avoid it? To try to get rid of it? To try to distract yourself from it? To pretend it isn't there, and try to go on with your daily life?

I guarantee you that, if given the choice, most people would prefer not to be experiencing chronic pain. So it is inevitable that our minds will do whatever it takes to create a separation between "us" and the pain. Although it is a natural, instinctive phenomenon, it is the exact opposite that we must do in order to heal it.

Remember that pain in Chinese Medicine translates into blocked energy or low energy flow. By distracting, ignoring or numbing ourselves from our pain sensations, we literally promote further blockage. On the other hand, when we pay attention to something, we promote energy flow to that "something". There is a Law of Attraction quote that goes, "Where

102

attention goes, energy flows, and results show". I love that quote because it is as true in the manifestation of health as it is in wealth and abundance.

For example, if your attention is focused on scarcity and lack, then you'll manifest, and notice, more scarcity and lack. If on the other hand, you focus on what you have and what you are grateful for, you manifest more things to have and be grateful for. It works like a charm when you turn it into an exercise to heal conflict between two people. Just to prove it to yourself, choose someone in your life that annoys you. For thirty days in a row, make a point to write down (and feel) at least ten things you appreciate about this person. Notice their strong points, not their weaknesses. If you start noticing their faults, train yourself to let those thoughts pass and re-focus your thoughts on their gifts. After all, we all have gifts. You just have to make an effort to look for and appreciate them. If you do this small exercise in earnest, you'll witness a dramatic change in the person's behavior towards you as well as how you feel about them.

In order to heal our pain, we often have to change our relationship with the pain. In other words, we need to change our perceptions. If we treat our pain as the "enemy", *what we resist will persist*. Part of mindfulness is learning acceptance rather than resistance for "what is".

What is Mindfulness?

I like what Jon Kabat-Zinn defines as mindfulness. He says that it is a state of pure awareness of what is, without judgment or reaction. In addition to the common reaction of avoidance and distraction that comes with experiencing chronic pain, many people end up feeling resignation or victimization. Mindfulness provides a different choice. You don't have to pretend that the pain is not there or try to distract yourself from it using common unconscious activities such as drugs, alcohol, television, and other addictive substances. On the other hand, you don't have to "pull yourself up by the bootstraps" and just suffer through the pain as if you are in the army. You don't have to prove to anyone that you are tough.

Mindfulness invites you to experience yourself and your body in a state of awareness of the present moment without resorting to the common ensuing judgments that we have all learned to have when we're in discomfort. Although our minds have been trained well in school when it comes to reading, writing, and math, there is no training in mindfulness.

Although there is no promise that the practice of mindfulness will cure your pain, it can. You see, when we resist what is, we re-pattern the same pain over and over again in our consciousness, thereby encouraging it to stay. Nothing really stays the same. Everything is always changing. But we can literally make things look and feel the same by thinking the same old thoughts over and over again. Mindfulness and meditation offer an opportunity to re-wire age-old patterns of resistance into new awareness and openness that can support you immensely in healing not only your body but your life.

What is Meditation?

According to Wikipedia, meditation can be defined as "a practice in which an individual trains the mind and/or induces a mode of consciousness to realize some benefit". There are many types of meditation practices but they all have one thing in common: training the mind. Some people use mindfulness and meditation to mean the same thing and others don't. The terminology is less important than your willingness to try some degree of mind training. Our minds are powerful attractors. We create our experiences through our minds and we are equally as capable of creating nirvana as we are of creating our own hell on earth. By making the effort to cultivate your mind using meditation, you can shift your entire perspective on life with as little effort as five minutes a day. Yes, just five minutes a day!

Here's the good news. It matters less the length of time you spend in meditation than it does the consistency with which you practice it. Like all things worthwhile achieving, meditation takes determination and discipline. I laughed out loud when I heard what Jon Kabat-Zinn says to his patients in his Mindfulness Based Stress Reduction Program: "You don't have to *like* the meditations; you just have to *do* them". When the patients in the program actually followed through on the meditation they were taught, they got great clinical results. Although meditation is not difficult per se, it does indeed require discipline. Over time, the state of mindfulness, however, can become a moment to moment meditation in the course of your daily life. That experience can be extremely rewarding and joyful.

Re-inhabiting Your Body

Before you start inviting all of your pain to the surface because now you think it is a good idea, allow yourself to first get accustomed to the notion that your attention has been elsewhere. In fact, it's been almost everywhere but fully present in your body. We'll discuss more about the practice of being present in the Spirit section of this book. For now, just be open to the possibility that your attention (and thus your energy) is not fully in your body.

In order for us to even try to encourage the body to self-heal, we need to re-inhabit our bodies. First, however, we need to feel safe so that we don't feel overwhelmed by our physical pain. Meditation and mindfulness practices are excellent ways to start re-inhabiting our bodies and learning to pay attention to ourselves without judgment or agenda.

In my personal experience, it is extremely challenging to stay present when the pain is intense. I remember trying to fall asleep one night as I experienced intense uterine cramping. As I paid attention to the pain, interestingly it would shift and even fade, but when it did so, I automatically began thinking of something else. My mind wouldn't stay focused on the pain. When the pain increased, it would remind me to pay attention again. Because I had refused to take drugs for the intense pain, this experience gave me ample respect for the power of mindfulness and meditation.

I have a confession to make. I like "easy", and I can be a bit lazy. That's why I use so many of the energy-based tools I'll be sharing later with you to *quickly* ease pain. Years ago, I would have been too embarrassed to admit something "human" like that. Mindfulness and meditation, however, take discipline and effort, and are not quick fixes by any means. They take time to learn and master. On the other hand, they can be really fun because you discover more about yourself in the process. Being mindful brings with it gifts of joy and clarity. If someone is extremely depressed or unmotivated due to chronic pain, it can be helpful to first diminish the intensity of the pain using some of the other energy tools in this book, then come back to the meditation and mindfulness practices.

There have been plenty of patients who have tried meditation, yoga and other mindfulness based practices and felt like failures. They complain that their anxiety is severe and they cannot concentrate. Thoughts spin in their minds like a whirling dervish and they cannot consciously "be" with them. Many can't sleep at night. They wake up with incessant unwanted thoughts that rule their life. Thus they feel that their yoga or meditation practices are not useful and they are frustrated with their "lack" of results.

My observation is that 100% of these types of patients have a severe brain imbalance (see Chapter 6). More and more people are experiencing these issues and it can be incredibly frustrating for the more "enlightened" patient to experience a lack of results from their meditative efforts. It isn't that their methods are wrong or useless; it is that their bio-electrical brain chemistry is so out of balance that they can't achieve the minimum amount of "success" with these beneficial practices.

When I've quickly been able to brain balance these patients, usually within a couple of weeks, their meditative practices soar to new heights. Their natural in-born abilities to pay attention, be present, without judgment, are reignited. The incessant thoughts are no longer turning in their heads and they can finally sleep at night. At this point, the meditation and mindfulness based practices are even more powerful. If someone's brain has a severe imbalance, it may be necessary to use strong energetic or biologic therapies to rebalance their brain patterns before she can follow through on meditative practices.

Meditation and mindfulness based practices have been a centuries-old strategy to healing mind, body and soul. In this day and age, we can now integrate more tools to enhance the benefits of this wise practice, especially in cases where severe stress has hampered the brain's ability to function normally. I encourage you to try a few of the mindfulness exercises in this chapter to get a feel for these practices and what they can do for your chronic pain and your overall enjoyment of life. If they resonate with you, I encourage you to pursue further training and study.

Mindfulness Meditation #1: Wellspring Meditation

In this meditation, we are going to have you experience (re-inhabit) your body through your breath. Breath is a common source of focus in yoga, meditation and mindfulness. I also call this the wellspring Chong ma meditation because you'll be breathing through the acupuncture channel Chong ma which is the meridian that runs through your central axis. If you imagine a globe (the kind you'd find in geography class) and spin it, the stake at the center of the globe would be the central axis. Your body has a meridian running right through the middle of it as well. In acupuncture, we often needle the points that activate this meridian for people who are energetically depleted. You can consciously activate this meridian through the breath in this exercise I'm about to teach you.

First, find a quiet place to sit comfortably with your back relatively straight. You may need a straight-backed chair if you're not used to supporting your spine in a meditation pose. Make sure that if you are short, your feet are not dangling from the chair. Choose a sitting position where your feet can touch the ground. Alternatively, you may feel comfortable sitting upon a meditation cushion or folded soft blankets in a cross-legged position. For this exercise it works better if you do not lie down, as the visualization can be a little trickier if you do. The important thing is to get comfortable, but not too comfortable so that you fall asleep.

If you happen to have some meditation music, you can play it at the same time and it may make this meditation even easier. Once you get some practice with this, you won't need extra paraphernalia to help you. I've even done it in the car while I'm stopped at a red light.

Next, once you're comfortable, close your eyes and focus on your natural breath. If you've never focused on your breath before, you might notice that you're breathing into your upper chest. This is a type of nervous breath. It is a habitual way of breathing that adults have been accustomed to because of stress and trauma. If you notice your shoulders and upper chest moving a lot while you breathe, see if you can breathe all the way down into your lower belly or pelvis. We call this belly breathing. It is also called yogic breathing. Breathing into your lower belly so that it expands and contracts gently helps you get into a calmer state of mind. You might wish to put one of your hands over your belly so that you can feel the expansion and contraction of this part of your body. Breathe slowly but naturally, without force or exertion.

Once you've established a natural breathing rhythm, we can now begin. On your next inhale, visualize that you're breathing in from the bottom of your tailbone or perineum (the area between the scrotum and the anus in a man or the area between the vagina and the anus in a woman) all the way up the center of your spine until it reaches the top of your head. When the breath reaches the top of your head, exhale: visualize it bursting out like a bubbling spring and washing over your entire body until it reaches the tips of your fingers and ends of your toes. Repeat this visualization over and over again with each breath. Most yoga teachers prefer their students to breathe in and out through their nostrils rather than through their mouths. If, however, you prefer to breathe out through your mouth, that's fine.

You may find that you feel energy or tingling throughout your body as you practice this meditation. That's great if you do, but don't be upset with yourself if you don't. Often, it takes some practice to "re-inhabit" your body i.e. to *be* energetically in your body, because chronic pain makes it tempting to "leave". You may also find that you get distracted and start thinking of something else. If you do, just let the thought go and return to focusing on your breathing and visualization.

During this meditation, our focus is not to specifically pay attention to the painful or non-painful areas of the body, but just to practice training the mind to move energy. It really is a form of Qi Gong, a healing exercise you'll learn more about in a later chapter.

As you do this wellspring meditation, you may notice a shift in how your body feels after the meditation. You may feel calmer or more energetic. You may feel less discomfort or you may not. It doesn't really matter as long as you let go of any preconceived ideas or judgments you may have. Just experience it. If you encounter any difficulty, just let it be there and don't judge it. Everything you experience is part of mindfulness if you pay attention to it.

Mindfulness Meditation #2: Intuitive Healing

This meditation can be done lying or sitting and also involves breath work. First, begin noticing your breath moving in and out. See if you can set your intention to breathe all the way down into your deep pelvis. This breathing pattern alone can be very energizing and healing for many people when done on a regular basis.

After you've established belly breathing at a comfortable pace, turn your attention to a body part that feels uncomfortable. If you have several, just pick one, preferably a spot that is not the most painful. As you continue to breathe steadily, turn your awareness to the area of discomfort and begin noticing the quality of what you feel there. If it helps, you can choose words to describe it, such as cold, hot, tight, etc. You may also note some emotions emanating from that area such as fear, anger, sadness, etc. Whatever it is, just accept it without judgment.

Intend to just "be" with these sensations for several breaths without trying to changing anything. Your intuition may suddenly give you additional insights during this time, but don't force it. At this point, you may wish to ask the area of discomfort what it needs or wants. I know it sounds funny asking your hip or your low back, "What do you want?" but you'd be surprised how often an answer just pops out of nowhere into your awareness. See if you can be open to whatever flows into your consciousness after you ask this question. Again, intend to accept whatever comes without judgment.

It never ceases to amaze me that even people who have never done formal meditation before often come up with "answers" to this question fairly quickly. If you're struggling or feeling like nothing is coming through, that's okay too. Sometimes, you just feel resistance and that in and of itself is telling you something of value. Examples of what may come up when you ask your painful body part what it wants include:

> *"I want to be loved."*
> *"I want warmth."*
> *"I need rest."*
> *"I want respect."*
> *"I need more attention."*
> *"I need more support."*
> *"I need more relaxation and fun."*
> *"I need reassurance that I'm safe."*

Imagine that you've established what you think your painful body part is asking for. Now with the breath, you can extend this particular meditation to "give" that body part what it is asking for energetically. If your hip, for example, is longing for security, imagine that with the next breath, you could inhale the *energy* of security. Imagine what that energy would feel like. As you exhale, breathe the energy of security into your painful hip. Repeat over and over again several times. Notice if anything shifts in how your hip feels. This breath work may or may not make an appreciable change in how your pain feels in the moment, but with repeated practice, you'd be surprised how often it does.

Your painful body part can give you loads of intuitive information about your life and what may best serve you or make you happy. Taken in this light, you can infer how your pain may change once you start addressing its needs in your everyday life. For example, if your shoulder tells you, "I need rest", check if that feels true to you. If it does, what choices do you have to honor that request?

I once had a patient with terrible recurring shoulder pain. I found out that Petra was doing lots of heavy labor on her property because her husband's mental illness prevented him from helping out in a meaningful way. It was obvious to me that her shoulder pain reflected severe resentment she harbored. Once I pointed out to her what her shoulder was trying to tell her, Petra began to make different choices in her life. She hired people to take over some of the heavy labor and focused her efforts on things she'd rather be doing instead. Her shoulder improved as did her outlook on life. To her surprise, her husband started pitching in with the yard work once she honored her shoulder's intuitive guidance to stop doing heavy labor.

How to Make Mindfulness and Meditation Work

Two of the questions most often asked of meditation or mindfulness practices are, "How long do I have to do this?" and "Do I have to do it every day?" Most mindfulness meditation gurus will instruct their students to do some form of meditation daily. The minimum time necessary for formal meditation to be effective is felt to be five to ten minutes a day. Neale Donald Walsch, author of the popular Conversations with God series, feels that ten second meditations done sporadically throughout the day, is more than enough to experience a shift.

There are huge benefits to a daily meditative practice, one being that your new "skill set" can be transferred to your everyday life in a meaningful way. Being mindful of your pain in a meditative practice may transfer to being more mindful of your other relationships. I can attest to experiencing joy and contentment through the practice of mindfulness, whether it is while talking to a friend, doing the dishes or analyzing an emotional reaction.

I encourage you to make a daily commitment to a mindfulness meditation practice for a month and see how that changes your life. If, for whatever reason it doesn't resonate with you, then honor it and move onto something that does.

Next, in the Body section, I'll give you energy tools and holistic strategies to get quick relief from your chronic pain. In the Spirit section, I'll introduce you to some fabulous spiritual practices that can help you create a joyful healing experience.

Chapter Summary

- Mindfulness and meditation are tools that can shift your perception of pain and dissolve the pain itself.
- Honor your current relationship with pain and learn from it.
- Mindfulness is a way you can tap into your intuitive guidance system to ask what your pain needs.
- Aside from pain relief, a daily meditation or mindfulness practice can benefit all facets of your life.

Section C

Your Body—Supporting Your Body's Self-Healing Mechanism

"Take care of your body. It is the only place you have to live."
-Jim Rohn

11

ACUPUNCTURE WITHOUT NEEDLES

Using "acupuncture pain patches", I can often achieve pain relief faster than I can with traditional acupuncture. That's good news since you're probably not an acupuncturist. What's even better news is that I can teach you how to use these pain relief patches so that you can do your own "acupuncture without needles" and get the same results that I'm getting. If you are ready to let go of your chronic pain right now, then read on because this technique is the fastest way I know how to get rid of pain. Even if you're skeptical because you have severe pain or your doctor has told you that you'll never get better, just try it. At least ninety percent of people with chronic pain that I've met respond to this technique the first time I teach it to them regardless of the laundry list of incurable diagnoses their doctors have given them.

IceWave Pain Relief Patches

In Chapter 6, I spoke about the LifeWave Y-Age Aeon patches that I use specifically for balancing the brain. In this chapter, I will show you how I use the Aeon patch as well as the LifeWave IceWave patches to relieve acute and chronic pain. The IceWave patches come in a set of two; one white and one tan. The white patch is more positively charged and the tan patch is more negatively charged, and when used together, they move energy in the body. The energy flows from negative to positive. In Eastern medical philosophy, pain is caused by a blockage of energy, so if we move energy through the blockage, then the pain symptoms subside.

The LifeWave patches work by reflecting and sending infra-red energy. They are a form of portable phototherapy, also known as light therapy. The specific spectrum of frequencies it reflects emanates from the nano-sized crystals within the patch. The crystals are embedded in a polyester membrane which is then surrounded by a waterproof seal. There is a medical grade adhesive on one side of the patch which is the side you'd adhere to your skin. Once these patches come into contact with your energy field, they "turn on" and begin reflecting specific bands of infra-red energy emanating from your body.

The IceWave patches have the effect of increasing energy flow between the white and tan patches. Research studies have proven the efficacy of these non-invasive patches to produce significant pain relief effects. The Aeon patches have the effect of decreasing the body's stress and inflammation.

There are three pain relief patching protocols that I will cover in this chapter. The first pain relief protocol is called the Clock Protocol and it uses LifeWave IceWave patches to relieve localized pain. The second protocol is my "shortcut" for localized pain relief using the LifeWave Y-Age Aeon patches. The third protocol uses LifeWave IceWave patches to relieve generalized pain, or whole-body pain. If you have pain in more than one area or joint in the body, you may wish to try the whole-body pain relief protocol. People with fibromyalgia who have the "hit by a truck" kind of pain throughout their bodies often respond well to the whole-body pain protocol. You can try both to see which works better. Generally, we don't recommend using more than two sets of IceWave patches at one time, unless you've been specifically trained in advanced uses of these patches. Please note that LifeWave does not claim that their patches can cure, treat or prevent any disease. The advice herein is to teach you how to use them to reduce or eliminate the symptom of pain.

General Guidelines when Using the Patches

1. Store the patches in a cool place away from strong electromagnetic fields, such as cell phones, and heat. I store my patches in a basket on top of my bathroom counter. They are about three feet away from overhead fluorescent lights. In the winter when the sun shines horizontally through the windows, I cover my packages with a terry cloth so that heat from the passive solar exposure won't deactivate my patches.

2. Do not carry your patches close to your body unless you are using them. They will become activated on exposure to your electromagnetic field. If you wish to carry them in your purse,

store them in the original packaging or purchase a metal wallet so that any body heat is reflected away from the patches.

3. Do not cut the patches in half and do not re-use them once the adhesive backing is removed.

4. Both the Y-Age patches and one of the IceWave pain patches are white in color so if you take them both out of their packaging, remember to label them on the back when you're doing the protocols below so you don't mix them up. I usually write "A" on the back of the Aeon patches and "IW" on the back of the IceWave patches.

5. Drink plenty of pure filtered water while using patches as they work better when you are fully hydrated. The signaling or communication system of the body is much more efficient if your cells are hydrated.

Materials You Will Need:

- One or two sets of LifeWave IceWave pain relief patches
- Optional: one or two LifeWave Y-Age Aeon anti-stress patches
- Tape that you can use to temporarily adhere the patches to your body. Clear tape, masking tape, or medical tape works just fine.
- Glass of water in case you need to hydrate
- A quiet setting so you're not distracted by television, telephone or other people
- Pen and paper to jot some notes

The LifeWave Clock Protocol for Localized Pain

If you have not been drinking water before testing this protocol, you may wish to drink 16 ounces of water before patching. It isn't necessary, but I find that many people are dehydrated and don't know it. If you regularly consume caffeinated beverages, such as coffee, then you'll actually urinate an excessive amount of fluid throughout the day and become dehydrated. Caffeine is a diuretic and can cause dehydration. If this is your first time doing this protocol, I recommend drinking a couple glasses of pure filtered water beforehand. Other than that, follow the instructions below. Check out my "how to patch" videos online.

1. Curl a piece of tape on the underside of each of the white and tan IceWave patches without taking the adhesive backing off.
2. Locate the most painful part of your body (see Figure 6) and rate the pain out of 10, with 1 being mildly painful and a 10 being unbearably painful.

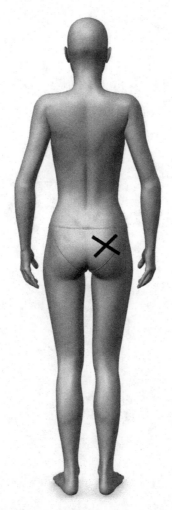

Figure 6: X indicates painful area

3. Take the TAN patch and stick it right over the most painful spot on your body. If it is inconvenient and you have tight-fitting clothing on, you can even stick the patch right on top of your clothes. It still works.

4. Take the WHITE patch now and stick it above the TAN patch anywhere from 1 inch to 3 inches away. This position is the 12 o'clock position, assuming the TAN patch represents the center of a clock (See Figure 7).

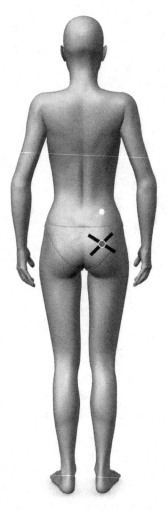

Figure 7: Tan patch on area of maximal pain

5. Wait 10–15 seconds, and then re-evaluate the pain level out of 10. If the pain is not significantly relieved (at least 50% reduced), then move the WHITE to approximately 3 o'clock relative to the TAN patch (see Figure 8).

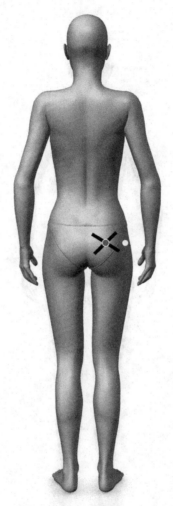

Figure 8: Tan patch on pain; White patch at 3 o'clock

6. Again wait 10-15 seconds, then re-evaluate your pain level. If the pain is not relieved to your satisfaction, then move the WHITE patch to the 6 o'clock position (see Figure 9). If the tape is losing stickiness at this point, just put a fresh piece of tape onto the back of the patch.

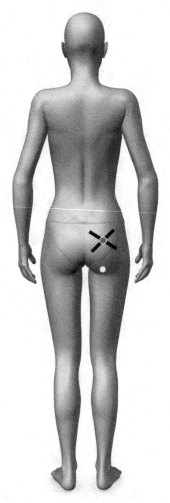

Figure 9: Tan patch on pain; White patch at 6 o'clock

7.   Again wait 10-15 seconds and if the pain is not relieved to your satisfaction then place the WHITE patch at 9 o'clock (see Figure 10).

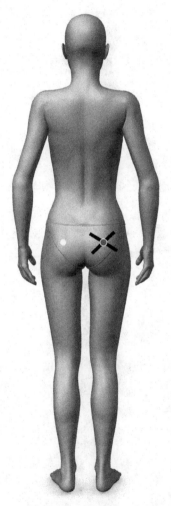

Figure 10: Tan patch on pain; White patch at 9 o'clock

8. If after 10-15 seconds your pain relief is not enough, they you can move the WHITE patch to the opposite side of the body. I call this technique "sandwiching" the pain (see Figure 11)

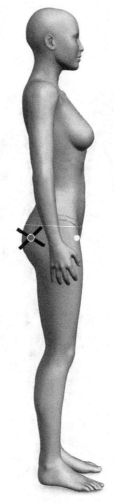

Figure 11: Sandwich the pain

9. If after 10-15 seconds, this is not satisfactory, then you can move both the TAN and the WHITE to either side of the pain. This is called Bracketing (see Figure 12) to see if that gives you better pain relief.

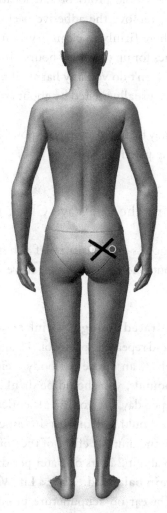

Figure 12: Bracket the pain

10. Lastly, if your pain is not at least 50% better with this protocol or if you wish to try for a greater degree of pain relief, you can do the whole Clock Protocol again with the WHITE patch in the center of the pain while moving the TAN patch around the clock.

11. After doing the whole protocol and locating the best IceWave patch positions, remove the adhesive backing from the IceWave patches and adhere firmly to clean dry skin.

12. Wear the patches for up to twelve hours. If you wear them longer than that, they won't do you any harm. The nano-crystals inside the patches have usually melted by about twelve hours so they are no longer active.

13. Remember to stay hydrated as much as possible to get the maximum benefit from the patches.

Tips for Success Using the LifeWave Clock Protocol

If you're not having success with pain relief using the LifeWave Clock Protocol, which is about one in ten people, there are usually four main reasons:

1. **You're not hydrated enough.** Drink an additional 16 ounces or more of water and repeat the protocol. Healthy water consumption is approximately ½ an ounce per body weight (lbs.) per day. So if you're 150 pounds, you should be drinking 75 ounces of pure filtered water per day. If you drink coffee, then for every cup you drink, you should add another 16 ounces of water per day to counterbalance the diuretic effect of the coffee. For most people, it works out to about 2 liters of water per day.

2. **You're not brain balanced.** Place a LifeWave Y-Age Aeon patch behind the right ear on acupuncture point Triple Burner 17 or any of the other brain balancing points and do the protocol again. Often the IceWave will then work to reduce the pain.

3. **You have significant mineral deficiencies.** The patches require minerals for their energy signaling mechanism to be effective. If you take a lot of medications, or eat a lot of processed food, or have been extremely weak and ill, you could have mineral deficiencies.

In this case, sometimes placing a few grains of unrefined Celtic sea salt, or Himalayan Crystal Salt, on your tongue can activate your system to respond to the patches. If it works, then you will likely benefit from a quality mineral supplement on a regular basis. I will share more on that in a later chapter.

4. **The patches aren't on the right location**. Sometimes pain isn't coming from where you are feeling it. We call that referred pain. This can be tricky so you might need the help of a trained LifeWave distributor to patch you. If this is the case and you don't have one near you, you can purchase the patches from one of my team members and she/he will help you personally.

It is unusual that someone does not respond to the IceWave pain relief patches and most often it is a hydration or brain balance problem. At times, because I like to be efficient, I will place a LifeWave Y-Age Aeon patch on the head behind the right ear (TB 17) *before* I start the clock protocol. If I get the pain relief I'm expecting, then I will remove the Aeon head patch and wait 30 seconds or so to see if the pain returns. If it does, then I know that the person requires the brain balancing effects of the Aeon patch.

The reason I use the point behind the ear is because it is more discreet. Any of the brain balancing points will work, but most people aren't going to be comfortable going to the grocery store with a patch in the middle of their forehead! Of course, you can always wear a headband or hat if you want to use any of the other brain balancing points. I personally love the point at the top of the head, GV 20. I call it my "happy point" because I get a sense of bliss and peace whenever I use it there.

One time while doing demonstrations at a health fair, I patched a woman named Justina. She had a painful shoulder that she could barely lift and it would sound "crunchy" the entire time she moved it. After discovering that she carried a cell phone with her wherever she went, I decide to patch her head with an Aeon patch and then patched her shoulder with the IceWave patches. Sure enough, she was able to lift her arm all the way up without any pain and the "crunchy" sounds disappeared. Pleased with the result, I decided to remove the Aeon from the head to see what would happen. Within seconds her pain began to return. It was clear from our little experiment that her brain balance was abnormal and she needed the Aeon patch on her head to achieve lasting pain relief.

Dr. Karen's Shortcut for Localized Pain Relief

Now that you know the LifeWave Clock protocol for pain using the IceWave patches, I want to share with you a little shortcut that I've found to be helpful when you don't have a lot of time or you don't have any IceWave patches available. This shortcut works best if you mainly have localized pain.

Take an Aeon patch and place it behind your right ear. Then take a second Aeon patch and place it over the pain spot on your body (see Figure 13). Make sure you're hydrated. Often within a few minutes, the pain will start easing away. It may take a little longer than the IceWave to relieve the pain, but both the Aeon and the IceWave patches reduce inflammation on contact, so often either work well. It is of course, always helpful to move energy, which is what the IceWave does, so I always recommend IceWave for pain relief if you have them on hand.

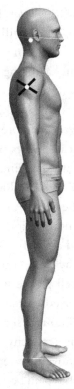

Figure 13: Aeon on head; Aeon on localized pain

On the LifeWave website, you will be able to see pictures of infra-red photographs of people in chronic pain. Areas of pain and inflammation show up as dark purple and red on the photographs, yet within minutes of patching these areas with either the IceWave patches or the Aeon patches, the colors shift to a cooler green and yellow. See Resources for links.

Whole Body Pain Patching Protocol

If you have pain in multiple areas of your body or you have the "hit by a truck" type of pain, also described as "flu-like" pain, then the Whole Body Pain Patching protocol may be particularly helpful. This protocol uses two sets of LifeWave IceWave patches. The addition of one LifeWave Y-Age Aeon patch is optional. Remember to hydrate yourself so that the patches will work better. If you're a visual learner like me, I have "how to patch" videos available free online for you to learn this protocol.

1. Assess your pain level out of 10, **1** being mild pain and **10** being unbearable pain.
2. *Optional:* Place an Aeon patch behind the right ear on Triple Burner 17 (Figure 14).

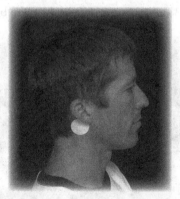

Figure 14: Aeon on Triple Burner 17

3. Take one set of IceWave patches and stick the WHITE patch on acupuncture point **Kidney 1** (KI 1) on the bottom of the RIGHT foot.

4. Take the TAN patch and stick it on KI 1 on the bottom of the LEFT foot (see Figure 15).

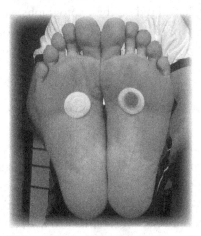

Figure 15: IceWave on Kidney 1

6. Wait approximately 15–30 seconds and re-evaluate your pain out of 10. See if you have at least 50% reduction in overall pain. If not, or if you desire more pain relief, continue with the protocol.

7. Using a second set of IceWave patches, using tape on the back of the patches, temporarily stick the WHITE patch to acupuncture point **Heart 3** (HT 3) on the inside of the RIGHT elbow and the TAN patch to HT 3 on the inside of the LEFT elbow (Figure 16).

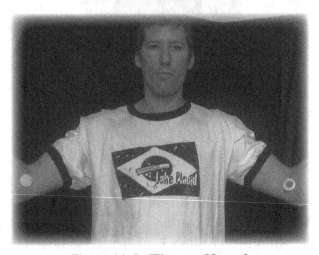

Figure 16: IceWave on Heart 3

8. Wait approximately 15-30 seconds to see if you've had any additional pain relief. If pain relief is not reduced to your satisfaction, you can then move the patches from the elbows to the wrist crease right above the thumb (see Figure 17). This point is **Lung 9** (LU 9). WHITE goes on the RIGHT and TAN on the LEFT.

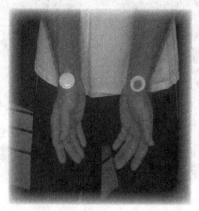

Figure 17: IceWave on Lung 9

9. Again wait approximately 15-30 seconds and re-evaluate the pain level. If at any time the tape on the back of the patches loses its stickiness, replace it with a fresh piece of tape before moving the patches again.

10. If you wish, move the patches again to another acupuncture point on the back side of the wrist approximately three finger widths up from the wrist crease, **Triple Burner 5** (TB 5), WHITE on RIGHT, TAN on LEFT. (See Figure 18).

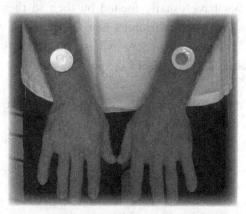

Figure 18: IceWave on Triple Burner 5

11. Wait 15-30 seconds and if you wish, move the patches from your wrist to the shoulder muscles on either side of your neck and put them on **Triple Burner 15** (TB 15) WHITE on RIGHT, TAN on LEFT. (See Figure 19).

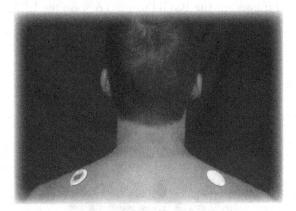

Figure 19: IceWave on Triple Burner 15

12. Decide which of the upper body acupuncture points worked best with the second set of IceWave patches, all the while having the first set on the bottom of both feet. Once you've located the best spot, remove the adhesive backing from the IceWave patches and adhere firmly to clean dry skin over the most effective acupuncture point.

13. Wear the patches for up to twelve hours. If you wear them longer than that, you won't do any harm. The nano-crystals inside the patches have usually melted by then so they are no longer active and you'll have to put a new set on if and when your pain returns. Remember to stay hydrated as much as possible to get the maximum benefit from the patches.

For how-to videos of the above protocols, go to my YouTube channel: www.YouTube.com/karenkanmd.

LifeWave Patches: Frequently Asked Questions

Question: What scientific evidence is there to prove these acupuncture patches work?

One of the things I really appreciate about the LifeWave company is its commitment to research. There are many energy-based products on the market (holographic discs, wands, pendants etc.), but if you look carefully, few are validated by quality research. Go to the Research page on the LifeWave website to view the most current research on these patch products. There are approximately sixty research studies to date involving LifeWave products from around the world. In Europe the Silent Nights patch product for sleep has been approved as a medical device for the treatment of insomnia. It may be a decade or more before energy technology like LifeWave will be approved for the treatment of a medical condition here in the United States by the pro-pharmaceutical Food and Drug Administration. Thankfully, the Europeans are more forward-thinking.

Question: Are there any side effects to wearing LifeWave patches?

Because LifeWave acupuncture patches increase the flow of energy in the body, the body can begin to heal itself by detoxifying. Detoxification symptoms are also known as healing reactions. Some people experience detoxification symptoms when they first begin using the patches as toxins are released from their storage places in the body in order to be excreted in the urine, feces or sweat. Symptoms are usually mild and can include fatigue, headaches, nasal stuffiness, loose stool, constipation, unusual body odor or rash. The most common symptoms seem to be headache and fatigue. Most of these symptoms resolve with additional hydration, but if they are more severe, LifeWave recommends removing the patches and wearing them for shorter periods of time until your body accommodates to them.

Question: Will I have to wear IceWave pain relief patches every day?

It may be necessary to wear the IceWave pain relief patches daily when you first start, as your body needs extra support to keep the energy channels open and clear. Often, after someone has been patching daily for several weeks, they will notice that their overall pain levels have diminished significantly and that they do not have to use the patches as often. I have found that patients who use both the LifeWave Y-Age Aeon and the IceWave patches together have a faster healing rate than with IceWave alone. The anti-stress and anti-inflammatory effects of the Aeon patches support the self-healing processes of the body, so the effect is more than just pain relief. In time, you may not need pain relief patches once the body self-heals the source of the pain.

Question: How soon will I get pain relief with the patches?

It should be fairly immediate. We are aiming for at least a 50% reduction in pain levels after patching. Many people get total pain relief, even from their first patching session. If you follow the instructions to the letter, you should be getting results. If you are the one in ten that doesn't, then contact your LifeWave distributor for help. With continued daily use, many people find that the level of pain diminishes over time and that their response to the patches is quicker or more complete. Occasionally, someone will get only a 50% reduction of pain within 10 seconds, but then over the next 20 to 60 minutes, will experience additional or complete pain relief.

Question: Will my pain be worse when I'm not wearing the patches?

Rarely, after an initial patching whereby the pain is significantly reduced or eliminated, a few people notice that when the patches wear off, their pain seems to return with a greater intensity. A plausible explanation for this "rebound" symptom is that the energy was flowing well with the patches on, and toxins were being kicked out. When the patches wore off, the channels became blocked again before all the toxins could be released. Pain is considered blocked energy in Eastern medicine. The body, preferring the open clear flow of energy, may temporarily give an increased pain signal. Don't be alarmed if this happens to you. With consistent patching, the body learns to keep the energy channels open and flowing. Occasionally toxins may be physically present in the painful area and the addition of the LifeWave Y-Age Glutathione patches may improve the body's response to IceWave. See below for more information on the Glutathione patch.

Question: LifeWave has other anti-aging patches available. Would those help my chronic pain?

LifeWave has three types of anti-aging patches on the market so far. You have already been introduced to the Y-Age Aeon patches which are designed to decrease stress and inflammation. Using the Aeon for brain balancing or pain is ideal.

One of the other anti-aging patches is called the Y-Age Glutathione patch. This patch is designed to stimulate your body's own production of glutathione, a master antioxidant that has an important role in detoxifying the body and supporting the body's immune system. As we age, glutathione levels often drop and it gets worse if we are taking glutathione-depleting pain medications such as acetaminophen (Tylenol®). Using the Y-Age Glutathione patch can help the body detoxify which in turn will keep the cells healthier and thus improve the body's overall function. Using them may amplify the pain relieving effect of the other patches. I have found that in my practice, the use of the Y-Age Glutathione patches helps to soften scars and other connective tissue issues. Scar tissue can be the cause of pain in many people, especially if they've had surgery.

The third anti-aging patch is called the Y-Age Carnosine patch. This patch is designed to stimulate the production of carnosine, another natural anti-oxidant in the body. Carnosine levels drop as we age, but the Carnosine patch is able to improve Carnosine levels very quickly. In various research studies on carnosine supplementation, carnosine has been shown to improve tissue and cellular repair. Along with the Glutathione patch, using the Carnosine patch on a regular basis has the added side benefit of improving skin quality. Fine lines and wrinkles improve as well as skin smoothness and suppleness. The Carnosine patches also seem to help my patients who have significant scar tissue in their bodies.

I personally use all three Y-Age patches to support my body in healing itself. I love what they do to support my organs, especially my skin organ! Here's a secret few people know. If your skin is healthy, it reflects the health of your internal organs. If your skin is unhealthy, that means your internal organs are in trouble.

Ever since I was a young child I had unhealthy skin. Even as an adult, I still had breakouts on my face and rough skin all over my arms and legs. I was so embarrassed by my skin that I used a ton of make-up to cover up the bumps and scars. Now, after using the Y-Age patches consistently, I no longer feel the need to wear make-up except for formal parties, photo/ video shoots and television. My skin is clearer, softer and smoother than it's ever been. On more than one occasion, I've been told by others that my skin is practically "glowing". How cool is that? Seriously, I'm telling the truth. Just ask my mom.

Once you have had success using the LifeWave IceWave pain patches and the Y-Age Aeon patches to reduce or eliminate your chronic pain symptoms, you may wish to try the other Y-Age patches, Glutathione and Carnosine, to see whether they work for you as well as they did for me.

Question: Will I get addicted to the patches?

Given the context of our drug-dependent society, this is an understandable question. However, it's sort of like asking whether you'd get addicted to organic food or brushing your teeth twice a day. The answer is no. Using the patches supports the body in a non-addictive way.

Still, you might be concerned that you might become dependent on the patches. Once your body gets used to the beneficial effects of eating organic food, for example, you will probably find conventional food tasteless and unattractive. Your body will know the difference. Likewise, once your body gets used to feeling good using the patches, it might not like going back to feeling bad. I have been using the LifeWave patches since 2005 and I can honestly say that my body is stronger and more flexible now than it was before I used the patches.

Please remember that the patches are not drugs. Nothing enters the body. They increase the flow of energy in the body which then balances the functions of the body. In a perfect world, we would live perfectly healthy lives and once our bodies return to a balanced state, we would never go out of balance again. But that isn't our reality. We are exposed to daily stresses that tip the scales towards illness and dis-ease. By using energy tools, such as the LifeWave acupuncture patches, we counterbalance these stresses in order to keep the energetic balance of the body.

Few people fully appreciate the amount of stress that our bodies are bombarded with, and until now, we had very few healing tools that could counteract that stress in a formidable way. The LifeWave acupuncture patches are an easy, affordable and effective energy tool that you can use to not only relieve pain within minutes, but also support the body in healing itself by reducing stress and inflammation.

Question: Can I wear the patches for more than twelve hours?

Yes, and doing so doesn't do any harm, but they become ineffective after approximately twelve hours of use on the body. If, for whatever reason you wish to use them for shorter than twelve hours, you can apply them to your body with medical tape and then remove them for future use as long as you do not remove the adhesive backing until you are ready to use them up for the rest of the twelve hours. Applying them to clean, dry skin will prevent skin irritations using this method.

Question: Can I re-use the patches?

Generally LifeWave does not recommend reusing the patches if the adhesive backing has been removed due to the risk of skin irritation. If you wish to use the patches for less than the recommended twelve hours, you may wish to use medical tape to adhere the patches on the temporarily on the skin. Alternatively, you may wish to affix the patches to tight-fitting clothing. Regardless of whether you remove the adhesive backing or not, the patches will only have a life span of approximately twelve hours on your body. Remember, the clock starts ticking the minute you place them on or near your body. Some people have erroneously assumed that if they remove only half of the adhesive backing that only half the patch is active. So let me clarify: the entire patch will "turn on" and the twelve hours will start when you place the patch on or near your body whether or not the adhesive backing is removed.

Question: How much do the patches cost?

Well, that depends. Let me tell you how it comes. The retail cost of thirty patches is approximately $90 US. The company has a preferred customer program that you can sign up for that automatically ships patches to you on a monthly basis for ten dollars less, so approximately $80 US. People wishing to become distributors can purchase the patches wholesale for as low as $50 for thirty patches after signing up. Thankfully for many people who are just looking for wholesale options, there is no pressure to "sell" these patches once you become a distributor. When you take into account how well these patches work compared to drugs or other therapies, they are a great value. Normally patients spend anywhere between $75 to $155 per acupuncture treatment. If LifeWave patches work as well or better than acupuncture for pain relief, it can be a huge savings for people.

Question: The patches sound kind of expensive, don't you think?

Whether you feel the cost is justified depends on your point of view. For people who value their health to a great degree, they feel the patches are reasonably priced because of how well they work and how much time they save by not having to go from doctor to doctor to get better. When I was interviewing an Olympic bobsled athlete who used the LifeWave Energy Enhancer patches, she felt that one set of patches (approximately $6 retail) worked better to sustain her energy and enhance her stamina than consuming three cans of Red Bull (a caffeinated energy drink that cost her a total of $7.50). Furthermore the yo-yo effect of stimulated, caffeinated energy did not lead to better athletic performance, and it had negative side effects. It's up to you. It's not for everyone, but for people desperate to get out of pain, I think it is worth a 30 day money-back guaranteed trial don't you? To see the other athletes that use LifeWave check out the MEDIA page on the LifeWave corporate website.

Question: Why not buy patches from discount stores such as Amazon or eBay?

The problems with buying LifeWave patches from discount stores are multifold. Firstly, the LifeWave company does not guarantee them if they are bought from outside the company. In other words, you can't return them for a full refund if they don't work for you. Secondly, LifeWave prohibits its distributors from reselling products online, which means that those that do are breaking the rules of ethical conduct. Do you really want to buy from someone who, when caught, is eventually going to get kicked out of the company? Thirdly, patches bought from Amazon or eBay may not have been properly stored (since they are heat-sensitive) or may have already expired. Fourthly, practically anyone can receive wholesale pricing that is lower than what is advertised on Amazon or eBay by signing up for a distributor wholesale account, so it isn't worthwhile to take chances with quality.

Lastly, and most importantly, the reason these patches are sold through distributors is so that customers receive personalized help, support and training. When you purchase patches from online discount stores, you don't get any support. The number one reason that people fail in using the patches is improper use. Having a distributor guide you through your first patching is invaluable. You can call the LifeWave company to find a well-trained distributor near you or I can connect you with one of my personally-trained team members. See Resources for links.

Question: What about the LifeWave Energy Enhancer patches? Would they help me too?

It depends. If in addition to experiencing chronic pain you also experience chronic tiredness, then yes, the LifeWave Energy Enhancer patches may be helpful. In my practice, I have found that using the Energy Enhancer patches on a regular basis has improved the balance of energy in the entire body and they help to support the stress–handling system of the body i.e. the adrenal glands and the nervous system.

In an earlier chapter, I mentioned that you must restore the energy in your energy battery in order to fully heal. Regular use of LifeWave Energy Enhancer patches is one way that I restore my own energy batteries. I find personally that using the Energy Enhancer patches daily helps my strength, stamina and focus. In addition, I'm much calmer while at the same time more productive. Like IceWave, the Energy Enhancer increases the flow of energy in the body, but even more so, it improves the balance of energy in your acupuncture meridians. Studies have shown that putting the Energy Enhancer patches on one acupuncture meridian quickly balances that meridian as well as many other meridians in the body. The more balanced your energy is, the healthier you'll become.

Question: I have trouble sleeping since having chronic pain. Would the LifeWave Silent Nights sleep patches help me?

Possibly. Quality sleep is vital in order for the body to repair and rejuvenate. If you have trouble falling asleep or staying asleep, the Silent Nights patches may help you. I will be devoting an entire chapter to sleep so stay tuned!

Chapter Summary

- Acupuncture without needles using LifeWave patches can deliver quick and non–invasive pain relief similar to acupuncture.
- The LifeWave Clock Protocol using IceWave patches can be used for localized pain relief.
- The LifeWave Whole Body Pain Relief protocol using two sets of IceWave patches can be used for generalized or whole body pain.
- Using the LifeWave Y–Age Aeon patch on the head can be added to the IceWave pain relief protocols for additional benefit.
- When you don't have IceWave available, you can use a LifeWave Y–Age Aeon patch on the area of pain and one on the head for brain balancing.
- LifeWave patches offer a truly energetic form of pain relief therapy that is extremely effective and easy to learn.

12

GET GROUNDED!

There is a natural health trend that is spreading like wildfire in the United States called Earthing, also known as grounding. The concept of Earthing is really simple, so I'll give you a little background first. Each of our bodies is electromagnetic in nature and thus we react to and respond to other electromagnetic energies in our environment. In the modern world, we are exposed to far more harmful than beneficial energy and it explains, in part, why so many people are suffering from chronic pain, disease and cancer. Unhealthy frequencies are given off by electrical devices and create a phenomenon called electrosmog or electropollution. Although you can't see it, many of us energy-sensitive people can feel it. Electrosmog is incredibly stressful to the body, causing it to shut down many of its self-healing mechanisms.

Exposure to electrosmog causes an excess of positively charged free radicals to accumulate in our bodies. In animal tissues, this reactivity can damage cells and is believed to accelerate the progression of cancer, cardiovascular disease, and age-related diseases. The end result is inflammation, which of course contributes to chronic pain. That is why you'll want to pay attention to how you can reduce free radicals levels in your body. Anti-oxidants such as glutathione, vitamin C, and beta-carotene are known to reduce free radicals in the body. Earthing is now another way you can get rid of excess free radicals and you can do it while you sleep!

Earthing is the epitome of the term "getting grounded". Literally, it means connecting our bare skin to mother earth. When our skin connects with the earth, the positively charged free radicals that are running amok in our bodies get neutralized by the relatively huge dose of negatively charged electrons that flow up from the earth. When this happens, free radical activity diminishes and the body can heal itself again. In the book Earthing, by Clint Ober, Stephen T. Sinatra, M.D. and Martin Zucker, several studies document the benefit of Earthing on the stress-handling system of the body. Stress hormones such as cortisone and youth hormones such as DHEA normalized in individuals who were "earthed" while they slept. Many people even had improved levels of melatonin, a hormone necessary for restful sleep.

Now at this point you're probably wondering if you're going to have to lie outside naked on the ground every night. The answer, thankfully, is no. Clint Ober, a former cable television executive, discovered a way for us to connect to mother earth's energy without having to go outside. He fabricated a simple Earthing sheet made of conductive material and a wire that connects to the grounding port in your electrical outlets. As long as the electricity in your house is properly grounded, just plugging in this sheet and lying on it at night has the same grounding effect as touching the earth with your bare skin.

Very old homes may not be properly grounded, but there are ways you can still use the grounding sheet. You can purchase the Earthing kit that allows you to string the wire outside your home through a small hole in your window or wall, and ground it to the earth using a metal rod. The Earthing company now markets several products available in different sizes and shapes so that you can "earth" or ground yourself practically anywhere as long as you're not moving. Go to www.earthing.com to view the different products available.

Earthing Naturally

The best way to earth is going outside and planting your bare feet on the ground. Walking barefoot, especially on the beach, is highly beneficial although I have to admit that this practice was highly discouraged in my household when I was growing up. My feet are pretty sensitive to rocks and prickly things, so I am just as likely to sit on my lawn chair on a beautiful day, plant my bare feet on the warm grass and read for hours. It is such a treat that I miss it during the winter months! For those of you who love going barefoot, now you have another reason to do it.

My patient Kaitlin is extremely sensitive. She can't stand going into shopping malls. The accumulated energy from a crowd of people coupled with the electromagnetic stress generated by security systems, computers and other electrical equipment leaves her anxious and exhausted. When I told her about Earthing, she realized that throughout her life, she had always loved sleeping on the ground. She loves to garden and will often just lie on the ground next to her flowers and nap. We both now realize that her sensitivity to everything can be transmuted through regular grounding.

The Benefits of Sleeping Grounded

When we sleep, are bodies are supposed to be restoring and rejuvenating. If you don't sleep well, you can't really heal. According to many experts, our energy fields are highly vulnerable to energy input while we are sleeping. Thus, if you have surrounded your bed with clock radios, cell phones or cordless phones, you are literally zapping your body with harmful energy as you sleep at night. I believe that the advent of wireless internet has created a whole generation of post-menopausal women with dysfunctional sleep cycles. Like I said before, if you don't sleep well, you can't really heal.

Being grounded at night while you sleep not only protects you to some degree from the negative influences of electrosmog; it allows your body to receive the beneficial electrons from the earth during a time of restoration and rejuvenation. There was an anecdotal case in the Earthing book that described an elderly man riddled with arthritis. He was practically bedridden, yet within a few weeks of sleeping on an Earthing bed sheet, he was able to get up and do things around the house. Months later, he had returned to functioning independently in society. In the Earthing book, you'll see thermal photographs of people with various pain conditions. Like with the LifeWave patches, the photos show that inflammation decreases dramatically after Earthing.

What I have found personally is that the Earthing sheet needs to be touching the painful body for optimal pain relief. Recovery bags have been used very successfully on athletes. Although more pricey than a half sheet, it envelopes almost your entire body. You can also purchase Earthing bands to go around your arms, legs or torso near painful areas of your body. Just remember to be careful not to trip on the wires if you get up in the middle of the night when the bands are on!

Earthing nightly is necessary to maintain pain relief and other benefits, such as improved sleep and hormonal regulation. The fitted bed sheets are of very high quality despite their conductive nature, and are perfect for both bed partners to Earth at night. They cost between $229 and $299 US. The half sheet, however, is perfect for single people or people who want a more affordable bed sheet. The cost is around $169, although most people choose the Earthing Premium Starter Kit for $199 that includes both a half sheet as well as a portable Earthing Universal Mat and outlet checker. I love using the Earthing Universal Mat while I work at the computer as I find that I feel pleasant energy flowing in my lower body when I have my bare feet on it. For people who use the computer a lot, I highly recommend investing in an Earthing Universal Mat.

Decreasing the stress response is another fantastic benefit of sleeping grounded. To take a look at what happens to stress hormones levels before and after sleeping grounded, you can go towww.KarenKan.com/earthsleep to see the color charts.

How to use the Earthing Sheet for Pain

Although I have found that the Earthing sheet relieves pain only when it is physically touching the painful body part, this is not the case for other people. Many people have the Earthing sheet just touching their bare legs at night while they sleep and they experience whole body pain relief. It is important not to have creams or lotions on your skin when you use the Earthing products as they may reduce the conductivity of the material. If I've used creams during the day, I'll take a damp, slightly soapy wash cloth and wipe myself down and dry myself off before lying on my Earthing sheet. The exception to this rule would be if you are using magnesium oil (see chapter on magnesium) since it isn't really oil, but a water-based solution of magnesium chloride salt (sea water) which would theoretically increase, rather than decrease, electrical conductance.

If you have more questions about how to properly use Earthing products, go to www.Earthing.com and click on the FAQs/Usage link.

Enhancing the Grounding Experience

Given my own sensitivity to electrosmog and geomagnetic earth activity (earthquakes, for example), I have found that Earthing works even better when I have enough minerals in my diet and I keep brain balanced during the day. When I've tested the Earthing Universal Mat in the office, I've documented that many people become brain balanced within thirty seconds of touching the mat. Unfortunately, once they are no longer touching the mat, their brain balance goes back to an unbalanced state. On my treatment table, I have an Earthing Universal Mat. Some patients have remarked that they feel calmer when they are touching the mat. Others have noticed that their feet don't get as cold while lying on the treatment table. A friend of mine who is a therapist notes that her patients are more open and relaxed when she works with them while they are "earthed".

When I have patients who come in who are not brain balanced, I will often stick a LifeWave Y-Age Aeon patch on their head. This ensures that they will benefit from their acupuncture treatments for a longer period of time. I highly recommend to all my patients that they sleep grounded at night and patch their heads during the day with the LifeWave Y-Age Aeon patches. This protocol seems to really amplify the improvements of using either product alone.

Grounding Shoes?

Granted, I'm not planning to walk around barefoot all the time, so I bought grounding flip flops for the summer. They are made of natural non-toxic rubber and have a grounding apparatus touching your foot at the Kidney 1 acupuncture point, one of the most important acupuncture points on the body. They are well-made, comfortable and sturdy. If you purchase a pair, just be careful to pick up your feet when you walk. Sometimes I drag my feet so once in a while the front of the shoe flips under and trips me.

Lately I've been wishing for an insole I can put in my shoe so I can feel grounded during the day when I'm indoors. I have a tendency to be sensitive to solar and lunar activity which indicates that I need more "earth" energy. Just recently, I found out about the VibesUP Divine Soles. These Divine Soles contain over 80 essential plant oils plus liquid crystal and gems including: Clear Quartz, Black Tourmaline, Rose Quartz, Amethyst, Blue Lace Agate, Moss Agate, Green Aventurine, Tigers eye, Rhodocrosite, Carnelian, Red Jasper, Banded Agate, Labradorite, Peridot, Smokey Quartz, Sunstone, Prenite, Dalmatian Jasper, Fancy Jasper, Selenite, Rutilated Quartz, Mookite, Lapis, Sodalite, Picture Jasper, and Obicular Jasper.

A friend of mine, who was in pain, put her feet on top of the Divine Soles and within minutes her pain diminished significantly. She then tried the LifeWave IceWave pain relief acupuncture patches on her feet using the whole body pain protocol which also diminished the pain. When used together with the insoles, she said her pain disappeared completely and that her whole body felt energetically solid and aligned.

Unlike the Earthing Universal Mat, which is plugged into your grounded electrical outlet, the Divine Soles are convenient in that they do not require any sort of wiring. It is likely that the spectrum of infra-red frequencies in the gems and oils will give you a different "grounded" feeling than being connected to the Earthing Universal Mat. Both are beneficial and the combination of sleeping earthed and walking around on Divine Soles is probably ideal. Keep in mind that the Divine Soles are thick enough that you may need to remove the original insoles in your shoes in order wear them comfortably. There are two versions: One is purple and the other is clear (for sandals). Both work similarly. You can find the Divine Soles at www.karenkan.com/vibesup.

Are there Side Effects to Grounding?

I can't really say there are many side effects to grounding, but there may be detoxification or healing reactions. A colleague of mine felt an uncomfortable feeling of energy shooting through her pelvis within minutes of touching an Earthing Universal Mat. Although she didn't feel this while walking barefoot outdoors, I couldn't explain why she reacted this way to the mat except possibly that it was "detoxifying" her body. What she did to acclimatize to the Earthing product was to sleep next to, but not touching, an Earthing sheet. Within a week, she was able to sleep with her body actually touching the sheet. My colleague is extremely energy sensitive. Gradually increasing her exposure to the "new" energy was the best approach.

Even in the Earthing book, it is recommended that people with chronic conditions may wish to gradually increase the amount of time Earthing in order to get used to the detoxifying effects. I would recommend that you ease slowly into using VibesUP Divine Soles as well. Energy therapies can be fairly potent. Anyone can enter a healing reactions with new therapies designed to help the body heal itself. Most reactions are mild and actually validate that the therapy is working. On occasion, however, more severe reactions require stopping or slowing down the therapy temporarily to let the body acclimatize.

Chapter Summary

- Earthing or grounding, especially while sleeping, is a fantastic way to manage chronic pain.
- Earthing decreases inflammation through decreasing the effects of free radicals.
- Earthing decreases the stress response and in some people helps to balance hormones.
- Earthing may actually help the body self-heal with continued daily use.
- The beneficial effects of Earthing are amplified when a person stays brain balanced and has enough dietary minerals.
- The beneficial effects of Earthing disappear if someone discontinues regular use of the Earthing products.
- The infra-red "earth" energy of the VibesUP Divine Soles may be helpful for you to feel more grounded while indoors during the day.

13

MAGNESIUM MIRACLES

As I was getting ready to write this chapter on magnesium, I got an urgent phone call from my mother. My father was dizzy, weak and nauseous. All he wanted to do was sleep, but my mother took his vitals. His blood pressure and pulse were dropping at an alarming rate. I told her to call 911 and luckily the heart attack was diagnosed by the cardiologist at the hospital. You have no idea how I wished that I could have been there, in the dire minutes and hours during and after the heart attack. Why? Because I would have doused my father in as much magnesium oil as he could stand. Magnesium is heart-saving in an acute heart attack. Many magnesium experts feel that it may even prevent heart attacks in certain people.

The Importance of Magnesium

So you might be wondering, what does magnesium have to do with chronic pain? Well, a lot. Magnesium, a mineral, is crucial for over 300 different biochemical reactions in the body. When depleted in the body, the health consequences are devastating. Magnesium is required to make ATP-the main source of energy for cells. If you are low on magnesium, you are low on energy, and all the body's processes become inefficient. Magnesium is also responsible for muscle relaxation, so if you suffer from stiff muscles, muscle spasms or trigger points, you likely have a magnesium deficiency. Magnesium is also important for proper nerve function.

In an earlier chapter, I mentioned the role of toxins in the development of chronic pain. Interestingly, magnesium is required for our cells to produce glutathione, a master antioxidant that helps us get rid of toxins. Thus magnesium is an important mineral necessary for detoxification and healing chronic pain. In the case of my father, the magnesium would have opened up his heart blood vessels and allowed more blood flow through his heart muscle, possibly preventing a full blown heart attack.

Have you ever had muscle spasms? They can be terribly painful. Most people assume that muscle spasms are "normal" if they've overworked their muscles. Muscle spasms are never normal. They are commonly caused by magnesium deficiency. Elite athletes who train very hard actually waste magnesium from their bodies, urinating excessive amounts of it, and thus become magnesium deficient despite a healthy diet. Muscle spasms can also be caused by potassium deficiency, and thanks to a scientific article I just read by magnesium expert Mildred Seelig, I now know that magnesium deficiency can cause potassium deficiency.

A study by Guy D. Abraham, MD showed a reversal of fibromyalgia pain and symptoms using 300-600 mg of magnesium and 1200-2400 mg of malic acid per day. Malic acid, an acid found in apples, is helpful for energy production. People with fibromyalgia not only have pain, they experience severe fatigue. Thus the combination of magnesium with malic acid has been found helpful in this particular chronic pain disorder. In my office, I actually use a combination magnesium-malic acid product made by Metagenics called Fibroplex. You can find it in health food stores under the commercial name, Ethical Nutrients Malic Magnesium.

How do you know if you're magnesium deficient? If you experience chronic pain, you probably are. If you'd like to see what your risk factors are, you might want to take the quiz at Ancient Minerals: http://www.ancient-minerals.com/magnesium-deficiency/need-more/.

Testing for Magnesium Deficiency

Traditional laboratory tests are inadequate to diagnose magnesium deficiency because they only measure the magnesium in the blood not in the cells. Your serum magnesium levels will rarely show an abnormality. Why? Because the body will steal magnesium from other parts of your body (even if you are deficient) in order to keep the serum magnesium levels in the normal range. If this didn't happen and your serum magnesium levels dropped, your heart might stop working! Thus the only people with "low" serum magnesium levels are people who are very sick, for example patients in intensive care. People who take multiple medications that cause magnesium deficiency are also at risk.

There are newer laboratory tests that can more accurately diagnose magnesium deficiency, but few are covered by insurance companies and most doctors don't know about them. Also, they are not widely available in all locales. Check out the Resources chapter for a link to these tests. Because laboratory testing is impractical, it is best to assume that you are probably magnesium deficient if you have significant risk factors.

Causes of Magnesium Deficiency

When I tell my patients they may be magnesium deficient, they often give me a blank stare. Reports published by the World Health Organization have estimated that three quarters of Americans do not meet the Recommended Daily Intake (RDI) of magnesium, yet the media hasn't educated the public about this fact, so it goes unnoticed. Half a century ago, the average daily intake was about 500 mg per day. Today it is about half that amount. Magnesium deficiency is a big problem especially in America. Most people are well aware of calcium deficiency so they often load up on calcium supplements to support their bone health. Doctors, like me, were taught in school that our patients should be taking up to 1500 mg of calcium per day to prevent osteoporosis. Sadly, we were never taught that magnesium, Vitamin D and Vitamin K are also needed to form healthy bone.

If one is consuming milk and other dairy products, calcium supplements can often exacerbate an already-existent magnesium deficiency. Calcification of soft tissues is arguably due to magnesium and/or Vitamin K deficiency; essentially, the body doesn't know what to do with the calcium it already has without proper magnesium and Vitamin K balance. Without sufficient magnesium, calcium can come out of solution and become solidified. Calcification of joints, arteries and tendons may not be due to just "overuse" or "aging" but the relative excess of calcium in the body. Worse than that for people with pain is the fact that calcium causes muscle contraction and magnesium causes muscle relaxation. Thus a relative excess of calcium may cause stiff, contracted muscles!

Why do you think that our diet is so low in magnesium these days? If you guessed "conventional farming" or the excessive processing of food, you are correct! In conventional farming where they grow monoculture produce, the soil is stripped of minerals and the fertilizers do not include the whole spectrum of minerals and micronutrients naturally found in nature. Conventional fertilizers make the fruits and vegetables grow very large, yet they are less nutritious than their organically grown counterparts. Magnesium is apparently one of the minerals most affected by the processing of food. If the majority of your meals come from boxes, bags, bottles, cans, or fast food restaurants, you're probably magnesium deficient.

Poor quality food contributes to excess acidity. This acidity then causes leaching of the body's stored minerals in order to buffer the pH of the blood. In other words, your body will steal magnesium from your bones in order to neutralize excessive acidity in your body caused by poor diet. Did you know that drinking soda puts you at a higher risk of developing osteoporosis?

There are other reasons besides poor nutrition that contributes to magnesium deficiency and thus pain in many people. One is stress. Magnesium is considered a natural stress reducer. Magnesium is used up during times of stress. The more stress you have, the more magnesium you require. And I'm not just talking about chronic emotional stress. Physical stress is equally important. Some of the elite athletes I work with have no idea that the intensity of their training can cause excessive magnesium losses through their urine. Not only do these athletes need more magnesium, they are depleting it at a faster rate than the average person! Yet, it is rare for me to meet a trainer or coach who tells their athletes that they need to take more magnesium.

One of the most common causes of magnesium deficiency I've noticed is pharmaceutical medications. Many medications deplete magnesium, including blood pressure reducers, anti-inflammatory steroids, birth control pills, hormone replacement, and diuretics ("fluid" pills). And just think, the more medications you take, the more you are at risk for magnesium deficiency. In addition to magnesium losses, many medications also promote nutritional deficiencies of other minerals and vitamins, particularly the B vitamins, Coenzyme Q-10, zinc and potassium.

How to Get More Magnesium

Eating whole nutritious foods is always a good strategy when it comes to healing anything, including chronic pain. According to USDA food charts (see link in Resources) the foods with the highest magnesium per typical serving are:

- Halibut
- Mackerel
- Boiled spinach
- Almonds

Foods with the highest magnesium per milligram, regardless of typical intake, are:

- Cocoa
- Almonds
- Cashews
- Pumpkin seeds

You may find that bran breakfast cereal is listed as having a lot of magnesium. Unfortunately, bran contains a lot of anti-nutrients that make the magnesium unavailable to the body, so I do not recommend it. Eating magnesium rich foods is a great start, but often it isn't enough for people in chronic pain. There exist several factors that can impair your ability to get magnesium from the foods you eat, including what we've mentioned before such as lowered magnesium availability in conventional food, excess stress and excess calcium. Dietary habits such as drinking sodas and carbonated beverages will also lower magnesium absorption from food.

If you have chronic pain, taking magnesium supplements is going to be crucial. If you have kidney disease, you may need to be more careful, so check with your doctor first. Oral magnesium comes in many forms. The type of magnesium that you'll find most commonly at the drug store is magnesium oxide. This form of magnesium is the least expensive. Clinical studies have shown, however, that only 4% of magnesium oxide is actually absorbed by the body-a very unimpressive amount. Nevertheless, studies using magnesium oxide have shown benefit. Magnesium oxide, although inexpensive, has a tendency to cause diarrhea more than any other form of oral magnesium, so I do not usually recommend it for my chronic pain patients unless they also suffer from constipation. I recommend magnesium amino acid chelates such as magnesium glycinate or taurate.

They are harder to find in drug stores but are available online, at the health food store or at a practitioner's office.

One day, one of my skating coaches woke up with a terrible crick in her neck. She could barely move or turn her head without excruciating pain. In addition to LifeWave patches, I recommended transdermal magnesium oil, a topical form of magnesium you can put right on the skin. She couldn't believe the difference in how she felt. Now, she is a big fan of transdermal magnesium and tells everyone to use it. She even uses it on her children's growing pains and she says it works like a charm. In the past, whenever I would recommend magnesium to my chronic pain patients, approximately half of them could not tolerate the oral form because it would cause diarrhea. Thanks to the research of Norm Shealy, MD on transdermal magnesium, I can now recommend a better-absorbed form of magnesium for chronic pain patients.

Chances are that you probably have never heard of magnesium lotion or magnesium oil. Because magnesium can cause diarrhea in some people, even if they are deficient in it, magnesium that can be absorbed through the skin has distinct advantages. In healing chronic pain, magnesium oil or lotion can be applied directly on the sites of pain, delivering the magnesium right to the painful muscle or joint without having to go through the digestive process. The Ancient Minerals brand of magnesium oil that I use is magnesium chloride from a pristine seawater source called Zechstein. It is devoid of impurities and toxins, so I feel very comfortable recommending it to patients.

Mark Sircus, O.M.D, who authored the book, Transdermal Magnesium, which was thoroughly eye-opening for me. In the book, he cites the many advantages of using transdermal magnesium, namely the ability to deliver magnesium ions directly into circulation via the skin. According to Dr. Sircus, oral forms of magnesium are beneficial as well, but require energy and enough chloride in the body for proper digestion and assimilation. Magnesium chloride bath salts used in a warm bath is an extremely relaxing and enjoyable experience. Epsom salts are a form of magnesium called magnesium sulfate. This form of magnesium can also be beneficial but it doesn't penetrate into the tissues as well as magnesium chloride.

Magnesium Dosing

For people experiencing chronic pain, especially if they have muscular pain or spasms, I'll recommend both transdermal magnesium as well as oral magnesium (if tolerated). Magnesium oil can feel stingy or itchy when you first use it so you may need to dilute it 50% with distilled water. Since magnesium relaxes the blood vessels, you'll often notice a warming sensation when you use it in areas of pain. I love this feeling.

Sometimes in the winter, I'll apply some magnesium oil or lotion to damp skin and then stand in front of the fireplace and use the heat to improve the penetration of the magnesium. Although its texture feels like oil, magnesium oil is just magnesium chloride in water. I usually tell my patients to start applying the oil to areas of pain once a day at first and then slowly work up to spraying it all over the body, sparing sensitive areas such as the nipples and genitals.

Dr. Carolyn Dean, author of Magnesium Miracle, recommends approximately 600 mg of transdermal magnesium. The Ancient Minerals brand of magnesium oil, which I exclusively use, contains 560 mg of elemental magnesium per teaspoon. Eight sprays equal approximately 100 mg of elemental magnesium or approximately 12.5 mg per spray. So if you spray eight sprays on each leg and arm, you're getting approximately 400 mg of elemental magnesium. If you add another eight sprays to the front and back of your torso, you'd get another 200 mg of elemental magnesium for a total of 600 mg. Transdermal magnesium takes about 30 minutes to penetrate the skin fully, so if it feels too itchy, you can always wash it off after that time.

Magnesium oil can sometimes make the skin feel dry during the winter months. The magnesium chloride is hygroscopic, meaning that it draws water to itself. Instead of using the oil, I will often use Ancient Minerals magnesium lotion instead. It does not contain methylparaben or other toxins that might be absorbed into the skin. The lotion isn't as potent as the oil, but it is generally well tolerated by most people, even children. One teaspoon contains approximately 185 mg of elemental magnesium which means that approximately 3 ¼ teaspoons per day on the skin should be adequate to give you 600 mg of elemental magnesium. The lotion isn't greasy at all and unlike the oil, doesn't feel as stingy or itchy. I will often use the lotion right after a hot shower in the morning and then apply magnesium oil to key areas in the evening before bed. If you're using a grounding bed sheet, however, you may wish to wash off the lotion before you go to bed. I don't bother washing off the oil because it isn't really oil and shouldn't disturb the conductivity of the grounding sheet. In fact, since it is actually made of sea water, it should be conductive.

The magnesium bath flakes are great for children and adults who love taking baths. Approximately one cup of Ancient Minerals bath flakes contains 15 grams (1500 mg) of elemental magnesium. Depending on the size of your tub, it is recommended to put between 1 to 3 cups (200 to 700 mL) of the bath flakes into warm water at approximately 108 degrees Fahrenheit (42 degrees Celsius). For more intense applications, you can put up to 8 pounds (3.6 kg) of magnesium bath flakes. I'll often use between 3 and 6 cups (700 to 1400 mL) in my large six foot soaking tub.

Since most people healing chronic pain require much greater amounts of magnesium to recover past losses, I'll often recommend taking oral magnesium in the form of magnesium glycinate or another magnesium amino acid chelate. Magnesium citrate is a relatively inexpensive form of magnesium easily found in pharmacies and health food stores. Although it causes more diarrhea than the chelates, it is a good option for many people. I use a simple muscle test to determine the ideal dose. Generally it is between 200 to 800 mg of magnesium per day in divided doses. Alternatively, you may wish to try subtle-energy enhanced ionic magnesium, which is arguably the most active and bioavailable form of magnesium on the market. I like Nutrilink Energy's Mag Force and use approximately one to three Tablespoons of this liquid at bedtime for people who dislike taking pills. Start with one capsule or tablet and then work your way up. If your bowels get too loose, then reduce the dose. If you have more frequent bowel movements, but they remain formed (log-like), then you don't have to change your dose.

The ideal number of daily bowel movements is about three to four a day-once in the morning and then after every meal. For many people this many bowel movements is a rarity. Most of my patients with chronic pain have only one daily bowel movement, and many are constipated. By taking magnesium orally, you not only help boost magnesium levels, you can relieve chronic constipation. When my chronic pain patients have healthier bowel function, they not only feel less pain, they often lose unwanted weight as well.

Dr. Dean recommends taking magnesium first thing in the morning and just before bed and somewhere late afternoon if you take a third dose because it is when we are most deficient. Most people feel relaxed when they take magnesium. Have a magnesium bath before bed and it might help you sleep. Rarely, and sometimes this happens to me, it can energize you, so you'll have to experiment to see what dosing time works best for you.

By using magnesium oil or lotion on painful areas and taking oral magnesium, you may notice an improvement in how your joints and muscles feel as soon as 48 hours. For some people who are severely deficient, it may take longer, but don't give up. It won't hurt you and will likely help you in the long run by energizing you, relaxing your muscles, improving sleep, and reducing stress. Here's an extra bonus. If you're using LifeWave patches, they will work even better when you have adequate amounts of magnesium in your body.

Chapter Summary

- Magnesium can help heal chronic pain by relaxing muscles, decreasing stress, increasing blood flow and improving energy and sleep.
- Without adequate magnesium, the body cannot detoxify efficiently; toxins contribute to chronic pain.
- Magnesium deficiency is common and is due to dietary factors, stress and modern food production and processing.
- Magnesium deficiency is difficult to diagnose using traditional blood tests and should be suspected if risk factors are present.
- More accurate magnesium tests are now available through specialized labs, but they are not usually covered by insurance nor are they widely available.
- Magnesium lotion or oil can be applied directly to painful areas to increase circulation and relax tense muscles.
- Magnesium supplementation, oral or transdermal, will help LifeWave patches work better to relieve pain and inflammation.

14

FOOD SENSITIVITIES AND PAIN

Lose the Grain, Lose the Pain

I can honestly tell you that a majority of patients who come to see me in the office are sensitive to gluten, a composite of proteins found in grains. These grains include barley, bulgur wheat, drum, einkorn, faro, graham, kamut, rye, semolina, spelt, triticale and whole wheat. Sensitivity to gluten causes inflammation in the body that can lead to all sorts of clinical problems including brain and nerve damage, diabetes, heart disease and intestinal leakage to name a few. Some experts like Dr. William Davies, cardiologist and author of the bestselling book, Wheat Belly, feel that the reasons so many of us are gluten sensitive is that the genetic code of wheat has been manipulated by man so drastically over such a short period of time that our bodies can't adapt.

The wheat that your grandparents used to bake their bread is genetically different from the wheat you currently buy at the grocery store. The gluten-content has increased dramatically over the last fifty years in particular because food manufacturers like the fluffy, elastic nature of high gluten-containing grains. Ancient species of wheat, such as Einkorn and Emmer, seem to be better tolerated, yet are not used commercially because they produce bread that is rather hard and dense. Furthermore, these grains are only available from specialty online stores.

Many experts feel that severe gluten intolerance can cause the destruction of the intestinal villi that are responsible for the proper absorption and assimilation of food. The end result is commonly known as Celiac Disease. The intestinal damage of Celiac disease may also lead to lactose intolerance and multiple food allergies. It is estimated that Celiac Disease affects approximately 1 in 133 people in the United States, yet fewer than 5% are diagnosed properly. In Europe, however, where the pharmaceutical industry doesn't have as much control over medical education, Celiac Disease is routinely diagnosed at a young age.

In the United States, most people suffer with various symptoms for well over a decade before being diagnosed, if at all. I remember that when I was in medical school, we thought of Celiac Disease as only affecting young children with diarrhea, abdominal pain and failure to thrive symptoms (weight loss). I didn't realize until recently that people don't have to have these symptoms in order to be diagnosed with Celiac Disease. In fact, many adults with Celiac Disease have constipation and weight gain.

Beyond Celiac Disease, there is a greater proportion of the population that is gluten-sensitive. It is easy to test for Celiac Disease today because we have blood tests that check for anti-bodies to gluten. Nonetheless, many people whose antibody tests are negative still have significant intolerances to gluten. More accurate testing for gluten sensitivity can be done via stool and saliva testing, but only two laboratories in the United States offer this testing and it may not be covered by health insurance companies.

ALCAT blood testing is another way to determine gluten sensitivity by observing the presence of an inflammatory reaction when your white blood cells are exposed to gluten. According to nutritionist and author, Shari Lieberman, in her book The Gluten Connection, if people used more accurate forms of gluten intolerance testing, such as stool and saliva, an estimated one third of the population would be diagnosed as gluten intolerant. That's a lot of people!

Thanks to some friends and colleagues who alerted me a few years ago to the possibility of gluten-intolerance in patients, I've begun to see great improvements in many of my chronic pain patients after they start a gluten-free diet. Now my motto is: if in doubt, stop gluten for a month and see how the pain responds. The most difficult aspect for people is that eating wheat is addictive. In the Wheat Belly book, Dr. Davis explains that once wheat is broken down and absorbed by our gut, a highly addictive component of wheat can attach itself to the opioid receptors in our brain (think morphine receptor). People can actually "get high" eating wheat, as if it were a drug, and can go through withdrawal once they stop. This is certainly the case with many people who simply crave wheat. Luckily the withdrawal symptoms of cravings and crankiness last usually no more than a week. I've found that if I can maintain brain balance in someone, he experiences fewer withdrawal symptoms. My patient Janice told me that when she eats wheat pasta, she can't stop eating, but when she eats rice pasta, she gets full very easily.

My significant other, James, was highly addicted to wheat. We didn't connect his flare-ups of joint pain and crankiness to wheat ingestion until I started noticing a pattern. Whenever we'd go out to eat and he'd order a gourmet sandwich, the next day he'd be in pain. He wasn't convinced about the gluten connection until he went without gluten for a solid week and then reintroduced it into his diet. The ensuing reactivation of massive joint and tendon pain convinced him to assiduously avoid eating gluten.

The other challenge with eating gluten-free is that the majority of processed food in America contains wheat or gluten, so unless you are on a strict whole food diet, which most of us aren't, you are at high risk of consuming some form of gluten. The obvious choices of crackers, cookies, cakes, bread, cereals and pasta are easily avoided. But things like ketchup, spices, sauces, cold cuts, soups, oatmeal and gravies often contain gluten or are processed in factories that also process gluten-containing products. The good news is that corporate America is realizing that many people are choosing to go gluten-free; so many companies are making an effort to sell products that do not contain gluten, such as gluten-free crackers, cake mixes, cereals, and snacks.

Please keep in mind that just because it says gluten-free on the package doesn't mean it is healthy for you. Processed food (food that comes in boxes, bags, cans, bottles, and jars etc.) are often devoid of nutrients and may have a lot of sugar, which can also contribute to inflammation in the long run. According to Dr. Davis, many commercial gluten free foods are made by replacing the wheat with cornstarch, rice starch, potato starch or tapioca starch which are gluten free but have a very high glycemic index and can cause weight gain and sugar dysregulation. Moreover, the cornstarch will often be made with genetically modified corn.

Taking wheat products out of a person's diet can be emotionally traumatic since eating wheat is seemingly culturally ingrained. I have to admit that it is a hard-sell in my office to convince my patients to cut out gluten. Many people naturally feel that as humans we've always eaten bread, so why should it be unhealthy? What they don't realize is that before the agricultural revolution, humans were actually taller and healthier and that eating grains is a relatively *recent* phenomenon in human history! Did you know that today's wheat has been mutated so much that it cannot survive in the wild? Wheat of today no longer resembles those tall golden stalks seen on cereal boxes. In fact, the stalks are much shorter (for better yield) and require plenty of fertilizers and pesticides in order to survive. The bottom line is that it is unnatural for our bodies to eat a lot of wheat.

Going Gluten-Free

Despite the growing body of evidence proving that eating grains like wheat is detrimental to our health, America's addiction to wheat is not going to end any time soon. There are wonderful books available on how to become gluten-free. Often people can tell a difference in their pain levels within one to four weeks of eliminating their gluten consumption. Not only that, it is common to lose between five and fifteen pounds in a month if you're overweight! Some people lose even more. I'm always amazed at how toxicity can cause unnatural weight gain in people.

If going gluten-free seems overwhelming, you can always start slowly by increasing your meat, fat, and vegetable intake and decreasing your grains. For example, you can forgo the morning toast and instead eat free-range organic eggs for breakfast. Your blood sugar levels won't yo-yo up and down as much, and you won't be consuming gluten. Unless you have an egg allergy, consuming pastured eggs for most people does not contribute to high cholesterol. Inflammation causes high cholesterol, not eggs or eating cholesterol alone. Toxic foods like wheat and sugar can cause inflammation which in turn causes high cholesterol. Don't be surprised if your cholesterol levels improve if you remove toxic food from your diet and replace it with whole foods. I'll discuss more about how nutrition can help your body heal in a later chapter.

Other Food Sensitivities

If you've gone gluten-free and nothing has changed with respect to your pain level, you may have other food intolerances or sensitivities. Food intolerances differ from food allergies in that the reaction is often not immediate. It can be delayed. It also does not cause hives, difficulty breathing or death, as would a true peanut allergy. The proteins in coffee tend to cross-react with gluten so many people who are gluten-free still have symptoms because they drink regular or decaf coffee. I'm not a big fan of coffee, so if in doubt, drink organic tea instead.

There are many reasons we often develop food intolerances, but some of the most common have to do with stress and inflammation of the gut (see Chapter on Healing the Gut). There are two ways I test for food sensitivities in my office. One is applied kinesiology. I can muscle test my patients with various foods and see if their energy system responds by blocking energy flow. When energy flow is blocked, the test muscle goes weak and it means the patient is intolerant to that food.

The other method is the ALCAT test. It is an objective blood test that quantifies the reaction of your white blood cells, the cells that are part of your immune system. Even if there is no allergic response, the white blood cells will respond with an inflammatory reaction when exposed to a food substance that you're intolerant to. By avoiding these foods and desensitizing yourself from them, and using a rotation diet, where you eat the same foods only one out of every four days, you can heal your inflammation and thus the underlying cause of your pain.

With the ALCAT test, you can check for intolerance to over 200 foods, molds, food additives and colorings, environmental chemicals, functional foods and even medicines. Gluten and wheat sensitivities are also tested in ALCAT and luckily, this test is available worldwide. Many health insurance companies cover this test, so it may be well worth doing if you're not getting better. For more information, go to www.ALCAT.com. Listen to the radio show interview I did with a functional medicine specialist who uses the ALCAT test in his practice to help people with chronic conditions.

Of the many possible foods a person can be sensitive to, the most common are wheat, dairy, eggs, soy, tree nuts, peanuts, shellfish and fish. I have found in my testing, that many people are developing sensitivity to corn. Jeffrey Smith, author of Seeds of Deception feels that this increasing sensitivity is due to the introduction of genetically modified corn into our diets which causes inflammation.

When it comes to pain, many Chinese medicine practitioners will ask their patients to eliminate dairy because it causes a condition of "dampness" in the joints. If you ask people suffering from arthritis whether the barometric pressure affects their joint pain, most will say yes. This is the manifestation of the Traditional Chinese diagnosis of excessive "dampness" in the body. Removing cow's milk and milk products such as cheese, ice cream, and yoghurt will often significantly reduce joint pain, as does removing sugary foods, which also cause "dampness".

If you're not willing to do testing to determine your food intolerances, it may be worth your while to remove at least sugar, wheat, dairy, and GMO foods (anything made with non-organic soy, corn, canola, sugar beets and cottonseed oil) from your diet for a month to see if your pain resolves. Alternatively, you can perform a desensitizing procedure for all possible intolerances to see if that helps. It's never a great idea to eat lots of wheat, sugar or dairy anyway, but at least if you are no longer intolerant to them, consuming them won't contribute to chronic pain.

Methods to Desensitize Yourself

If you're convinced you may have gluten intolerance or you've tested positive on the stool test, saliva test or ALCAT test, then you may wish to desensitize yourself. Although still considered obscure to mainstream medicine, NAET (Nambudripad's Allergy Elimination Technique) is a well-known method of desensitizing allergies and intolerances. This method was developed by an acupuncturist and it uses a blend of selective energy balancing, testing and treatment procedures from acupuncture/ acupressure, allopathy, chiropractic, nutritional, and kinesiological disciplines of medicine.

According to the NAET website, it is recommended to desensitize one allergen at a time although I know of colleagues who do more than one allergen at a time. Nevertheless, it can take upwards of twenty or more visits to desensitize someone from multiple allergens. The nice thing about the NAET procedure is that there aren't any fancy blood tests or stool tests to be undertaken to prove or disprove an allergy. The practitioner uses applied kinesiology (muscle testing) to determine intolerance and to confirm clearing of the same intolerance after the procedure is completed.

A business colleague of mine, Gretchen Uhe, learned the NAET process to clear her children of multiple allergens. She recently discovered, however, that she can accomplish the same desensitizing effect using acupuncture patches. When she told me about her discovery, I was intrigued because of my own issues with chronic constipation due to multiple food sensitivities. The procedure with the patches is simpler and easier than NAET and seems to be just as effective. With NAET the clearance of allergies lasts a lifetime for most people. Although this method pioneered by Gretchen Uhe is relatively new, it seems to also produce long lasting results in removing symptoms of intolerance.

Here's a disclaimer: NAET and the Uhe Method have not been rigorously studied using conventional scientific methods. Although the Uhe Method utilizes LifeWave acupuncture patches, the LifeWave company will not endorse this technique until adequate clinical studies have been undertaken. Furthermore, neither technique can claim that it "cures" allergies. However, my extensive personal research with patients has proven the latter's effectiveness in ameliorating allergic and intolerance symptoms. Compared with "allergy shots" offered by conventional medicine, the Uhe Method is faster and more effective. Since it is harmless to try these non-invasive methods to reduce the symptoms of allergy or intolerance, you might as well try them for non-life threatening conditions.

As of this writing, I am currently using the Uhe Method on as many people as possible, and I'm impressed by the results. My own personal results have been spectacular. I have successfully desensitized myself from gluten, corn, dairy, and soy. I'm finally having great bowel movements without having to take a slew of herbal and homeopathic remedies. A few days after doing the Uhe Method, I went to the movie theater and ate popcorn, which normally constipates me for days. I was delighted that there were no negative effects from it and I have continued to perform the Uhe Method on any new foods that I discover I'm sensitive to. The Uhe Desensitizing Method has made travelling and eating out easier for me and I'm very grateful for it.

My friend Shana is extremely sensitive to gluten. So are her two young children. Before using the Uhe Method, traveling was challenging because they had to bring all their own food. Eating in restaurants was out of the question, lest one of the children suffered an adverse reaction. After doing the Uhe Method, Shana was thrilled that she could "cheat" on her gluten-free diet and eat a whole slice of chocolate cake without any intolerance symptoms! Now her whole family can enjoy a restaurant meal when they are travelling without worrying about anyone getting sick.

To learn the Uhe Method you can take a one hour class. It is available online at www.UheMethod.com. If you think you're gluten intolerant or you'd like to desensitize yourself to possible gluten intolerance, I recommend you take the time to learn this method. You may need someone at home to test you "before" you do the Uhe Method so you can verify what you're sensitive to, and then "after" so you can make sure you're clear of the sensitivity. If you have any known sensitivities besides gluten or dairy, this technique can really help. For a more detailed sensitivity analysis, invest in an ALCAT test. It can give you a fairly accurate assessment of the substances you may be reacting to. The list can be surprisingly long for those of us who have had intestinal issues. In the chapter on healing the gut, it will make sense why some people stay in a chronic state of inflammation and why taking anti-inflammatory medications (NSAIDs) can make matters worse in the long run.

We've also discovered that many people can be desensitized to their environments including their bedroom, their cars, electromagnetic fields, and volatile organic chemicals (VOC's). Any of these sensitivities can contribute to chronic pain. My partner James went to work one day when pipes were being installed into the plumbing system of a new house. He said the smell was so awful that he felt nauseated and had to leave the room after just ten seconds of exposure. That night, we used the Uhe Method to desensitize him to the VOC's. The next day, he was able to work several hours in the same room without feeling bad. In fact, he took a huge whiff of the stuff just to test his tolerance. It must've been a funny sight to his co-worker! James was tickled pink that he was no longer sensitive to the chemical smell.

When allergies or intolerances are connected to past trapped emotions, they can be more challenging to clear. I've used the Emotion Code to assess whether there are any trapped emotions that need clearing in order to clear the allergic reaction. Often there is. If you have difficulty clearing your sensitivities using NAET or the Uhe Method, you may wish to try the Emotion Code as well. Often sugar and gluten sensitivities (as well as sugar addiction) are associated with trapped emotions. See Resources for links.

Determine Your Sensitivities

Before you do the Uhe Method, you'll want to determine what sensitivities you actually have. There are three ways you can determine your sensitivities.

The first two don't cost anything. The first way is to do an elimination diet. In an elimination diet, you eliminate the common allergens from your diet and eat strictly whole foods for a few weeks to clean your system. Then you slowly reintroduce the potential "allergens" one at a time, every four days or so, to determine whether or not you have reactions to them. Reactions can be varied so you have to pay attention to how your body feels. Upset stomach, diarrhea and constipation are pretty easy symptoms to spot, but skin rashes, brain fog, insomnia, pain, anxiety, or emotional irritability may also be sensitivity symptoms.

The second way you can determine what you're sensitive to is to learn basic muscle testing. Gretchen Uhe teaches this in her online class. It isn't hard but takes a bit of practice. I use it in the office almost daily because it is a quick way to tap into the body's own intuitive guidance system. When your body's energy field comes in contact with a substance that you're sensitive to, your energy flow becomes blocked and your muscle test will become weak. Alternatively, when your body's energy field comes into contact with a substance that you're not sensitive to, your muscle test will remain strong.

I've done this sort of testing with my patients to demonstrate the harmfulness of cell phones. First I do the muscle test when they are not holding the cell phone. I push down on their outstretched arm, and in a healthy individual, the arm tests strong. In muscle-testing vernacular, this muscle is now locked (strong). Then I have them hold the cell phone in one hand and repeat the muscle testing. Suddenly, their muscle weakens and their outstretched arm "unlocks". Some people are so surprised that they actually gasp. Try as they might to keep their outstretched arm strong, they cannot withstand the relatively light pressure I exert when I tell them to resist. Why? Because cell phone radiation is weakening their energy field. I love doing this demonstration on children and teenagers because it shows them that without a shadow of a doubt, cell phone radiation is harmful.

You can have some fun with this once you get some practice with muscle testing your friends and family members. Here's a caveat though. Both of you need to be well hydrated. Ideally, being brain balanced improves the accuracy of the muscle testing as well. If in doubt, place a LifeWave Y-Age Aeon patch behind the right ear on the mastoid bone (Triple Burner 17) on yourself and on the person you're testing.

Here is a simple guide of how you can use muscle testing to determine if someone is allergic or sensitive to something. If you are not sensitive to it, your arm will remain strong. If you are sensitive to it, your arm will go weak.

1. Hydrate yourself and the person you are testing.
2. Ask the subject to pick an arm he wishes to use for the testing. Ask if there are any shoulder injuries and avoid using the side that is injured.
3. Have the subject stretch out his arm in front of himself and lock the elbow. I find that people are stronger if they make a first with the thumb facing up towards the sky.
4. Stand to the side of the person being tested rather than in front of him or behind him. Place your fingertips gently over the person's outstretched wrist above the wrist bone. If the subject is young, weak or fragile, you can place your fingertips closer to the elbow, thereby decreasing the fulcrum.
5. Tell him that when you say "Resist", he is to resist your downward pressure, matching your pressure so that his arm remains locked in one position.
6. Gradually press down on the arm slowly increasing the pressure over the count of three. If the arm is strong, or locked, there will not be any "give". If the arm weakens or becomes unlocked, that means that his energy field is weakened or blocked. A normal response for everyone is that the arm remains locked when you're testing him in the clear, that is, without the test substance touching his body.
7. Once you've determined that the person you're testing has a normal locked muscle in the clear, have him hold the test substance next to his chest. Alternatively, you can ask him to say the allergen out loud, such as "wheat". Immediately retest. If he becomes unlocked, that means that he is sensitive to that substance. *NOTE:* do not use the actual test substance on someone with known severe life-threatening reactions to things like peanuts.
8. If you're not sure of the result, you can retest the person with and without the test substance. If he consistently unlocks when this

allergen is within his energy field, then that means he is sensitive to it.

9. You can repeat this testing with several different potential foods or environmental substances.

Tips for Muscle Testing

When first learning muscle testing, it is best to see if the person is testable. Ask him to say his name. For example, "My name is John". The muscle test should be locked. Then ask him to say a false name, such as, "My name is Bob". The muscle test should then become unlocked. Once you've determined that this works, then you can go ahead to muscle test various test substances.

The basic substances you'll want to test first are the ones listed below.

- Gluten or Wheat
- Salt (test table salt, sea salt, Celtic Sea Salt, Himalayan Crystal Salt)
- Legumes/Peanuts/Soy
- Sugar
- Tree Nuts
- Nightshade vegetables (eggplant, potatoes, peppers)
- Corn (test genetically modified and non GMO)
- Dairy (yogurt, ice cream, butter, milk, cheese)
- Artificial sweeteners (aspartame, neotame, sucralose, saccharin)
- Monosodium glutamate (autolyzed yeast extract, torula yeast)
- Food coloring
- Food preservatives
- Nitrites (found in processed food)
- Mushrooms
- Eggs
- Fish
- Shellfish
- Alcohol: red wine, white wine, hard liquor, beer
- Caffeine
- Coffee (decaf and regular)

• Cinnamon

Sometimes a person will have intolerance to conventionally grown corn, for example, but not have intolerance to organic corn. Because of this, feel free to experiment whether the organic or non-organic varieties make a difference to your body. Keep in mind that just because you might not have intolerance to MSG, it doesn't mean that it is healthy for you. It just means that your body doesn't react negatively to it.

Please note that if you don't have a sample of the substance with you, you can always try muscle testing using an energetic representation of the substance. For example, you can write the name of the substance down on a small card and have the subject hold the card next to his chest while muscle testing. Alternatively, you can have the subject say the name of the substance, such as "eggs".

Lastly, you can even have the subject say an entire sentence before muscle testing him, such as "Eating wheat is for my highest and greatest good". Please note that if you're using this sentence, the person will muscle test weak if he is sensitive to wheat. Once you've determined what you're sensitive to, you can use the Uhe Method to desensitize yourself. To learn this method, please go to www.UheMethod.com.

We've had several anecdotal stories from doctors who have used the Uhe Method to desensitize themselves from life-threatening allergic reactions. I do *not* recommend that anyone do this method with the offending allergen present and certainly not without the participation of a licensed medical doctor (with access to epinephrine) because of the risk of death.

How to Make the Desensitizing Last

After doing NAET or the Uhe Method, most people will become permanently desensitized if they do the following:

• Avoid eating too much sugary food and/or junk food
• Keep their bodies more alkaline and less acidic (see Chapter 18)
• Eat a whole food diet and decrease or eliminate processed foods
• Stay brain balanced

Having the actual substance next to your body when you do the Uhe Method is the most effective, especially when the substance comes in many different frequencies, such as gluten. There are hundreds of different types of gluten-containing flours. If you can't stand avoiding gluten entirely, at least you can desensitize yourself from the gluten-containing foods you absolutely love. If you don't love it, just forget about it. Gluten-containing carbohydrates aren't required for optimal nutrition.

Chapter Summary

- Wheat and wheat products are not easily tolerated by up to a third of Americans most likely due to the shifts in the genetic composition of the wheat over the last 50 years.
- Wheat can cause significant inflammation in the body leading to pain and other problems like high cholesterol.
- Dairy is the other common food that many people in chronic pain are sensitive to.
- Removing gluten/wheat products, as well as sugar and dairy, from your diet may resolve the underlying cause of pain.
- Stool, saliva and ALCAT testing may be helpful in determining specific food sensitivities such as gluten and dairy.
- Muscle testing is an inexpensive way you can determine food and other sensitivities. Although it takes practice, it is well worth learning.
- NAET, Uhe Method and Emotion Code are techniques to diminish or eliminate your symptoms of food sensitivity.

15

HEALING THROUGH HYDRATION

Hydration is one of most underrated natural treatments known. Proper cellular hydration means that the cells in your body can both absorb nutrients and expel cellular waste. If the cells are dry and shriveled, this healthy exchange doesn't occur and the body ages. Although it seems simple to follow the rule of drinking eight to ten glasses of water a day, or half an ounce of water per pound of body weight, many people who do are still dehydrated. While on a family cruise, I had my cellular hydration measured by a personal trainer using a bioimpedance machine. Despite my heavy consumption of water, I was still dehydrated. I suspect that the quality of the water aboard the cruise ship was vastly different from my purified well water that I have access to at home.

Apparently the type of water we are drinking has an effect on its ability to penetrate into our cells. One of my favorite health books of all time is Water & Salt, a truly beautiful book, written by German physician, Dr. Barbara Hendel. After reading this book, it finally made sense how important water is. Apparently it is a conduit of information and thus without proper hydration, cell signaling, and thus cell function is severely impaired. The type of water that our cells recognize as "healthy" is water that has maintained a crystalline structure. This type of water is also called structured water or may be referred to as revitalized water. Even though water is just chemically H_2O, there are vast differences in the structure of these H_2O molecules depending on where the water comes from.

Until I read Dr. Hendel's book, I had no idea that water flowing through 200 feet of straight metal pipe could become devitalized, which means that every single modern household is expressing devitalized water from the tap. Once devitalized, the water then becomes a foreign entity to the cells. To make matters worse, people assume that their water is "good" once they use a quality water filter or distiller to get rid of contaminants such as heavy metals, pesticides, herbicides, bacteria, fluoride, and chlorine disinfection by-products.

Unfortunately, getting rid of toxins from the water is only half the battle. The water left over from various methods of filtering and distilling still leaves the water devitalized and literally alien in structure from the water that our bodies crave. Just because you may have removed the pesticide residue from your water doesn't mean that the energy vibration of that pesticide residue is removed. This is probably the hardest concept for the average lay person to understand. Toxins can leave energetic footprints of where they have been, even though they have been mechanically removed.

Our cells respond negatively to the energy of a toxic chemical as well as to the toxic chemical itself. That is the reason why it would be highly beneficial to revitalize or restructure your water to its original pristine state. Think for a moment about how pure water looks as it's rushing down a mountain. Notice how the water never travels in a straight line? It is unnatural for it to do so. Water travels in spirals and curves. This spiraling action helps water retain its crystalline structure. There are ways in which you can restructure your water, but before we get to that, let me share with you some other things about the way we drink our water that affects its hydration potential.

Many of us switched from plastic reusable water bottles to stainless steel water bottles because of the toxins leaching from plastic. Some plastics are known to leach toxins called xenoestrogens which have hormone-disruptive effects on the body. Unfortunately water stored in stainless steel quickly loses its structure and becomes devitalized according to popular natural health expert David Wolfe. I don't know about you, but I have found that even my deep well water starts to taste funny when I use stainless steel water bottles. There is one exception, and that is a stainless steel water flask that has been programmed with scalar energy. I have only tried one, from a company called Fusion Excel. Even water from a public fountain tastes fairly good after being in the $110 Fusion Excel Quantum Flask.

I bought one for my mom and she carries it everywhere with her because she said that everything she puts in it, hot or cold, tastes good. As far as I know, it is the only such product that has its technology scientifically validated by Dr. Masaru Emoto himself, the scientist responsible for discovering that water's crystalline structure can be changed when exposed to negative or positive frequencies. I've dented mine several times by dropping it out of my purse or skating bag, but it still works. The most difficult challenge is purchasing an authenticated flask because there have been many "copycat" companies that sell facsimiles that don't work. Furthermore, as of this writing, the Fusion Excel company has gone out of business so they no longer provide authentication services if you buy a flask elsewhere.

If you don't have a water bottle or flask that can re-energize your water on-the-go, your best bet is to carry revitalized water in a glass water bottle. If crystal water bottles ever became practical, they would be the ideal choice! As for glass, there are several on the market that either come with a neoprene protective sleeve or have a protective outer shell to prevent breakage. A newer option: VibesUP created an "earth-nurtured" wrap that wraps around any size water bottle in order to protect it and infuse the water with infra-red earth energy. See Resources for links.

Distillation is supposedly one of the best methods of getting rid of fluoride in municipal tap water. Most people have grown up believing that fluoride in the water is good for our bones and teeth. Nothing could be further from the truth. Jeff Green is an activist in the movement to eliminate toxic fluoride from our water supply. This movement has been active for the past 15 years! Apparently, the declassified files of the Manhattan Project and the Atomic Energy Commission show that the original motivation for promoting fluoride and water fluoridation in the United States was to protect the bomb and aluminum industries from lawsuits from farmers. The farmers suffered massive losses in herd deaths and orchard destruction after the fluoride industrial waste was released into the environment.

Instead of paying large sums of money for proper disposal, a plan was formulated to market water fluoridation to the public and disperse the toxic waste throughout the country. The scheme worked and for the last fifty plus years, municipalities have been paying to have their water fluoridated. To make matters worse, the fluoride waste from the phosphate fertilizer industry is even more toxic (in the form of hydrofluorosilicic acid) and shockingly, it does not have to be filtered or purified prior to being shipped and dumped into municipal water supplies. Studies on the health effects and safety of fluoride have always used pharmaceutical grade fluoride-not the far more toxic hydrofluorosilicic acid from the phosphate fertilizer industry. In studies that have included hydrofluorosilicic acid, it was found that its use increases lead accumulation in blood up to seven times. It also increases lead absorption in bones and teeth. To learn more, see the Resources link of Jeff Green's interview with Dr. Mercola on YouTube.

I'm lucky in that I don't have to drink fluoridated water because I have well water, but remember what I said before? Even if you remove the fluoride through distillation, you still have dead water. Bottled water is no better, because most of it is filtered tap water. Not only that, distillation removes many health-giving minerals from water. It seems like a no-win situation doesn't it? But it doesn't' have to be. If you have a natural spring near your home, you may be in luck. The older the spring, the better the water, according to Dr. Hendel. Furthermore, unless there is a long straight pipe from the spring to the access point, the water will be naturally vortexed by the time you put it in a bottle.

Water Carries Energetic Information

So far, I think I've made it clear that regular tap water is probably not that healthy for you and clean spring or clean well water are better choices. What I haven't shared, however, is water's role as an information carrier. Vital water, i.e. structured water, has the ability to store information. Many energy medicine experts agree that the blueprint for all of the body's various processes resides in the energy field. This field of energy can be changed, tapped into and manipulated for healing purposes. Water acts as a communication super highway for energy and thus can be a conduit between the energy field and our cells. In the 1960's, scientist Bernard Grad did an experiment showing that a salt water solution that received "healing" by a healer was able to hasten plant growth instead of retard it as expected. Later studies showed that plain glasses of water that were held by psychotic patients in a psychiatric institution actually retarded plant growth. Thus, water is able to store energetic information.

How to Revitalize Your Water

There are many ways to revitalize your water. I'll share with you the ones I know, but keep in mind that there are many others. If you have municipal tap water, it is a good idea to first filter or distill your water to get rid of the contaminants. Once you revitalize your water, the negative energy left over from the contaminants will be neutralized.

Quantum StirWand

The Quantum Age StirWand is a pocket-sized device with which you can stir your water. What impressed me about this wand is that it increases hydration in the body by an average of 23.5% and it increases blood oxygen levels by 9.6% according to a study conducted by Fenestra Research Laboratory. Just stirring your water with this space-age looking device for 20 seconds revitalizes it. According to the website, the StirWand is a simple combination of specific granulated mineral stones encapsulated within a fountain pen-sized enclosure of medical grade polycarbonate plastic. Its primary function is to increase the hydration potential of water. There are several varieties of wands. Some are for daytime use and some for nighttime use. Others can be used 24/7. The advantage of the StirWand is its portability. The disadvantage is that you cannot easily stir water that is already in a water bottle without first pouring it out into a glass.

The StirWand will immediately change the taste of your water for the better. Just beware that if you use the StirWand on sweet or carbonated drinks, it will flatten it, so I don't recommend using it for this purpose. You may think that the change in taste is "psychological", but I have a funny wedding story to tell you about the StirWand. At my cousin Diana's wedding, as part of the bridal party, I was sitting at the head table. During a break in the festivities, I walked over to where James was sitting and noticed he wasn't there. I thought that it would be kind of me to revitalize the water in his glass, so I stirred it around for twenty seconds with the StirWand (much to the amusement of my brother-in-law!). A little while later James marched up to the head table and said to me "Honey, why did you StirWand my Sprite? It's FLAT!" Apparently, I had mistaken his glass of clear colored soda for water and the StirWand had completely changed the taste!

If you go out to eat a lot at restaurants, having a StirWand with you is particularly handy. StirWands have polycarbonate shells and are unbreakable when dropped. Each wand comes with its own polycarbonate case and costs approximately $90.

Willard Water®

Another great way to revitalize or restructure your water is adding Willard Catalyst Water. Decades ago, Dr. Willard, a chemist, discovered a way to make water wetter. During a complex and patented chemical process, the CAW micelle was created. It is an electrically charged colloidal particle that is the core ingredient in Willard Water®. This CAW micelle causes the formation of a catalyst that alters the structure of water. After you put ¾ of a teaspoon of Willard Water® into a bottle of water and shake the bottle vigorously, you'll notice that the bubbles formed are smaller and they last much longer than those found in a regular shaken bottle of water. I love doing this demonstration for my patients. It's almost as if the water has soap in it, but it doesn't.

The Willard Water® somehow acts as a surfactant, reducing the size of the clusters of water molecules. The new water structure easily penetrates into cells, thus bringing in nutrients and expelling out waste more effectively. According to their website, research has shown that subjects drinking Dr. Willard's Water® had little or no undigested nutrients in their urine or feces. That means that their bodies had absorbed far more of the vitamins and minerals needed to maintain optimal health. Willard Water® also seems to increase the pH of acidic water by up to two points, which may also help our bodies to self-heal.

I have a patient, Larry, who suffered from many different health challenges. He had big swollen legs and was on a high dose of a diuretic (water-releasing pill) medication. He was also told by his regular doctor that he needed to restrict drinking fluids. Larry "cheated" daily by drinking extra sips of fluid because he felt thirsty all the time. He hated not being able to drink whatever and whenever he wanted. The swelling in his legs indicated that fluid was accumulating outside of his cells instead of hydrating the cells themselves. The diuretic medication did nothing to prevent the leakage of fluid out of the cells and instead worsened the dehydration. As well, it depleted him of important minerals such as potassium and magnesium.

After seeing Larry for the first time in the office, I realized that the first order of business to jumpstart his healing was to rehydrate his shrunken cells. I sent him home with Willard Water®. Within a week, his swollen legs remarkably decreased in size and he felt less thirsty. Not surprisingly, some of his other symptoms, including back pain, seemed to ease as well.

Other benefits of Willard Water® include its antioxidant and free radical scavenging abilities. To use Willard Water®, just add ¼ to ½ teaspoon to 8 ounces of fluid, 1 ½ teaspoons to a quart of liquid, or 2 tablespoons (1 oz.) to a gallon of water. A sixteen ounce bottle of Willard Water® costs approximately $30. If you don't mind the brownish color, purchase the Willard Water® Ultimate to get some extra minerals in your body but follow the directions because the dosing is different. Most people prefer the clear Willard Water® for aesthetic reasons, but it is up to you.

Crystal Energy

Crystal Energy is a patented product by Phi Sciences. Like Willard Water®, it makes the water wetter so that nutrients can penetrate the cell and toxins can be removed. In addition, the nano-sized spheres of silica can trap heavy metals, making them easier for the body to remove. Although I haven't used Crystal Energy myself, David Wolfe uses it in all the water he drinks. There are many published studies on the Phi Sciences website, but I couldn't find any human clinical studies. Even so, given the molecular structure of Crystal Energy, it makes sense why it improves hydration. One drop of Crystal Energy revitalizes one ounce of water. A four ounce bottle of Crystal Energy costs around $45.

Crystal Stones

An inexpensive way to revitalize dead water is to immerse rough-cut crystal stones in a glass pitcher of water over night. Stones like quartz, amethyst, rose crystal, sodalite, calcite and fluorite can be purchased for $20 and can be reused over and over again. The difficulty in using this inexpensive method is that you can only revitalize one pitcher of water every eight hours. The second challenge is being extra careful not to break your glass pitcher as you empty it! The third challenge is that you must remember to wash your stones weekly and recharge your stones monthly as they will absorb negative energy and literally become "full". Clear quartz is said not to require recharging, but other stones do. Most people leave the stones outdoors for twenty four hours to allow them to absorb natural piezoelectric and solar frequencies. Because I broke one glass pitcher already, I decided to use other ways to revitalize my water.

Vortexing & Remineralization

Vortexing the water and adding minerals can help to revitalize the water. There are some machines with various magnetic or energetic devices that vortex the water for you. As I mentioned before, the water coming through your tap is devitalized because of the straight pipe it must travel through. Apparently just shaking your water bottle vigorously doesn't do enough to "hold" the water structure. Believe me, I've tried!

Recently, there are some products on the market that attach onto the piping in your home and can recreate the vortexing effect of natural falling water. One of these products is called the Vortex Water Revitalizer. According to the website, when your water flows through the Revitalizer, it passes through a double-spiral flow form inside it. This flow form creates a powerful vortexing action just like vortices found in nature. Through this vortexing action, the water is restructured on a molecular level, once again revitalized. The cost of a whole house Revitalizer ranges from about $400 to $1500 depending on the model, and carries a sixty-day money-back guarantee. Check out Resources for links. There are other similar products available and you can find them by searching the internet.

Water Charging Flasks & Water Bottles

As I mentioned before, I carry my Fusion Excel Quantum Flask with me everywhere I go. It is relatively expensive for a water bottle and unfortunately, as I stated before, there are many counterfeit flasks that look exactly the same and which are readily available for purchase online. It is important to get the original flask that has been validated by Dr.

Emoto's research. This flask includes with it a special card and code. Unfortunately, you can't validate your purchase any longer because the parent company went bankrupt in early 2012. That being said, it is likely that a new company may be formed in the future given the popularity of this technology in Asia.

VibesUP is an American company that claims that its products can shift substances such as food and water to resonate at higher vibrations. The handsome Earth on the Bottom water bottles contain essential oils, liquid crystal and 10 gemstones (also known for their therapeutic abilities) on the bottom to re-energize your water. The VibesUP formula has been approved for patenting in over 20 countries. One of the ways to verify that you have a product that works is by tasting the water before and after being placed in the flask or water bottle. If the taste has changed for the better, then you know you have the real deal. To learn more about VibesUP or its creator, Kaitlyn Keyt, listen to the radio show we did together. See Resources for the link.

The SourxeII

Another way to revitalize your water is a method I use almost daily. It uses a computer software program that can reportedly wipe clean the energetic memory of any container of water you choose, and then recharge it with the energy of positive intentions such as love, abundance, and health. This program is called The SourxeII. Because it seemed too good to be true, I personally interviewed energy healer and computer programmer Peter Schenk, the creator of this software. He was on my radio show, not once, but twice! After trying the SourxeII myself, I'm convinced it works.

Not only does my water taste more pleasant and "softer" after charging it, but also I've personally witnessed some miraculous intentions coming true in my life. Sadly, I have no scientific "evidence", like crystal pictures of before and after charging, to show you because they were unavailable at the time this chapter was written. For more information, check out the radio shows I did with Peter Schenk in Resources. After you do your own research, you can decide for yourself whether you'd like to try this software. The software retails for $197 and carries a thirty day money-back guarantee.

Mineralizing Your Water

Many health gurus suggest putting a pinch of Himalayan Crystal salt in filtered or distilled water, to replenish the minerals removed in the purification process. A study conducted at the University of Graz in Austria found that people who drank water containing Himalayan crystal salt daily experienced improvement in respiratory conditions, organ functions, and connective tissues. Participants also reported sleeping better and having more energy. The study noted a boost in the ability to achieve higher levels of concentration. Some of the study participants stated they lost unwanted weight while others involved in the study showed enhanced hair and nail growth. The Himalayan Crystal salt used in studies written about in Dr. Hendel's book, Water & Salt, contains 84 minerals and trace elements, which are thought to be extremely beneficial to the body.

Unlike pure Himalayan Crystal salt, most commercial sea salt is stripped of its minerals during the purification process. Himalayan Crystal salt does not require purification because it is from a source not exposed to sea pollution as sea salt is. Unrefined Celtic sea salt, unlike most sea salt sold in stores, is gray/brown in color and clearly contains lots of minerals. Unfortunately, I could not find any clinical studies on the direct health benefits of ingesting Celtic Sea salt versus the studies available for Himalayan Crystal salt. However, there is plenty of evidence pointing to poorer health outcomes when people restrict their salt intake, according to health expert Dr. David Brownstein in his book, Salt Your Way to Health.

Lowering salt intake does not seem to help most people with high blood pressure, but we do know that mineral deficiencies make it worse. If you have been told to limit your salt intake due to high blood pressure, Dr. Brownstein recommends that you avoid regular table salt as much as possible, as it can harm your health. On the other hand, consider trying small amounts of Himalayan Crystal salt to see if it affects your blood pressure one way or the other. There are other ways to get your required daily minerals, as I'll discuss in a later chapter, but a pinch of Himalayan Crystal salt will help "hold" the energetic vitality of water.

The Future of Water

It won't be long when the general public, sick of succumbing to chronic diseases and pain, realizes that the daily tap water they drink is so contaminated and "dead" that they'll willingly pay for alternative solutions to revitalize their water. However, that day has not yet arrived. You, on the other hand, are ahead of the crowd by picking up this book and reading it. Now you know that the quality of water you put into your body is not just about "hydration" alone, but about the energy fields that govern all body processes that rely on a good carrier of information. I'm sure that I will have more to share on the latest cutting edge technology to revitalize water as time goes on. If you've signed up for my Book Bonuses, I'll keep you up to date on what I discover.

Check out the Resource chapter for links to some of the products I've listed in this chapter.

Chapter Summary

- Hydration is crucial to healing, allowing nutrients to flow into the cells and waste products to flow out.
- Water has the ability to store energy or information and thus plays an important role in the communication system of our bodies.
- Water from the tap or purchased in a bottle is often dead water and needs to be revitalized in order for your body's cells to become hydrated properly.
- Energy imprints of toxins stay in the water long after you've removed the toxin unless the water is revitalized.
- There are many ways to revitalize your water, some more expensive than others.
- Adding a pinch of Himalayan Crystal salt to your water may help to hold the vibration of revitalized water and replace minerals lost in the water purification process.

16

HEAL THE GUT

Leaky Gut and Pain

Shortly after Christmas, I got an urgent phone call from my mother. She had only a few days before leaving on a three-week cruise with my father. She told me on the phone that she had suddenly felt a shooting pain in her buttock and leg after twisting to pick up something. It was sciatica, and she remembered my dad having something similar happen to him years ago. Nothing like this had happened to her before and she didn't have a history of herniated discs. She was in agony, barely able to get in and out of bed. She called me to ask what she should do.

One of the things James, my partner, reminded me to ask her was how many wheat products had she eaten in the days prior to her sudden "sciatica". Since it was the Christmas holidays, my mother's friend had apparently baked a scrumptious coffee cake for her. My mother devoured several delicious pieces over two days. Rarely does my mother eat cake, but this was an exception. I only had a few days to get my mother functional before her trip, otherwise she would have to cancel it.

The first thing I told my mom was to abstain from eating anything made with wheat. Given that I was highly sensitive to gluten, I suspected she was as well. I asked her to sleep on the Earthing bed sheet at night with it touching her lower back and hip. I also started her on magnesium citrate (the type she could find easily at the drugstore). I taught her how to use the LifeWave Y-Age Aeon patch and IceWave pain patches on her pain, and within a few days she had remarkably recovered. She started the cruise in a wheelchair, just to be on the safe side, but not long after, she was making waves on the dance floor. Other people on the cruise couldn't believe what a miracle "healing" my mom experienced, and some even thought she was pretending to be disabled just to get special treatment!

I can't tell you how many times I've seen patients in my office with acute low back pain whose pain symptoms were brought on by their consumption of gluten or sugar. Gluten-sensitive people, about a third of the population, have what is commonly called "leaky gut" whereby the lining of the intestines become so inflamed over years of ingesting gluten, that they literally become extra permeable. Think of the gut wall becoming like a sieve. Not a pretty picture right? Imagine partially digested liquid intestinal contents leaking out into the pelvis causing inflammation of nearby organs and structures like bones, nerves and fascia.

Many people have indigestion, bloating, diarrhea or constipation and have no idea that their condition is literally causing their chronic pain. And it's not just low back pain. Inflammatory substances can penetrate the blood vessels and lymph and can literally inflame other organs and joints throughout the body . . . even the brain. Leaky Gut Syndrome is rampant and finally conventional medicine is beginning to recognize its significance in chronic immune problems.

Healing Leaky Gut Syndrome will not only help heal chronic pain, but will help heal any chronic disease you may also suffer from. Most people would agree that the immune system is pretty important, wouldn't they? Well, did you know that over 70% of immune system cells actually reside in the intestines? In acupuncture school we were taught that "dampness" in the body predisposes people to all sorts of chronic health problems. A common symptom of dampness is nasal congestion and allergies. At first I didn't understand how "dampness" in the abdomen could be connected to nasal symptoms, but after learning about Leaky Gut Syndrome, it all began to make sense.

Immune System & Pain

I'm now going to explain as simply as I can how your intestinal health is related to chronic pain. The immune system has checks and balances so that foreign invaders get quickly destroyed and removed, yet your own normal cells are left alone to thrive. The cells of the immune system are ever on the alert for foreign invaders. When it senses a foreign molecule (not "self"), the immune system gets into "full combat mode" to aggressively get rid of the invader. Protein molecules are pretty big so when you ingest food and fluids, the protein is broken down into smaller components. Assuming you have healthy digestive function, you shouldn't respond to food as allergens unless you have a genetic predisposition. Foreign invaders such as parasites, viruses and bacteria are also pretty big and the immune system normally recognizes them quickly (by reading the proteins they have on their cells) and gets rid of them.

Chronic inflammation in the intestines can be caused by repeated exposure to foods such as gluten (in gluten-sensitive individuals), sugar, genetically modified foods and food additives. Antibiotics and other drugs like birth control pills can also upset the natural balance of the intestines. Antibiotics are known for destroying the population of healthy organisms found in the intestines, also called gut flora. I explain to my patients that healthy gut flora is like having a large army of soldiers protecting the gut wall, ready to destroy invaders, such as rogue bacteria, before they have a chance to do any damage. They are an important part of the immune system. Prescription and non-prescription medications, poor eating habits, and stress can wipe out this army and leave the intestinal wall susceptible to damage. As you can imagine, stress makes any unhealthy situation even worse.

Without protection, the walls of the intestines develop "leakiness". When this happens, partially digested food and other proteins can leak into the bloodstream where they aren't supposed to be. The interior of the body isn't used to these proteins and immediately recognizes them as foreign invaders, mounting a full scale inflammatory immune response. Here's the problem: some of these partially digested proteins resemble components of our own cells! Remember, these large proteins weren't supposed to get absorbed into the body before being fully digested in the first place. The immune system then not only begins creating an immune response to the leaky gut components but also to our own tissues. In the integrative medicine world, leaky gut is considered to be a major cause of or contributor to autoimmune diseases. There isn't a patient that I've treated with an autoimmune disease who does not also have some form of Leaky Gut Syndrome.

Even if you do not have a full-blown autoimmune disease like Lupus, Multiple Sclerosis or Celiac Disease, you may suffer from allergies. Chronic nasal congestion from allergies is just a symptom of the immune system working overtime against something it considers foreign to the body. A healthy gut will prevent many airborne allergens from entering the body and causing the immune system to overreact.

However, in the case of Leaky Gut Syndrome, all sorts of allergens can penetrate into the interior of the body and set off a full scale allergic or autoimmune reaction. Leaky gut is likely the cause of many food allergies as well.

So how do Leaky Gut Syndrome and its sequelae cause chronic pain? As you've learned in earlier chapters, chronic inflammation underlies most chronic pain as well as most chronic diseases. Having your immune system work overtime against what it considers to be foreign invaders due to leaky gut causes widespread inflammation through the entire body. In the process of getting rid of foreign invaders, the immune system creates an inflammatory reaction. This inflammation is actually healthy if it is indeed fighting a true invader such as a flu virus, but it is supposed to be short-lived. Unfortunately in the case of Leaky Gut Syndrome, the inflammation continues until the gut is healed and the balance of gut flora is restored. This chronic inflammation can cause pain that you just can't get rid of easily. Also, it is felt that this inflammation can literally damage our joints and tighten our muscles.

Four Vicious Cycles

Allergies are the first in the vicious cycles that people with leaky gut have to contend with. As I described above, the immune system just isn't used to dealing with an onslaught of foreign proteins that normally would stay within the confines of the intestines. The second vicious cycle that is set up with Leaky Gut Syndrome is malnutrition. Elizabeth Lipski PhD, in her book Digestive Wellness describes the primary cause of mal-absorption with a leaky gut: The small intestinal villi become inflamed and thus prevent small nutrients and food molecules from being absorbed. Villi are small fingerlike projections in the small intestine. Villi have a large surface area to absorb nutrients. When they are destroyed, not only are nutrients not properly absorbed, but also the gut fluid leaks between the cells of the intestines before being processed.

Nutrients are supposed to be taken in through the intestinal cells themselves. It seems that the leakier the intestinal wall, the less nutrition is absorbed by the intestinal cells. Without proper nutrients, not only do other parts of the body have difficulty healing but so does the metabolically-demanding intestinal wall itself. A symptom of nutritional deprivation is overeating. Most of the obese people in America are malnourished. They may eat a lot, but either the quality of what they eat is poor or they just aren't absorbing nutrients effectively.

The third vicious cycle in leaky gut is the overgrowth of "bad" bacteria, yeast, fungus and parasites in the intestines. In Digestive Wellness, Dr. Lipski discusses bacteria translocation, whereby "bad" bacteria normally associated with the intestines make their way into the bloodstream through the leaky gut and colonize other parts of the body causing inflammation and pain. Blastocystis hominis, a bacterium that causes GI problems, has been found in the synovial fluid of arthritic patients. This condition is called dysbiosis. Without the "army" of healthy gut flora protecting it, the moist warm environment of the intestines can harbor all sorts of foreign invaders that cause chronic disease.

Sometimes I can easily tell if someone has an imbalance of intestinal organisms by asking one question: "Do you have sugar cravings?" Often, if not always, my patients with uncontrollable sugar cravings have intestinal dysbiosis. The overgrowth of yeast, such as Candida, love to be fed a diet of easily digestible energy, so they'll literally signal the body to crave sugar. My patients often feel guilty when they can't stop eating sugar, but when I explain to them that it is the extra five to seven pounds of dysbiotic organisms living in their gut which are making them crave sugar; they have an easier time letting go of their guilt. Also, when they feel like reaching for a candy bar, they think twice about feeding the opportunistic organisms growing in their bellies.

The fourth vicious cycle of having Leaky Gut Syndrome is stress on the organs of detoxification, specifically the liver. The liver is often overworked trying to get rid of toxic molecules. In the process, the liver creates free radicals which in turn get released into the bile and this damages the gut further. When your liver is sluggish, you feel sluggish. You may also have poor skin health, chronic pain and low energy.

Do You Have Leaky Gut?

There are many risk factors for having greater intestinal permeability, i.e. leaky gut. Check the list below and see how many risk factors you may have:

- ☐ You've taken or are currently taking non-steroidal anti-inflammatory drugs (NSAIDs) such as ibuprofen, naproxen, aspirin etc.
- ☐ You have been on antibiotics in the past.
- ☐ You've taken or are currently taking drugs for acid reflux (GERD) such as omeprazole or ranitidine.
- ☐ You've taken or are currently taking drugs to lower cholesterol.
- ☐ You've taken or are currently taking steroids such as prednisone.
- ☐ You've taken or are currently taking oral contraceptive pills.
- ☐ You eat quite a bit of grain, including wheat (gluten) and corn (genetically modified).
- ☐ You are addicted to sugar or carbohydrates (not including fruits and vegetables).
- ☐ You consume acidic beverages such as coffee and soda.
- ☐ You eat processed food on a regular basis.
- ☐ You have or have had lots of stress in your life.
- ☐ You don't get enough sleep.
- ☐ You eat while driving, working or watching television.
- ☐ You are a vegan who eats grains, but no fish, eggs, or animal protein.

There are many symptoms associated with leaky gut and the list is rather exhaustive. You can view this list online at http://www.leakygut.co.uk/symptoms.htm. Here is a partial list of symptoms:

Intestinal Symptoms:

- • Abdominal pain (chronic)
- • Abdominal Bloating
- • Indigestion

- Excessive flatulence
- Constipation (hard or infrequent stool)
- Heartburn
- Diarrhea
- Gluten intolerance (celiac disease)
- Anxiety or depression
- Chronic fatigue
- Seeing undigested food in your stool

Non-Intestinal Symptoms:

- Insomnia
- Malnutrition
- Migraines
- Muscle cramps
- Multiple chemical sensitivities
- Muscle or join pain
- Myofascial pain
- Mood swings
- Poor immunity
- Recurrent vaginal infections
- Recurrent skin rashes
- Brittle nails
- Hair loss
- Swollen lymph glands
- Food allergies/sensitivities
- Brain "fog"

There are a couple of different laboratory tests for Leaky Gut Syndrome that you can ask for if you really want hard proof. That being said, I don't often order the tests for two reasons. Firstly, I can usually diagnose leaky gut through my patient's history. The grand majority of my patients with chronic pain have some degree of gut dysfunction, so I usually just proceed with treatment. Secondly, my patients are concerned that their health insurance may or may not cover the cost of the testing. If you really want to know and if you have an open-minded gastroenterologist or family doctor in your area, you may want to ask her if she could test you. Here are two different kinds of tests you can do. Keep in mind that not all laboratories are allowed to test patients from all 52 states, so you'll have to contact the lab to find out.

Leaky Gut Test # 1—Intestinal Permeability Test

This is the simpler of the two lab tests. This test requires that the client consume a mixture of two sugars (Lactulose and Mannitol). A urine sample is then collected and examined to determine the sugars your gut absorbed. In a healthy gut, Mannitol is easily absorbed whereas Lactulose is only slightly absorbed. If you have leaky gut (i.e. increased intestinal permeability) the Lactulose is easily absorbed through the large leaking gap junctions of the intestinal wall and it shows up in the urine.

This test can be ordered from Genova Diagnostics:
www.genovadiagnostics.com

Leaky Gut Test # 2—Intestinal Barrier Function Test

This is the more comprehensive of the two tests. Through a saliva sample, it assesses the level of secretory immunoglobulin A (sIgA) and the levels of free IgA and IgM (antibodies) your body is making against combined dietary proteins (wheat/gliadin, corn, soy, cow's milk, egg); aerobic bacteria (Escherichia coli and E. enterococcus); anaerobic bacteria (Bacteroides fragilis and Clostridium perfringens); Candida albicans yeast. The levels of the measured antibodies determine what stage of leaky gut development you are currently in.

I know that was a lot of big words, but basically this test checks your immune system for antibodies against dietary proteins, and can give you a feel for what foods you're currently reacting to (thanks to your leaky gut). If you avoid the foods that are giving you trouble while you heal your gut, your path to pain relief will be much faster.

The test can be ordered at Biohealth Diagnostics:
www.intestinalbarriertest.com

Strategies to Heal the Gut

Even if you don't think you have full blown Leaky Gut Syndrome, I bet you that you have at least some degree of intestinal dysfunction. Why? Because you are in chronic pain. Remember how important brain balance and the nervous system are in the healing response? Well, the intestines happen to have their own nervous system! It is called the enteric nervous system and it houses 100 million nerves. So if the gut is out of balance, your nervous system is out of balance too. Below are the main strategies to get this "second brain" back into balance so that you can heal your chronic pain from the inside out.

Strategy 1: Brain Balance

I probably sound like a broken record, but I'm going to say it again. Make sure you are brain balanced. Without balancing your nervous system, your other efforts will be wasted. If you haven't read the chapter on brain balancing, please do that now.

Strategy 2: Hydrate

Drink at least ½ your body weight in ounces of water throughout the day and decrease your dependency on dehydrating fluids such as caffeinated beverages. In overweight adults, that amount might be too much unless you are also taking diuretic medications or drinking caffeinated beverages. For most healthy adults, the right amount is about 2 Liters per day or about ½ a gallon. Drinking revitalized water will help the water and nutrients enter the cells and let toxins escape out of the cells.

Strategy 3: Optimize Nutrition

Eat nutritious whole foods and minimize processed foods that typically come in cans, bags, bottles, and boxes. Whole foods such as fresh fruits and vegetables, local meat, fowl and eggs, fish, seafood are ideal. Grains, like wheat, have less nutritional content than other whole foods and can contribute to leaky gut, so I don't recommend them. I know the USDA food pyramid endorses whole grains but you actually don't need them. It has been definitively shown in anthropological fossil records that hunter-gatherer humans were taller, healthier and had perfect teeth, until the agricultural revolution began.

The Paleolithic diet is a whole food diet based on the diet of our healthier ancestors who ate lean meat, healthy oils, vegetables, fruits, nuts and seeds. Grains, dairy and sugar are very recent additions to our original ancestral diet. According to researcher, Loren Cordain, PhD, who has spent the better part of his life researching the Paleolithic diet, the introduction of grains and dairy into our diets caused shortened stature, poorer dentition and the onset of chronic diseases in our society. You don't have to give up grains completely, but if you do eat grains, I'd recommend sprouted organic grains. The sprouting process eliminates the "anti-nutrients" naturally found in grain and makes the grain more digestible and more nutritious for the body.

If you have a lot of abdominal symptoms, it may be prudent to go "grain-free", not just gluten-free. You see, if the walls of the small intestine are damaged, the villi get squashed. A great visual aid is imagining your intestines going from shag carpeting to linoleum flooring. When these villi get destroyed, you then become unable to digest disaccharides. Disaccharides are sugar molecules in sets of two. Glucose is a single sugar molecule, called a monosaccharide, and is easy to digest so it does not need to be broken down any further in the intestinal villi. Many grain products, including rice, end up as disaccharides in your small intestines. For example, even though rice is gluten-free, some people can continue to have problems with their intestines when they eat it. Often these people have inflammatory bowel disease (IBD) like Crohns, a serious health condition that sometime requires hospitalization or surgery in its late stages.

Dairy foods such as yoghurt, cheese, milk and ice cream cause "dampness" in the intestines in many people so I would avoid these as well. Do not eat dairy if you're constipated. Also, there is some debate over whether pasteurization and homogenization of commercial dairy products cause detrimental changes in their nutritional content.

Raw milk enthusiasts will argue that much of the Vitamin C and iodine are destroyed in the pasteurization process and that the calcium in milk becomes less soluble, leading to problems with digestion and assimilation. They also argue that fresh, raw milk from a local farm is much more healthful and does not increase the risk of food-borne infection. Although I do not eat much dairy because I have found it causes weight gain in my body, I haven't had the benefit of raw milk. Those who I know who culture raw milk into healthy yoghurt, whey and kefir, swear by its healing properties. After seeing what raw and pasteurized milk look like under the microscope, it is clear that the two are not the "same" as government food agencies would have us assume.

Soy has been all the rage in America, especially among vegans and vegetarians. It appears in all sorts of processed foods. Unfortunately, most if not all of the soy found in America is genetically modified. GMO's have been found to be harmful in laboratory studies and sadly, the scientists who have reported these findings have been ostracized and their reputations tarnished because of the negative impact of their findings on corporate interests. Furthermore, soy and other legumes such as beans and lentils contain anti-nutrients that make the nutrients in them less available to the human body.

I'm sure vegetarians aren't going to be very happy with me for saying this, but I'm not a proponent of a vegetarian diet that consists mostly of grains and legumes. Vegans, who don't eat fish, eggs or dairy, tend to have nutrient deficiencies, the most common of which is Vitamin B12, a vitamin that is plentiful in eggs, dairy and meat (including seafood). There is a misconception that in Asian countries, soy consumption is large, but the truth is that soy is consumed as a condiment and mostly in its unprocessed and fermented form. The exception would be vegetarian Buddhist monks who eat soy instead of meat thereby decreasing their testosterone levels. Because of the food processing industry, Americans consume far more soy than their Asian counterparts and this is worrisome.

You can't go wrong by increasing your intake of whole fresh fruits and vegetables. Quick frozen vegetables can contain more vitamins than fresh vegetables that have had to travel thousands of miles before they end up in your grocery aisle. Ideally organic and/or locally grown produce is best because we don't want to add more toxins to your body in the form of pesticides and herbicides. In Northern climates, eating fresh local produce may be challenging, but during the summer months, local farmers' markets are the best place to get good quality food, including meat.

Eating raw foods is becoming increasing popular as a healthy way to eat. A dentist in the 1930's, Weston A. Price, went on a journey to research what factors determined good dental health. He travelled to remote areas of the world, untouched by Western civilization and made the astonishing discovery that bad dentition is a result of nutrient deficiencies rather than a result of genetics. In the remote tribes he researched, Dr. Price analyzed the foods eaten by their society as compared to those eaten by modern American society.

He found that, in comparison to the American diet of his day, their diet provided at least four times the water-soluble vitamins, minerals including calcium, and at least ten times the fat-soluble vitamins, from animal foods such as butter, fish eggs, shellfish, organ meats, eggs and animal fats. All of the indigenous tribes he studied cooked their food, but they also ate a portion of their food raw. Seeds, grains and nuts were soaked, fermented or sprouted to remove anti-nutrients before being consumed raw. Grains that contained gluten were always soaked or fermented and often baked into sourdough breads or cooked as breakfast porridges.

The people of these indigenous cultures were the picture of health. They had wide dental arches and they were devoid of dental caries. They had fine bodies that did not suffer from the chronic diseases we suffer from in Western society. In the tribes that consumed dairy, it was always unprocessed and raw.

Raw food is not a popular prescription in Chinese medicine. It is felt in Chinese medicine that if there isn't enough "fire" or energy in the digestive system, eating raw food would be stressful and the patient would suffer from digestive complaints like diarrhea, abdominal pain and bloating. I remember my grandmother balking at the thought of eating raw salad when she first visited us in Canada during my childhood.

If you're wondering whether eating mostly raw or cooked is best for you, I recommend that you try both and see what feels the best. If raw food like salad or fruit gives you an inordinate amount of gas, intestinal discomfort or diarrhea, then you may have to hold off on eating it, especially in the colder climates, until your digestive system becomes stronger. Alternatively, adding some digestive enzymes in the form of a supplement may be helpful. You should never see chunks of undigested food in your stool if you're chewing properly and you are digesting properly.

Ginger is used in Chinese medicine to increase the digestive "fire" of the stomach to encourage good digestion, so if you like ginger, cook with it more often or add it to your juice if you're juicing. In the past, I wasn't able to tolerate salad, but lately I've been craving it. I'm happy to report that my intestines have healed to the point that I can now eat most raw vegetables and salads without a problem. Sushi is something that I've never had a problem digesting, so I often purchase low-mercury fish via mail order from Vital Choice Seafood. When I eat raw nuts and seeds, I try to eat organic varieties that have been properly soaked, sprouted and dried to remove the anti-nutrients, such as those sold by Beyond Organic.

Lastly, make sure you chew your food well. As a child I was an extremely slow eater, but while in medical school, I got into the bad habit of rushing through my meals. I remember wolfing down my meals in the cafeteria at the hospital so that I could answer my beeper, get to the next class or attend to my hospital rounds. I still have the bad habit of reading while I eat breakfast, but one of my daily intentions is a eating more mindfully. Recently, I've begun counting the number of times I'm chewing a piece of food, just for fun. Interestingly, I've found this practice rather enjoyable because I pay attention to the flavor and texture of my meal rather than my "To-Do" list.

I had no idea that my lack of chewing over the years had contributed to my digestive problems. I used to eat a lot in the car until I heard that nutrient absorption is diminished. Of course, eating while driving is probably somewhat dangerous, but more importantly, you aren't getting the most out of your meal. Energy flows where your attention goes so if you're paying attention to your food as you eat, you'll get greater benefit from it. Take it from me, chew your food well and eat slowly. The job of the teeth is to increase the surface area of the food so that the stomach and intestines can digest food more easily. According to Dr. Lipski, saliva contains enzymes that break down carbohydrates and fat. Saliva also reabsorbs nitrates from foods which then get converted to nitric oxide, a substance that helps to reduce inflammation throughout the body.

Strategy 4: Avoid GMO Foods

Genetically modified organisms (GMO) have made their way into our diets over the last ten years. Under the guise of feeding more of the world's population, GMO foods were created so that our crops could be sprayed with pesticides without killing off the crop. BT Toxin in corn actually makes the bellies of insects explode. Ingestion of this corn by livestock has resulted in gut inflammation. Unbeknownst to most Americans, genetically modified organisms have not been studied long term (greater than 90 days) in animals until very recently.

In a study released in 2012, rats fed GMO corn for eighteen months succumbed to cancerous tumors and early death. GMO expert, Jeffrey Smith, author of Seeds of Deception and creator of the film, Genetic Roulette, feels that there is undeniable evidence that GMO foods are outright dangerous to humans and should be banned from the marketplace. In Europe, overwhelming consumer concern over GMO dangers resulted in Europeans rejecting it without the European government having to reject it first. With knowledge of the truth, consumers have an important role in determining what ends up on their dinner table.

As of this writing, in the United States, GMO foods still do not have to be labeled. The average American is still innocently unaware of the dangers of GMO corn, soy, canola, sugar beets and cottonseed oil in their everyday food products. However, thanks to many passionate grassroots organizations including the Institute for Responsible Technology, Just Label It, and others, we may soon see GMO foods banished from America. In the meantime, do your best to avoid all corn, soy, and canola that is not labeled organic. Even health food stores such as Whole Foods and Trader Joe's have not eliminated GMO foods from their shelves although consumer pressure may soon change this policy in the near future. It is your responsibility to be aware and informed. GMO foods can cause all sorts of allergies, gastrointestinal symptoms, unwanted weight gain, and immune problems to name a few. Avoiding GMOs can reduce or eliminate many health problems, as documented by Jeffrey Smith, including Leaky Gut Syndrome.

Strategy 5: Starve Opportunistic Infections

A common finding with most of my patient with longstanding leaky gut problems contributing to chronic pain is the harboring of parasites, yeast and "bad" bacteria in their intestines. An overgrowth of these organisms contributes to malnutrition and ongoing inflammation. They are called "opportunistic" only because they cannot survive in a healthy gut environment that has a good number of healthy bacteria (flora) protecting it. These detrimental organisms can only flourish at "opportune" times when the intestinal wall is inflamed and damaged and when there are not enough healthy flora to keep their numbers in check.

When I talk to my young patients about their tummies, I tell them that if they have too many "bad" guys living in their bellies, they will stay sick. So I encourage them to starve the bad guys and feed the good guys (the healthy bacteria). The best way to starve the opportunistic organisms is to abstain from eating damp and sugary foods. Non-beneficial yeast, mold and fungi tend to love eating damp foods such as dairy, alcohol, sugar and carbohydrates like bread. Often fermented foods made with bacteria and yeast, like kombucha, may be problematic as well in certain people. In order to starve them so they do not continue to multiply, it is important to avoid eating sugar at all costs. Of course, there are natural sugars found in fruits and vegetables that you can still eat, but avoid processed foods including fruit juices because of the high sugar content.

One of the most common ingredients in processed food is corn syrup, also known as high-fructose corn syrup. The reason it is in so many processed foods is that it is cheap to make and it is highly addictive. Try asking for a tour of a factory that makes high-fructose corn syrup. Unless you're an industry insider, you'll never be granted one because the process is so toxic that the companies don't want people to actually witness how this artificial sugar is made. Furthermore, much of the corn in America is genetically modified, meaning that it contains a pesticide gene in it. If the label says "corn syrup", you can safely assume that it is made from genetically modified corn. There are absolutely no human studies showing the safety of these genetically modified organisms (GMOs) and yet they are allowed to be sold for human consumption. Apparently the safety of Americans is not as important as corporate profits.

Not only is sugar great "food" for opportunistic organisms to thrive on and take over your intestines, its ingestion via processed food can increase the rate of aging through a process called glycation. Excessive amounts of sugar in our diet causes our cells to age through a complex series of reactions in the body that produce advanced glycation end products (AGEs). Obviously prematurely aging cells will contribute to chronic pain and will prevent your body from healing. I won't go into the biochemical details of exactly what happens to produce AGE's, but just know that AGE's and the associated inflammatory reactions in the body are implicated in many chronic diseases including diabetes, Alzheimer's Disease, cardiovascular disease, and cataracts.

Back in the 1700 and 1800's America's sugar consumption was around 4 pounds per person per year. Guess what it is today? It is over 130 pounds per person per year and it keeps rising each year according to the USDA! Most people have no idea that the soda that they are drinking or that the non-fat gluten-free cookies they are consuming might have massive amounts of sugar in them. Processed food labeled "sugar free" isn't a whole lot better because they are still devoid of nutrients that are found in whole organic food plus they may contain potentially toxic artificial sweeteners such as aspartame.

Going "cold turkey" on processed food may be difficult for a lot of people. Even I like to enjoy crackers from time to time, although I try to buy gluten-free crackers made from flax seed rather than sugary grains. Just make small consistent changes in your diet over time. You don't have to incorporate all of my suggestions all at once. Just pick the most detrimental nutritional habit you may have and start changing that a little at a time. After your body has "withdrawn" from "bad" food and you start feeding it nutritiously dense whole food, you'll find you don't miss processed food at all. It is the first couple of weeks that are the most challenging. For example, if you're a diet soda junky, consider switching to soda with natural sugar (not high fructose corn syrup) first. Then you can start to decrease how much you drink and replace it with something fun and yummy like carbonated water with lime and stevia.

Eventually you can increase your non-carbonated water intake and increase your natural water intake. You may even wish to invest in a good quality juicer to make your own delicious and healthy juices from organic produce. I absolutely love my masticating juicer because it juices the fruits and vegetables relatively slowly (five minutes versus five seconds for centrifugal high speed juicers) and the juice keeps fresh for 72 hours. I find that adding freshly made juice to my diet has made me less hungry and more energetic. It is probably due to the high concentration of minerals in the juice. If the body receives and can absorb more nutrients, it becomes less hungry. That's what I've found in practice.

Strategy 6: Promote Healthy Intestinal Flora

While you're starving the "bad" intestinal organisms in your gut, you'll want to replace them with "good" organisms: beneficial bacteria or yeast. Healthy flora, as they are also referred to, help destroy unhealthy organisms, thus reducing their negative impact on the intestines. While many people argue that they get probiotics by eating yoghurt on a daily basis, in practice, this is often not enough. In addition, most commercial yoghurts are fat free and thus devoid of Vitamin A. They are also laden with sugar and artificial flavors or sweeteners, so they are not the healthiest of choices. As mentioned before, the "dampness" in the intestines can be worsened by pasteurized dairy products. The average yoghurt contains between one and four billion CFU's (colony forming units) of probiotics per serving. Yet, in most of my patients with leaky gut and chronic pain, they require upwards of 20 to 120 billion CFU's of probiotics per day to restore intestinal balance.

Instead of store-bought yoghurt, I often prescribe probiotic supplements. Probiotics contain beneficial bacteria or yeast that can re-colonize the intestines and help repair leaky gut. Certain folks have access to raw cultured dairy products which they can try instead since the culturing process uses probiotics. Raw dairy is difficult to come by unless you happen to live in a state or country where it is legal to sell it in stores. Some people choose to make their own raw cultured kefir or whey. In Chinese medicine, patients are asked to avoid dairy because it can often worsen joint and muscle pain. If you're a dairy fan, you'll just have to try live without it for a month and see if you notice a difference.

As far as taking probiotic supplements, there are many different brands available and some are better than others. What you're looking for is a brand that contains human strains of healthy organisms or have been validated in clinical studies using real people. In the office I use muscle testing as a simple tool to help determine which probiotic brand would be most beneficial for each patient. After several months to a year, I repeat the muscle test in case the body wants a different combination of probiotics. Some quality brands I've used in my office which are also available at health food stores or online include Culturelle®, RAW Probiotics by Garden of Life®, Prescript-Assist™, and Ethical Nutrients™ Intestinal Care DF (Dairy Free). In the office, I also use Genestra™ HMF Replete and Integrative Therapeutics™ Enterogenic Intensive 100 (100 billion per capsule). Available in pharmacies only is a brand called VSL#3® which contains over 112 billion CFU's per capsule, which is approved to treat inflammatory bowel diseases such as Crohns and Ulcerative Colitis as well as irritable bowel syndrome.

I recommend that you abstain from eating sugary foods in general, but especially while you're trying to rebalance the organisms in your intestines. If you continue to eat sugary foods while you use probiotics, you will both be feeding and killing off the "bad" organisms at the same time. This is not ideal because you can suffer from what is referred to as a die-off reaction. For example, if you've been eating ice cream every evening and feeding the "bad" yeast in your intestines and then proceed to kill them off with probiotics, you'll be left with a large amount of dead yeast remnants in your bowels, which could lead to all sorts of symptoms. Die-off symptoms could include lethargy, constipation, diarrhea, headaches, irritability, skin rashes, low grade fever and worsening of joint and muscle pain. It may be prudent to start with a lower dose of probiotics and work your way up to the higher doses over time while you continue to refine and improve your diet.

Strategy 7: Treat Constipation

If you have constipation, I can guarantee that it is contributing to your chronic pain. When your colon is backed up, it cannot process all the toxins flooding into it, so the toxins overwhelm other detoxification organs such as the liver and kidneys. The colon usually is responsible for dealing with the bulk of toxins that we are in contact with daily, so if it isn't working properly, the liver can become sluggish in its function. A sluggish liver is often the cause of chronic pain. When the bowels and liver aren't functioning optimally, you can bet that the other detoxification organs are also stressed: the lymph and kidneys. When the toxins cannot be removed effectively

Guide to Healing Chronic Pain

from the lymph into the kidneys for excretion, they can hang around the body's tissues and cause muscle and joint pain. The skin, which is one of the largest detoxification organs we have, uses sweat to detoxify us. But if the skin exhibits rashes and diseases, it means that the colon, liver, kidneys, and lymph have all become overwhelmed and the body has no choice but to try to detoxify through the skin.

I know from personal experience that constipation causes joint and body aches. Whenever I would become constipated, which was a common occurrence until I desensitized myself from my food intolerances, my muscle trigger points would start to ache and my joints would stiffen. When my bowels improved, my pain levels dropped almost immediately.

So what is considered constipation? Well, the ideal number of bowel movements you should have daily is between three and four. The first bowel movement is in the morning before breakfast and the rest is within an hour of eating a meal. For most people, they are shocked to hear this. Personally, I'm happy if I "go" once a day given my long history of constipation. If you do not have a bowel movement at least once a day, then you're in big trouble. Not only is your detoxification system backed up, you can't heal your body if you're constipated. Clearing constipation is vital.

Your bowel movements should be relatively soft, easy to pass and formed, like a snake. This is a type IV stool according to the Bristol University's Stool Scale. If you can pass 12 inches or more of stool in one sitting, that is superb and ideal. If you have small "rabbit pellets", Type I stool, you are severely constipated and need treatment for constipation. If you don't have constipation but have diarrhea instead, Type V to VII stool) you're not out of the woods either. Diarrhea is NEVER normal and you may have chronic leaky gut or nutritional malabsorption issues. See Resources for the link to the Bristol Stool Scale.

Here are some guidelines to treating constipation:

1. Make sure you're hydrating with approximately half your body weight in ounces of pure water daily or approximately 2 Liters.
2. Eat vegetables at every meal, some raw if tolerated.
3. Eat enough healthy fats and oils which include pastured butter, coconut oil, olive oil, and grass-fed animal fat.
4. Take a good quality probiotics daily.
5. Avoid eating sugar, dairy and gluten.

197

6. Avoid caffeinated drinks as they contribute to dehydration.
7. Take extra magnesium (see Magnesium Miracle chapter).
8. If the above fail, use a simple, magnesium-based bowel cleansing kit such as Enzymatic Therapy's™ Simple Cleanse or Whole Body Cleanse. Although it isn't the strongest cleanse on the market, it is safe for most people and non-habit forming for long term use.
9. Test for food intolerance and do the Uhe Method to desensitize yourself from these intolerances.

If constipation persists despite your best efforts, it may mean that you have a low or underactive thyroid condition. I find hypothyroidism very common in women, especially after the age of forty. However men can become hypothyroid as well. If you have some or most of the hypothyroid symptoms below, you may wish to get tested for it.

- Fatigue
- Sluggishness
- Increased sensitivity to cold
- Constipation
- Pale, dry skin
- A puffy face
- Hoarse voice
- An elevated blood cholesterol level
- Unexplained weight gain
- Muscle aches, tenderness and stiffness
- Pain, stiffness or swelling in your joints
- Muscle weakness
- Heavier than normal menstrual periods
- Brittle fingernails and hair
- Depression

The laboratory tests I usually ask for are: Free T4, Free T3 (active form of thyroid) and TSH. I look to see if the Free T4 and T3 are in the upper normal range and if the TSH is in the low normal range, all of which are desirable. If your lab results are "normal" yet you display symptoms of low thyroid, you may wish to check if you're iodine deficient. According to Dr. David Brownstein, an expert in the holistic treatment of thyroid disorders, approximately 96% of his patients are iodine deficient. Those with thyroid disorders almost always are low in iodine. A simple 24-hour iodine loading test can be done (as long as you don't mind collecting your urine for 24 hours) to determine whether you are deficient or not. It only costs about $50 US, not including the iodine tablet you have to take, and your insurance may even cover it. I use Doctors Data, the only laboratory that is permitted to do testing in my state of New York. Dr. Brownstein uses Hakala Labs.

Sometimes when the thyroid lab tests are in the normal range, my patients are still experiencing hypothyroidism. Even if their thyroid production is adequate, their tissues can be less sensitive to it. Alternatively, the hypothalamus gland, one of the master glands of the brain, can be weak or unbalanced, thus affecting thyroid function.

Strategy 8: Desensitize Food Intolerances

Please read the chapter on Food Sensitivities. It is ideal to both recognize and avoid the foods that cause sensitivity reactions in your body as well as desensitize yourself from them. Sensitivity reactions cause chronic inflammation in the body, which contributes to chronic pain. Avoiding the foods that cause this inflammation will help your intestines heal. By desensitizing your body as well, using NAET or the Uhe Method, you'll turn down the excessive reaction that occurs, so you'll minimize or eliminate your symptoms.

Strategy 9: Support Your Detoxification Organs

Once your colon is working better, the other detoxification organs can then be relieved of the extra burden they've been carrying. If you're no longer constipated but you feel that the detoxification organs need some support after years or decades of stress, you may wish to try the LifeWave Y-Age Glutathione and Carnosine patches on specific acupuncture points that support those organs. The LifeWave patches have been proven in clinical studies to improve organ function.

I have found that the liver is usually extremely stressed in most of my patients and that can contribute to chronic pain. As long as someone is not constipated, I like to recommend the LifeWave Y-Age Glutathione patches on the right Liver 3 acupuncture point, which is on top of the foot. Glutathione is a very powerful antioxidant molecule that the body makes to help detoxify itself. Glutathione recharges other antioxidants such as Vitamins A, C, and E, so that is why it is referred to as the "master" antioxidant of the body. Unfortunately as we age, our ability to make glutathione diminishes. That's where the LifeWave Y-Age Glutathione patches come in. When placed on acupuncture points, the patch stimulates the body to produce more glutathione. Unlike medicinal patches, there is no glutathione actually inside the patches. They work instead by signaling the body's own glutathione production mechanism. How elegant is that? Because glutathione is used up quickly in the body, I recommend using the Y-Age Glutathione patches daily if tolerated. It is the most efficient, least expensive way to increase your glutathione levels compared with using supplements, creams or intravenous injections.

The LifeWave Y-Age Carnosine patches help to repair connective tissue and cellular DNA. Carnosine is an antioxidant. In mouse studies, carnosine supplementation improved longevity by 30%. If you have chronic pain, you likely have tissue that need repairing so I recommend these patches for long term use to support the body's self-healing mechanism. Like glutathione, carnosine production declines with age. By normalizing carnosine production in the body, the cells have the opportunity to return to a more youthful state. Placing the carnosine patch on any of the acupuncture points listed in the LifeWave brochure or handbook is effective in supporting the organs of detoxification. Some people even put the carnosine patch over areas of chronic degeneration to diminish pain. I recommend using the carnosine patches every night while you sleep because that is the time that your body regenerates itself. They last twelve hours so you can put them on sometime after dinner and wear them overnight.

In many of my patients with chronic pain, I've found a set of acupuncture points on their upper chest that can become really sensitive. These points are Kidney 27, on either side of the breast bone, up near where it connects to the collar bone. If these points are sore, it invariably means that their lymphatic flow is blocked and the toxins cannot escape through the urine. If toxins can't flow easily from the lymph, they will settle in your muscles and bones and cause chronic pain. The body has to detoxify these toxins in order for your chronic pain to disappear for good. If you push on the Kidney 27 points on your own chest and they are sore, it probably means you also have blocked lymphatic flow contributing to your chronic pain. Rubbing these points several times a day may help open up the flow of lymph.

A licensed massage therapist specializing in lymphatic drainage would also be able to help you unblock the lymph. My lymphatic specialist would usually take upwards of 30 or 40 minutes to unblock my lymph channels, especially if I was suffering from constipation. One day, she decided to experiment with putting LifeWave Energy Enhancer patches on Kidney 27, the white patch on the right and the tan patch on the left. To her amazement, the lymph channel opened up within five minutes. From that point forward, I've recommended that patients with tender Kidney 27 points patch themselves daily on this specific acupuncture point with LifeWave Energy Enhancer Patches until which time the points are no longer sore. I have found that not only do people experience more energy, they also have diminished all-over body pain as well. Kidney 27 in Traditional Chinese Medicine acupuncture is used to treat adrenal exhaustion.

One of my patients, Steven, had extremely tender Kidney 27 points. He shot me a look of anguish when I pressed on them! After I instructed him to use LifeWave Energy Enhancer patches on this point, he lost eight pounds within 24 hours! Steven was "water-logged" with sluggish lymph containing toxins that could not escape the body until we treated those points. I can tell you he has felt a whole lot better since and those acupuncture points aren't very sore any more.

There are some supplements that help the body's detoxification organs function better. Some of the best ones I've used were created by doctors for doctors and are thus not available for the general public, so I won't name them here. Milk thistle is well known for supporting the liver. Usually if I use it, my patients muscle test for between 200 and 500 mg per day in divided doses. It is very safe, so I don't hesitate to recommend it. L-Glutamine in doses around 3000 mg a day or more has been used successfully to heal the lining of the intestines. If you're really interested in taking supplements, it would be a good idea to connect with a holistic physician, herbalist, holistic nutritionist, or naturopath who is comfortable at evaluating you for supplements. I muscle test each patient who might benefit from taking supplements because I have found muscle testing to be the most useful way to evaluate their appropriateness.

Pain Relief with Gut Healing

At this point you might be wondering how quickly you're going to see results in pain relief once you decide to start healing your intestines. I have to admit that the gut doesn't heal overnight, so you'll have to be patient and persistent. Understand, however, that by doing what it takes to heal the intestines, you'll be doing your entire body a favor, not just your muscles and joints! Your skin will be clearer and younger. Your mind will be brighter, happier and more focused. You'll likely enjoy your life more because you feel so much better.

For many people, just getting rid of chronic constipation relieves a large proportion of their chronic pain. If they have blocked lymphatic flow due to a sluggish set of detoxification organs, unblocking this flow helps tremendously in getting rid of chronic achy joint and muscle pain.

If you prefer a step-by-step eating guide to cure Leaky Gut, check out the radio interview I did with Leaky Gut expert Karen Brimeyer about her program. See Resources for links.

Chapter Summary

- Chronic pain can be caused by a condition known as Leaky Gut Syndrome.
- Healing Leaky Gut can restore the body's ability to heal from chronic inflammation and allergic reactions.
- The gut is a second "nervous system" and if it is out of balance, so is your nervous system, which can keep you in pain.
- Strategies to heal the gut and reduce chronic pain include brain balancing, hydration, optimizing nutrition, starving opportunistic infections, promoting healthy intestinal flora, reducing food sensitivities and/or their reactions, eliminating constipation and supporting the detoxification organs.
- Blocked lymphatic flow can cause achy chronic joint and muscle pain. By checking acupuncture point Kidney 27 for tenderness and then treating it with acupressure or LifeWave Energy Enhancer patches, you can help to encourage the free flow of lymph.

17

REDUCE EMF STRESS

I was giving a free presentation on stress to the local Rotary club and I asked the audience members to name some of the common stressors each of us face on a daily basis. Many named job, marital or family stress. Interestingly, none named electromagnetic stress as a culprit in our ill health. Toxins in our environment such as those found in air, food, water, household cleaners, and skin care products were also not recognized as stressors. Most people thought stress meant mental and emotional stress. They had no idea that there were other stressors that can profoundly influence our health. Electromagnetic stress is a topic that I'm passionate about because this type of stress is more prevalent than ever and will only increase as new electronic products are produced and more powerful mobile phone towers are erected.

Electromagnetic fields (EMF) in the form of electropollution may be the number one cause of stress in all of us who live in the modern world. The reason it is so important is because few of us have the ability to avoid EMF radiation if we live with electricity, cell phones, wireless internet and computers. Even if you don't own or use a cell phone or wireless internet, your neighbors or coworkers probably do and you'll still be negatively affected. If you've read my chapter on balancing the brain, you already know that it is vital to maintain brain balance in order to get rid of chronic pain for good. What I've found in my practice is that almost every new patient I meet owns a cell phone or uses a cordless phone on a regular basis. Most have wireless internet in their homes. Electropollution causes brain imbalances in many people.

In addition to brain imbalances, the constant stress from EMF exposure causes an energy drain on the body. When the body doesn't have enough energy, it will be in survival mode, not healing mode. When you can generate and keep as much energy as you can, you will start filling up your energy battery, a necessary prerequisite to healing the body. Energy drains from any source including electropollution, need to be minimized, in order for you to heal.

In America, the importance of money and convenience far outweigh the importance of health, as witnessed by our lack of concern over the growing number of studies showing that wireless microwave radiation has significant detrimental health effects. In 2009 France issued a ban on advertising cellular phones to children due to the studies showing brain dysfunction in children even with minimal exposure to cell phone radiation. There was no such ban here in America and in fact, it is rare to see any news on cell phone radiation dangers at all. Why? Because corporate interests and the advertising dollars they represent are more important to the media than health interests here in America. A point of fact: the World Health Organization in 2011 announced that it now considers cell phone radiation a potential carcinogen (cancer causing); yet the majority of the public is ignorant of that announcement. Instead, people read about how taking vitamins may be harmful to one's health. Dr. Mercola, arguably the most popular natural health advocate online, feels that the public can often be misinformed by the media. Check Resources for a link to his article.

Camilla Rees is a leading health educator who is well versed in health issues and in medicine. She is very adamant about our need to better protect ourselves from increasingly invasive electromagnetic fields. She is co-author, with Magda Havas, PhD, of Public Health SOS: The Shadow Side of the Wireless Revolution. Microwave radiation, especially the frequency used by cellular phones, has been proven to create DNA damage; yet regulatory agencies only consider the potential damage to humans via heat transfer. That's bad news for us cell phone users because we can have a false sense of security about the safety of using these devices.

The public attitude has been: "If the government allows the sale of cell phones, it must mean they are safe". Nothing could be further from the truth. When the cell phone industry was just blossoming, federal regulators did not require cell phone manufacturers to prove that these devices were safe, only that they did not heat the head too much. The incorrect assumption was that if the head is not heated, then there is no damage done to the body. We now know that this assumption is incorrect. Many studies by various scientists worldwide have come to the conclusion that there are non-thermal changes to those exposed to microwave radiation that may cause serious long-term health consequences. Go to the electromagnetic health website for more information.

In addition to cell phones, the following devices also radiate harmful microwave radiation: cordless phones, baby monitors, wireless (Wi-Fi) internet routers, wireless laptop computers, wireless-enabled book readers/ tablets, and of course microwave ovens. Even if you don't own any of these devices, I'm sure the people around you do. You can be negatively affected by someone's cell phone even if you are standing a few feet away from him/ her. And what about other types of electromagnetic radiation, like those from appliances, lighting, clocks, computers, cars, planes and electrical wiring in buildings? They all affect our body's energy field whether we feel it or not. The electricity in our walls oscillates at a similar frequency as our nervous system and thus can create chronic stress in our bodies.

Think about the cumulative stress of all the EMF that surrounds us in our modern life. Isn't it a wonder why so many people feel on edge much of the time? It can be especially frustrating for people who like to live more "green" to discover that energy-saving devices like compact fluorescent light bulbs emanate more EMF than regular incandescent bulbs.

There is growing concern over Smart Meters. These are a type of electrical meter that records consumption of electrical energy at regular intervals many times a day and reports the results back to the utility company for monitoring and billing purposes. Unlike home energy monitors, Smart Meters can gather data for remote reporting. Thus, health advocates are genuinely concerned of the dangers associated with higher levels of EMF that families are unknowingly exposed to. Unlike your cell phone, Smart Meters can't be turned off, thus exposing the home occupants to a constant level of harmful radiation 24/7.

Smart Meters are being installed in homes and businesses in Canada, USA, Australia and Europe. If you've been affected by this and want to know your rights and how to challenge those installations, go to www.smartmeterdangers.org.

Strategies to Minimize EMF Stress

There are practical and not-so-practical ways of minimizing your exposure to EMF stress and its negative effects on your nervous system. The not-so-practical ways include living in a cave away from city dwellers and not using any electronic devices. Just kidding. Seriously speaking, it is almost impossible for most of us to avoid EMF stress completely, so I'll share some of the successful strategies I use and recommend to my patients.

Grounding/Earthing

When your body is literally grounded to Mother Earth, either by connecting your bare skin with the earth outside or by touching a grounding/Earthing Universal Mat, your body is more resilient to the negative effects of EMF. I notice that when I am working long hours on the computer, I never get tired anymore because my bare feet are touching a grounding mat the whole time. Of course, you can't be physically grounded 100% of the time, so use other strategies as well. I highly recommend sleeping grounded on an Earthing bed sheet so that you are protected during the time when your body's energy is most vulnerable.

Wireless EMF Protection

Since I've become hypersensitive to EMF over the years, I am very grateful to have some pretty nifty protection devices for my electronics. Before using these devices, I'd develop severe fatigue and migraines from prolonged cell phone exposure. If I slept in a hotel with wireless internet, I'd wake up achy and sore all over. Now, in addition to travelling with my grounding bed sheet, I use several other products to protect myself.

For cell phones, I recommend the Quantum Cell (EarthCalm), the Matrix 2 for smartphones (LifeWave) or the EMF Transformer (Energy Tools International). The Quantum Cell grounds the negative energy emanating from the phone, creating a protective "bubble" around you. If you use the Quantum Cell on your phone, you won't need a separate protection device if you use a Bluetooth or headset. The LifeWave Matrix 2 technology takes an entirely different approach and re-radiates the microwave radiation emitted from the phone via Matrix 2's special antenna design thereby reducing harmful radiation by up to 98% in independent studies. The Energy Tools International EMF Transformer has been shown in brain mapping studies to prevent brain imbalances during cell phone use.

Please be aware that there are a plethora of cell phone protection devices on the market. Some are made of stones, holographic discs or plastic. Few, if any, have any decent scientific studies validating their effectiveness, so for safety reasons, I would recommend that you purchase the ones I recommend in this chapter.

For cordless phones, I recommend the EarthCalm Quantum Cell on the phone base. The EarthCalm Omega Wi-Fi fits in your wireless router to create a bubble of wireless protection throughout your entire house. The EarthCalm Torus is larger than the Quantum Cell and is appropriate for laptops and tablet devices such as the iPad. The EarthCalm products do not shield the EMF but rather "ground" the frequency to match that of the earth. Using them may feel different from grounding outside in your bare feet, but they work to calm your stress handling system as evidenced by the studies done on them.

Because of major wiring problems in my house, it was more practical for me to install wireless internet service. I can assure you that I didn't let the technician turn it on until I had the EarthCalm Omega Wi-Fi securely in place! The next day when I woke up, I was pleased to discover that I didn't have any EMF-related achiness or pain. Turning your wireless router off while you sleep may reduce your EMF exposure, but keep in mind that the electropollution that it creates lingers in your home even after turning off the device.

Home and Office EMF Protection

Many years ago, I bought some Graham-Stetzer Filters that filter the dirty electricity in my office. When I used an EMF meter on the outlets in one of my rooms, it was a whopping 1700 G (Gauss). I put one of the filters in that outlet and it brought the number down to under 100 G. The healthy ideal is 60 G or less. Although I felt really good about using these filters at work, the problem was that they would constantly emit a crackling and popping sound. In fact, it was so stressfully annoying, one patient asked me *"Is the place gonna blow?"* In addition, the filter would take up an outlet so I had to plug in my medical equipment elsewhere.

Then I got a call from Greenwave Filters who offered me a 30-day trial use of their newly designed EMF filters. They were four for $99. I agreed and much to my surprise, they worked just as well, if not better (since I used two per room) and they were completely silent. In addition, I didn't lose an outlet because their filters allow you to plug any device into it. I can honestly say that the office feels calmer energetically since I began using the Greenwave filters.

In addition to Greenwave filters for the office, I use a product made by Energy Tools International called Clean Sweep. It is an energized water product that you can spray to neutralize negative energy frequencies. I spray each of my treatment rooms after every patient because people often detoxify their negative energies during treatment and I don't want the next patient to be exposed to them. Clean Sweep also neutralizes electropollution as well, at least for a while, until it builds up again.

A study done by Energy Tools International demonstrated that irradiated cells in a Petri dish healed much better in a room that was energetically "clean" as compared to a room that was not. In this study, over 80% of these cells survived in the "clean" room and only about 10% survived in the "dirty" room. Given the results of this study, we can deduce that people probably don't heal well when they are living/working in energetically dirty environments.

Not only does electropollution create "dirty" energy, so do negative human emotions and stress. Thus hospitals are one of the worst places to truly heal because they are filled with electro-polluting devices as well as the energetic remnants of thousands of sick people. I would highly recommend that you consider "clearing" the energetic pollution from your bedroom and home on a regular basis using Clean Sweep. You may have heard of the herb sage being used by Native Americans. It is used traditionally to cleanse the mind of negative spirits and impurities. Burning sage is still a common practice with people wishing to clear their homes of negative energy. I use Clean Sweep in my office because it is a faster and there is no smell.

I had a new patient once who was referred to me because she was at the end stages of her pregnancy and her blood pressure was high. Her obstetrician was trying to convince her to induce labor early. After interviewing her, and before I did any acupuncture, I measured her blood pressure. To her amazement, it was normal. She told me that her blood pressure had been consistently high for over two weeks. I can't prove it, but I'm guessing that it was the combination of Greenwave Filters and Clean Sweep in my treatment room that calmed the body's stress response down so much so that the blood pressure normalized. I couldn't convince her to measure or reduce her EMF exposure and thus her blood pressure remained elevated at home.

One of the products I've invested in is a whole house EMF protection product called the EarthCalm Scalar Home Protection unit. It has three pieces that plug into one of the outlets of your house. As long as the wiring in your house connects to only one electrical box, this unit will protect the entire house. Unlike individual Stetzer filters, however, the Scalar Home Protection unit does not filter dirty electricity. Instead, it grounds the frequency from a harmful one to frequency beneficial one. What I have found personally is that my entire house seems "calmer" ever since I began using this product.

I purchased this product before I heard about Greenwave filters, the latter of which you have to purchase for every room in your house. The main advantage of the Scalar Home Protection unit is that you protect the entire house with one unit. The main disadvantage is that chronically ill or sensitive folks will tend to go through detoxification symptoms and may need to acclimatize to the unit by using it for shorter periods of time and building up to full time use as tolerated. In my household it took about two and a half months before we installed the final piece of the unit. The advantage of the Greenwave filters is that there is no such detoxification response that I've noticed.

Personal EMF Protection

I decided to purchase a personal protector that would protect me from low frequency (such as electronics) as well as high frequency radiation (such as cell phone radiation) while I was away from home. There are many personal protectors on the market but alas few have been clinically tested in rigorous scientific studies. Since I had such great personal results with the EarthCalm products, I decided to get their Nova Resonator Pendant after trying some other products that didn't seem to be strong enough for me. I believe this pendant has helped me "survive" high EMF environments such as movie theatres and airports.

If you think you have as much EMF sensitivity as I do, I would highly recommend that you consider wearing a Nova Resonator Pendant as well as using the LifeWave Y-Age Aeon patches for stress relief and LifeWave Energy Enhancer patches for energy support. The combination has made life outside my home not only tolerable, but enjoyable.

Just a quick note about children. More schools in America are adopting computers in the classroom and wireless internet. EarthCalm also makes a Nova Resonator personal protection device for children, so remember to protect your children as well as yourself. When children are stressed, they misbehave, become moody or lose focus.

EMF Protection for your Car

EarthCalm now makes a device called the Voyager to help reduce EMF stress when you're driving in your car. This is particularly important if you own a hybrid car because of the high EMFs created by the battery and computer. The Earthing company also makes an Earthing mat for your car, but I found the EarthCalm Voyager more effective. Before using the Voyager, no matter what I did or how many EMF protection devices I had on, I would always get sleepy during long car rides. Since applying the Voyager to the car, I haven't felt that way, so I'm sold on its effectiveness.

Other EMF Reduction Options

If you're not willing to invest in so many EMF protection devices, then you can make some other choices. For example, instead of having cordless phones in your home, you can switch them to landline phones. Remove any electronic devices from your bedroom so that you're not bombarded with extra EMF while you are sleeping, the time when your energy field is most vulnerable. Never sleep next to a clock radio. Battery operated clocks are preferred. Also never use your cell phone as an alarm clock unless you've configured it to airplane mode or have one of the protection devices I've mentioned above.

If you read in bed, swap the energy efficient compact fluorescent light bulb for an incandescent one or get one of the more expensive compact LED bulbs that are both green and healthier for you. Instead of having wireless internet, you can choose to use a hard-wired connection. If you insist on having a television in your bedroom, which I strongly discourage, unplug it and any other attached device from its power source before retiring to bed. Then Clean Sweep your bedroom before you sleep.

You really shouldn't use a cell phone if you're not willing to get a protection device for it. Like I said before, it messes up people's brain balance more than anything else I've seen with the exception of closed head injuries. If there is one message I'll repeat over and over again it is this: brain balance is vital to the body's self-healing mechanisms.

A Bluetooth or headset does not offer adequate protection because the cell phone is still close to your body and the radiation is still entering your brain. An air-tube headset prevents the EMF from directly transmitting into your brain, so it has advantages over Bluetooth and regular wired headsets, but an unprotected cell phone is still radiating other parts of your body. That being said, you can minimize your EMF exposure even if you don't use a protection device, by following these recommendations:

✗ Avoid talking on your cell phone in the car because the EMF bounces off the metal and amplifies it.
✗ Avoid charging your cell phone in the car.
✗ Turn off your cell phone when you're in the car or when you're not using it.
✗ Use a landline phone and turn off your cell phone when you're at home.
✗ Do not carry your cell phone on your person, such as in a pocket but instead carry it as far away from your body as possible.
✗ Do not allow children to use an unprotected cell phone.
✓ Talk for short periods of time only and hold the phone as far away from your head as practical during the call or use the speakerphone feature.
✓ Avoid using the phone in an area with poor cell phone coverage because the radiation is higher.
✓ Use text messaging more often than calling if safe to do so.
✓ Do not talk on the cell phone when around children and pets, both of whom are extra sensitive to radiation due to their smaller body mass.

For links to the products I've listed in this chapter, go to Resources.

Chapter Summary

- Electromagnetic stress (EMF), electropollution are significant sources of stress and can cause chronic pain.
- There are many ways you can avoid or diminish the negative consequences of EMF exposure.
- For cell phone radiation protection, invest in the EarthCalm Quantum Cell, the LifeWave Matrix 2 or the Energy Tools International EMF Transformer.
- For Cordless phone protection, use the EarthCalm Quantum Cell.
- For protection from wireless internet (Wi-Fi) use a EarthCalm Omega Wi-Fi device in your router.
- For laptop protection, use the EarthCalm Torus.
- For driving protection use the EarthCalm Voyager device.
- For whole house protection from low frequency radiation use the EarthCalm Scalar Home Protection unit, or for sensitive folks, get Stetzer-type (e.g. Greenwave) filters for each room.
- Clean Sweep is an energy tool in the form of a water-based spray you can use to clean the energy in any space.

18

EAT WELL. FEEL GREAT.

Why Nutrition is Important

I'm always amazed how many people treat their cars better than they treat their bodies. I've had my share of abusing my body, especially with the fast-food, no-sleep habits I learned in medical school. Most people I know think they know what eating healthy is supposed to look like. Several years ago, I was in the supermarket when I bumped into my friend, two-time Olympic Figure Skating Gold Medalist, Oleg Protopopov and his wife Ludmila. Oleg happened to look in my shopping cart and saw that among the fruits and vegetables, I had pre-made pasta and sauce in there. He shook his head sadly at me and said in his thick Russian accent, *"You're a doctor. You should know better. This isn't good for you."* Needless to say, I was flabbergasted at the time because I really thought eating low fat, vegetarian pasta was healthy. Years later, I laugh every time I think of that incident because Oleg was right. I had no idea what eating healthy really meant.

Although there is no excuse for the inadequate nutritional training in medical schools, the average person hears the same old spiel about eating healthy. Some of it is good, like the advice to eat fewer processed foods, but some of it is downright harmful, like the advice to eat low fat. Slick advertising, medical mythology, and governmental ignorance have perpetuated poor nutritional habits in America. I'm not here to force you to eat the way I eat. On the contrary, I'm here to educate you on the basics of what your body needs to heal your chronic pain. Your optimal diet might be quite different from mine but certain basics will be the same if we're both eating "healthy".

Without adequate fuel such as carbohydrates, fats and proteins, the body cannot produce energy and repair itself. Your Qi (energy) battery will be low. Most people understand this. Adequate amounts of vitamins and minerals are hard to come by even with a whole food diet because of the chronic depletion of nutrients from our soil. Nutrients in food help to fuel many of the processes necessary for proper function of the cells including cellular communication, energy production, detoxification, cellular repair, and cellular growth to name a few. If you feed your body crappy food (excuse the terminology), your body will not perform as it was intended to, and that can lead to chronic pain.

Although an entire book could be written just on nutrition, this chapter is going to focus on some basics to get you started. I'm guessing that most people who are looking for a holistic approach to healing chronic pain understand that there are few "quick fixes" in life and are thus willing to make the necessary holistic changes in their lifestyle in order to heal. If you're a processed food addict, on the other hand, some of these suggestions may seem alien, so I'm going to divide my pain relief nutritional guidelines into three different "levels" of sophistication: Pain Relief Basic, Intermediate, and Advanced. You can read each one and decide which "level" you feel like committing to. Any change in the right direction is better than nothing, so please don't feel you have to adopt everything at once. What I suggest is that you try what resonates with you first and see how it feels in your body, then "level up", as the computer gamers would say, when you are ready for a greater commitment.

Nutrition Myths

Let's start with debunking some nutritional myths which have become "truths" that almost every person, at least in America, has learned through school, media and their doctors. As an allopathically-trained physician, I absolutely loved medical school. Nutrition seemed boring in comparison to learning about the latest drugs and surgery. I would have made an excellent surgeon, and a compassionate one at that, save for the fact that I'm not a morning person and dislike getting up at 5AM. Thankfully, my being trained in family medicine made me more open to holistic ways of treating illness. Unfortunately, I really didn't get any practical education in nutrition until I sought it out because of my own chronic pain and gut issues. So I'm going to share with you a few nutritional myths that even I once believed so you understand the reasons for my recommendations that follow.

Nutrition Myth #1: Eating Low Fat is Good for You

I still remember telling my father, who has diabetes and high cholesterol, that the best diet for him would be a low fat diet. Doctors had learned in medical school that this was the best type of diet for people with high cholesterol and heart disease. It sounds reasonable, doesn't it, that eating low fat, especially low saturated fat, would be healthy? Obesity is an ever-increasing problem in America and even young children are being diagnosed regularly with Type II diabetes. This type of diabetes, caused by obesity, used to be called "adult-onset" diabetes. If more and more people are getting fat, it seems to make sense that we should cut down on our fat consumption. Or does it?

Most of the saturated fat consumed in America is from animal products, so we were told years ago to tell our patients to decrease consumption of red meat and saturated fat. But here's the problem: I assumed that the scientific data on this advice was solid, i.e. that countries with high saturated meat-filled diets all had worse levels of heart disease. Shockingly, this assumption was wrong.

Apparently, the widely-touted study conducted by biochemist Ansel Keyes excluded data from countries that had low rates of heart disease despite high fat consumption and countries with high rates of heart disease with low fat consumption. Now, this famous study from the 1950's takes center stage in the controversial but highly entertaining movie, Fat Head. This movie explains in graphical ways, how Keyes had data from 22 different countries, but he conveniently threw out data from countries that didn't match his hypothesis. Nevertheless, via political alliances, the scientific community eventually adopted his lipid hypothesis of heart disease.

The alarming rate of obesity really sky-rocketed once Americans were told to eat "low fat". Want to know why Americans are fatter than people are in most other first world countries? I believe it is because of several factors. Factor number one is that nowhere in the world is there a higher consumption of processed food than there is in North America. Americans consuming processed food eat plenty of empty calories devoid of nutrients. The body, thus being starved of nutrients, hungers for more, and thus calorie consumption rises to meet the perceived starvation. This is a great way for corporate food manufacturers to guarantee giant profits.

One of my patients, a snack food distributor, once told me that his buddy, a corporate food insider, revealed that food companies add additives like maltodextrin in processed food in order to make people addicted to it. I've heard this from many other reliable sources, so I'm not surprised. No wonder people in France, who consume high fat diets consisting of meat, butter, dairy and cream have half the heart disease rates of Americans. They just don't eat as much packaged food as we do.

Factor number two may be the fact that Americans consume large amounts of sugar, a fairly addictive substance in its own right. Many experts now believe that excessive sugar consumption leads to an overabundance of insulin secretion by the pancreas, causing it to wear out and promote Type II diabetes and Metabolic Syndrome. Obese people with Metabolic Syndrome have a higher risk of Type II diabetes, heart disease and stroke. The U.S. sweetener market is the largest and most diverse in the world. The United States is the largest consumer of sweeteners, including high fructose corn syrup, and is one of the largest global sugar importers. In the 1700's Americans consumed approximately 4 pounds of sugar per capita per year. Now consumption has grown to over 130 pounds of sweetener per capita per year.

Sometimes it is obvious where the sugar is coming from. Foods like cookies, cakes, candy, ice cream, brownies and syrup are easily spotted as sugar-rich. Sugar and other sweeteners such as high fructose corn syrup in prepared foods such as ketchup, canned vegetables and fruit, and peanut butter can make up 25% of our sugar consumption. Fruit juice is also loaded with sugar. Here's where it gets sneaky though. Packaged "low fat" foods are often high in hidden sugar in order to make it tasty. Marketed as healthy, low fat processed food can be just as high in calories as regular fat versions and consumers wouldn't know otherwise because they assume low fat must be good.

Factor three involved in the growing obesity problems in America may be the fact that toxins that we ingest or absorb through our skin and lungs are so prevalent that the body is ill-equipped to get rid of them fast enough, so it has to store these toxins in the safest place possible where they'll do less damage. So where are these toxins commonly stored? You guessed it! In our fat. In other words, we actually "need" to be fatter to store all the toxins that would otherwise damage major organs like the brain or kidneys.

One of the basic problems of eating low fat, aside from the consumption of sugar-laden products many American turn to, is the body's requirement for adequate fat in order to keep cells functioning properly. Fat is required for cellular membranes and the absorption and assimilation of fat-soluble vitamins. The following is an excerpt from the Weston A. Price article on understanding fats (reproduced with permission):

> Contrary to the accepted view, which is not scientifically based, saturated fats do not clog arteries or cause heart disease. In fact, the preferred food for the heart is saturated fat; and saturated fats lower a substance called Lp(a), which is a very accurate marker for proneness to heart disease.
>
> Saturated fats play many important roles in the body chemistry. They strengthen the immune system and are involved in inter-cellular communication, which means they protect us against cancer. They help the receptors on our cell membranes work properly, including receptors for insulin, thereby protecting us against diabetes. The lungs cannot function without saturated fats, which is why children given butter and full-fat milk have much less asthma than children given reduced-fat milk and margarine. Saturated fats are also involved in kidney function and hormone production.
>
> Saturated fats are required for the nervous system to function properly, and over half the fat in the brain is saturated. Saturated fats also help suppress inflammation. Finally, saturated animal fats carry the vital fat-soluble Vitamins A, D and K2, which we need in large amounts to be healthy.
>
> Human beings have been consuming saturated fats from animal products, milk products and the tropical oils for thousands of years; it is the advent of modern processed vegetable oil that is associated with the epidemic of modern degenerative disease, not the consumption of saturated fats.

Saturated fats, found in animal meat and tropical oils such as coconut oil and palm oil, play an important role in the healthy function of our body's cells. Saturated fatty acids constitute at least 50% of the cell membranes and give our cells necessary stiffness and integrity. Calcium consumption in America is high due to the perception that it prevents and treats osteoporosis. However, in order for calcium to be effectively incorporated into the skeletal structure, at least 50% of the dietary fats should be saturated. Certain saturated fats are the preferred food for the heart, which is why the fat around the heart muscle is highly saturated and the heart draws on this reserve of fat in times of stress. Lastly, short- and medium-chain saturated fatty acids protect us against harmful microorganisms in the digestive tract.

Nutrition Myth #2: Eating Red Meat is Bad for You

Along the lines of the lipid hypothesis and the idea that eating saturated fat from meat sources is bad for you, the National Cancer Institute (NCI) published a study in 2011 in the Archives of Internal Medicine that revealed that people who ate more meat, both red and white, had a higher risk of dying than those who ate less. Unfortunately, because the study was observational (not a true controlled experiment), the folks eating the most red meat were also the least physically active, the most likely to smoke, and the least likely to take a multivitamin. They also had higher body mass index (BMI), higher alcohol intake, and a trend towards less healthy non-red-meat food choices. The researchers tried to "adjust" mathematically for these factors, but it is still an artificial statistical method which cannot truly take into account the gravity of other unhealthy lifestyle factors. There is a great article link in Resources explaining why the NCI study may not be relevant to you.

On the other hand, there are other studies that reveal that vegetarians live longer lives than meat eaters. So what are the problems with eating meat? Plenty . . . if you eat conventionally-raised meat. If it isn't the saturated fat or the higher cholesterol content of meat, what is it? The answer lies in the type of food that conventionally-raised animals eat themselves: genetically modified corn feed laced with hormones and antibiotics. GMO corn is not only toxic because it is genetically modified, but corn itself is basically turned into sugar in order to fatten up the animals it is fed to. Fat is a great storage place for toxins, so where do you think the antibiotics, GMO toxins and hormones end up? On our dinner plate and waistlines, if we're not careful.

To my knowledge, there has never been a prospective study (a controlled experiment) whereby vegetarians are compared to meat eaters who only eat local organic meat and eggs. Local, grass-fed, pastured animals produce meat that is much leaner and contains higher levels of beneficial Omega-3s than does conventionally-produced meat. In addition, the meat is more alkaline and less acidic, something that is beneficial for the body. Meat is one of the most nutrient-dense forms of food available. The B vitamins, fat-soluble Vitamins A and D, and minerals like zinc, to name a few, are much more concentrated in meat and are more easily assimilated than those found in plant food.

If you're a vegetarian for humanitarian reasons, I'm not going to try to convince you to start eating meat, but if you are vegetarian only for health reasons, I want you to reconsider. If you choose to stick with vegetarianism, you have to make sure you make up for the lack of amino acids, good fats (including saturated fat) and fat-soluble vitamins found in meat. In addition, Vitamin B_{12} is often lacking in vegan diets, so consulting a holistic nutritionist is a must. I've seen some teenagers become vegetarians because they think it is the morally hip thing to do, only to fill their tummies with chips, salsa, crackers, cereal and granola bars, instead of whole foods like vegetables, greens, and sprouted legumes, nuts and seeds.

A great film to purchase for your wellness library is C.J. Hunt's *The Perfect Human Diet*. Using anthropological bone studies, scientists discovered that humans in the Paleolithic age were devoid of chronic diseases like arthritis for millions of years. Their enlarging body and brain size correlated with their nutritional intake of primarily animal-based food. It wasn't until approximately 10,000 years ago when grains and dairy were introduced that chronic disease became apparent and humans began shrinking in size.

When it comes to chronic pain, what I've noticed is that people who also have chronic stress on their adrenal glands (stress organs), seem to have less pain when they eat more healthy sources of animal foods. According to my traditional Chinese medicine colleagues, patients found deficient in Qi and Blood, need the higher and more easily assimilated forms of energy found in animal food. For patients who are willing to eat fish, I often recommend wild salmon and sardines.

Wild Alaskan sockeye salmon from Vital Choice, where I buy my sushi-grade fish, is rich in healthy Omega-3s and an antioxidant called astaxanthin. Astaxanthin gives salmon its red hue. Farmed salmon do not eat what nature provides, so they have to be given synthetic astaxanthin in order to produce the red color in the meat. Otherwise, the flesh turns out gray. Farmed salmon have more marbling (in other words are fattier) than wild salmon, but don't be fooled that the extra fat is better.

Farm-raised salmon have been found to have much higher levels of PCBs, dioxin, and other toxic cancer-causing chemicals than wild salmon, according to a recent study. Salmon raised in farms in Northern Europe had the highest contaminant levels. This was followed by salmon raised in North America and Chile. The reason for the higher toxin levels is thought to be because of the feed used in fish farms. Farm-raised salmon also have more antibiotics administered by weight compared to any other kind of livestock. In addition, farm-raised salmon do not have the same omega 3:6 profile as wild salmon. Farm-raised fish contain considerably higher levels of omega 6 fatty acids, the kind that apparently we consume too much of relative to omega 3's. This imbalance can promote inflammation.

I can really taste the difference between real wild Alaskan salmon and farmed salmon. The former tastes fresh and succulent, while the latter tastes greasy.

Nutritional Myth #3: You Should Eat Whole Grains

The base of the former USDA's food pyramid is the recommendation of 6-11 servings of grains, preferably whole grains. Americans were taught that the basis of a healthy diet was the consumptions of grains such as wheat, corn and rice. What most people fail to realize is that with the advent of the agricultural revolution, which was fairly recent in human history, people actually became shorter and less healthy when they began eating grains regularly. Today, Americans who are health conscious often make sure they eat whole grains in the form of whole grain toast, cereal or pasta. However, eating grains is not required for optimal health. As I've alluded to in previous chapters, wheat is responsible for much of our inflammatory disorders including chronic joint and muscle pain.

Did you know that two slices of whole wheat bread, although more nutritious than white bread, raise blood sugar more than a candy bar, according to Dr. William Davis, author of Wheat Belly? Recurrent high blood sugars make the pancreas work extra hard and may lead to Type II Diabetes and obesity. The Glycemic Index and Glycemic Load are tools you can search for on the internet. The ability of a particular food to raise the blood sugar is called the glycemic index. The higher the index, the more the pancreas has to work to produce insulin to control the blood sugar levels. Glucose, the simplest molecule of sugar, has a value of 100, so it is the standard to which other foods are compared. A typical candy bar has a moderate glycemic index of 41, whereas wheat bread has a high index of 72. The glycemic load, however, accounts for how much carbohydrate is in the food. A GL greater than 20 is considered high; a GL of 11–19 is considered medium; and a GL of 10 or less is considered low. Carrots, for example, have a high glycemic index but a low glycemic load. In other words you'd have to eat one and a half pounds of carrots at one time to get your blood sugar to spike as much as it does by your consuming a piece of whole grain toast. Few people eat that many carrots at once!

Most of our processed foods contain grains in the form of wheat, oats, and corn. Most of the corn produced in this country is genetically modified, as is the soy, so it would be best to stay away from products containing corn unless it is labeled non-GMO corn. Even many cereals marketed to gluten-free consumers sold in health food stores contain genetically modified corn, so you have to be vigilant if you want to remove toxic food from your diet so your body can heal itself.

Many people erroneously believe that they must consume whole grains to get their daily intake of fiber. Whole fruits and vegetables, however, contain more fiber than grains, are more filling, and do not spike the blood sugar. Eating grains can cause excessive insulin secretion by the pancreas, resulting in a lowering of blood sugar and an unnatural increase in hunger. People who have to eat every two to three hours, because of hypoglycemia (low blood sugar), feel much better when they remove grains from their diets. By adding in more meat protein and saturated fat, their blood sugar stabilizes and they are less ravenous.

Wheat is actually addictive according to William Davis, MD, author of Wheat Belly. You can actually experience withdrawal symptoms when you stop eating wheat that include temporary weakness, irritability, and brain fog. Luckily this only lasts about a week and if you eat more nutritious vegetable-based carbohydrates during this time and remain brain balanced with LifeWave Y-Age Aeon patches, the withdrawal will be a whole lot easier I find.

I'm not necessarily recommending that you must cut out all grains because it can be challenging to say the least given our cultural habits, but getting rid of the most inflammatory of the bunch, wheat (and other gluten-containing grains) and GMO corn, will do a lot to help your body heal from chronic pain. Sprouted lower or non-glutinous grains such as sprouted brown rice, quinoa and millet are preferred and are now available either at your local health food store or online. The traditional way of preparing grains, such as soaking and fermenting them in order to neutralize anti-nutrients such as phytates, are much healthier choices.

According to Sally Fallon, co-author of Nourishing Traditions: The Cookbook that Challenges Politically Correct Nutrition and the Diet Dictocrats, whole rice and whole millet contain lower amounts of phytates than do other grains so it is not absolutely necessary to soak them. However, they should be gently cooked for at least two hours in a high-mineral, gelatinous broth. This will neutralize some of the phytates they do contain and provide additional minerals to compensate for those that are still bound. The gelatin in the broth will greatly facilitate digestion. Check out the www.HealthyHomeEconomist.com website on how to make healthy bone broth.

If you have a lot of abdominal discomfort or significant leaky gut symptoms (see Chapter 16 on Heal the Gut), then going completely grain-free, at least for several months, may improve your chronic pain symptoms much quicker.

Nutritional Myth #4: Milk is Good for You

Practically everyone in North America has seen the Got Milk? campaigns using famous celebrities and athletes. Like most doctors, I recommended dairy products for most of my patients so they would get enough calcium in their diet to prevent osteoporosis. I didn't know, however, that other nutrients are necessary for healthy bone to be formed, including magnesium, fat-soluble Vitamins D and K. The Wulzen Factor, discovered by researcher Rosalind Wulzen, is a compound present in raw animal fat. This "anti-stiffness" factor protects humans and animals from calcification of the joints i.e. degenerative arthritis. It also protects against hardening of the arteries, calcification of the pineal gland and cataracts. Calves fed pasteurized milk or skim milk not only do not thrive, they develop joint stiffness! Their symptoms are reversed when raw butterfat is added back into their diet. Pasteurization destroys the Wulzen factor which is present only in raw butter, cream and whole milk. The Wulzen factor is another reason why we shouldn't be eating dairy if it is pasteurized and/or fat-skimmed.

Dairy products are considered "too damp" by traditional Chinese Medicine practitioners and can lead to joint pain, intestinal overgrowth and sinus congestion, but I wonder if raw dairy that is cultured with probiotic organisms has the same negative effect. I doubt it. Jordan Rubin, founder of Garden of Life and Beyond Organic, suffered from a life threatening intestinal illness at the young age of 21 and might have died if it weren't for a holistic nutritionist who taught him how to eat whole foods, healthy meat and raw cultured dairy (which was easy to obtain in California). If raw dairy is truly too dangerous for human consumption, then Jordan Rubin should be dead by now because he drank the stuff like it was going out of style. Instead, he quickly regained his health and in forty days put on 29 pounds to his sickly 110 pound frame. In addition to probiotic supplements, Jordan owes much of his intestinal healing to the consumption of raw full-fat cultured dairy from pasture-raised animals. Cultured dairy is made with probiotics, beneficial organisms that proliferate in the intestines. For a great resource to learn more about raw milk and to connect with raw dairy farmers in the USA and Canada, go to www.realmilk.com.

Where I live, raw cultured dairy is not legal to sell in stores, so honestly, I haven't tried it. Dairy is definitely "damp-inducing" for most of my patients and thus contributes to achy joints and muscles. If, however, raw cultured dairy was available, I'd definitely try it to see how my body would react. Jordan Rubin's Beyond Organic company sells raw cheese and low-temperature pasteurized whole milk from pastured green-fed, green-finished cows. I'm not sure that raw milk enthusiasts would endorse any sort of pasteurization, even low temperature, but we do know that the beneficial enzymes in milk are not killed using this method. Check out the

Resources chapter to view an article showing microscopic photos of raw milk versus low temperature pasteurized milk and decide for yourself.

Just in case you're worried about being calcium deficient, you should know that magnesium deficiency is by and large much more prevalent than calcium deficiency. Because the relative ratio of these two minerals in your body is so important, magnesium deficiency actually upsets the body's ability to use calcium properly. There is plenty of calcium in vegetables, so if your diet contains plenty of whole food, you needn't worry about calcium deficiency. I make bone broth almost every weekend in order to get the bone-building minerals and co-factors naturally found in animal bones. Worry more about getting enough magnesium.

Nutritional Myth #5: Caffeine is harmless

According to Traditional Chinese Medicine teachings, caffeine stresses the kidney organ. It also stresses the adrenal glands which produce the flight or fight reaction through neurotransmitters such as adrenaline. When these organs are stressed, it can actually weaken the corresponding muscle groups that are on the same neurological circuit. The psoas muscle, also called the hip flexor, is often unbalanced or weakened due to caffeine-related imbalances in the kidney organ according to holistic chiropractor, Dr. Bradley Nelson, creator of the Body Code Healing System. Dr. Nelson, who has literally seen thousands of people with back pain over his seventeen years in practice, feels that caffeine is the number one toxic substance contributing to chronic back pain.

Aside from causing pain, caffeine revs up your fight or flight response, literally draining your Qi (energy) stores. If you're one of these people who think it's great that you don't get stimulated by caffeine, think again. If you're not feeling stimulated and the caffeine is not disturbing your sleep, it means that your stress-handling system is already exhausted and is now in the danger zone. I find that once I get my patients off caffeine for a month or more, they regain the ability to produce the proper neurochemicals in response to caffeine. In other words, they start feeling jittery again (adrenaline rush) whenever they consume caffeine.

Lastly, the protein in coffee is the most common cross-reactor to gluten. Because it is the protein in the coffee that is the trigger, switching to decaf coffee does not solve the problem if you're like the one-in-three people who are gluten-sensitive.

Nutrition Advice All Experts Agree On

Depending on which expert's advice you choose to follow, it can be challenging to decide between a mostly plant-based diet, versus an omnivorous diet that includes meat because the studies are sometimes contradictory. All the experts, vegetarian or non-vegetarian, however, agree on some basic things that I want you to pay close attention to. Here are the recommendations:

- Eat little or no processed food.
- Eliminate excess sugar/sweetener consumption.
- Avoid soda.
- Avoid food with toxins such as pesticides, herbicides.
- Avoid food additives and chemicals such as MSG, aspartame, neotame, sucralose, food colorings, artificial flavors etc.
- Eat more whole foods, including more fruits and vegetables.
- Avoid fast food which is laden with sugar, rancid oils and additives.
- Avoid fried foods because the oil used to cook them is rancid.
- Avoid table salt because it is highly processed and devoid of minerals.
- Reduce consumptions of "white" refined carbohydrates, including anything made with white flour, white sugar and white rice.
- Fats like extra virgin olive oil, organic flaxseed oil and avocados are good for you.
- Raw foods, if your digestion can handle it, contain more "energy" or "Qi" than cooked foods, so include some in your diet, especially during the warmer months.
- Take a daily quality multivitamin/mineral supplement (preferably whole food variety).

Pain Relief Nutritional Guidelines

Now, let's see what you're willing to change in your diet in order to help your body heal faster. Below are three levels of dietary recommendations. The first level, Pain Relief Basic, is the simplest and the Pain Relief Advanced is the most challenging. Even if you know intuitively that you'd benefit the most from following the Advanced guidelines, don't beat yourself up if you really feel too overwhelmed or stressed to follow it right now. Do what you can. Any small amount of positive change can work wonders. When you're ready, you can move to the next level.

Pain Relief Basic Level

Start at this level if you don't understand the difference between processed food and whole food. Processed food is food that has been manufactured from its natural state into something that is often sold in bags, boxes, jars, cans and fancy cartons. Highly processed foods have much of the mineral nutrition taken out of it during processing. Some processed foods are more highly processed than others. You can tell often by the number of ingredients listed and whether you can pronounce them easily. For example, take ice cream. One brand may only have three or four ingredients such as cream, sugar, and vanilla, whereas another brand may have twenty ingredients including highly processed sugars such as high fructose corn syrup, soy (likely genetically modified), artificial flavors and colorings.

At this level, we will focus on minimizing the crappy . . . er, I mean, non-nutritious food and on increasing the more nutrient-dense foods. The food "avoid" list is longer than the "eat" list at this level because we need to make sure you're not poisoning your body when your goal is to heal your body from chronic pain. Read the list below and check off what strategies you're willing to undertake right now to improve your diet at this level:

Basic Level Avoid List:

- ☐ Artificial coloring
- ☐ Artificial flavors
- ☐ Monosodium glutamate (MSG, torula yeast, yeast extract)
- ☐ Products with artificial sweeteners including aspartame, neotame, saccharin and sucralose
- ☐ Products that contain high fructose corn syrup, corn syrup
- ☐ Soda of any type
- ☐ Junk food
- ☐ Pre-made foods in grocery stores such as TV dinners, coleslaw, breaded chicken, potato salad etc.
- ☐ Sugary foods especially those made with grains: cookies, cakes, pies, brownies etc.
- ☐ Processed food, especially if not made with certified organic ingredients
- ☐ White foods such as white bread, white sugar, white flour, white rice
- ☐ Non-organic junk food in general
- ☐ Foods containing trans-fats like margarines or fake buttery spreads. Look for words such as "partially hydrogenated" or "hydrogenated"
- ☐ Table salt
- ☐ Microwaving your food

Microwaving destroys the energetic structure of food and makes it "dead" so it becomes a foreign toxin that the body has to get rid of. Instead, bake, steam, lightly sauté your food. Reheating your food in a small toaster oven is also safe.

Basic Level Eating Guidelines:

- ☐ Eat more whole food, less processed food.
- ☐ Eat a variety of seasonal fruit and vegetables.
- ☐ Eat a colorful variety of vegetables daily, at least during lunch and dinner.

☐ Add more leafy greens to your diet, including raw if your digestion is hearty and can handle it.

☐ Eat more fish containing an abundance of beneficial Omega-3 oils like salmon and sardines.

☐ Chew your food deliberately and slowly.

☐ Sit while you're eating and focus on your meal.

☐ Use real raw honey that has never been heated (not for babies), stevia, maple syrup, coconut sap sugar, or unprocessed cane sugar as a sweetener if you need one, instead of white sugar or artificial sweeteners.

☐ Drink at least half your weight in ounces of purified water daily.

☐ Replace flavored drinks with healthy green tea, preferably organic.

Pain Relief Intermediate Level

Once you are comfortable with most of the guidelines in the Basic level, you are ready to move up to the intermediate level. Now that you have minimized your intake of processed foods, you can start being pickier about what you put in your body. At this level, we want to avoid toxins like pesticides, herbicides, antibiotics and hormones in our food. Conventionally-raised cattle are raised in tight quartered feed lots, standing in their own excrement for weeks on end. The animals are not allowed to pasture and feed on greens, their natural diet. Instead they are fed corn, a grain that is most often genetically modified, in order to fatten them up much faster than normal. The starchiness of the corn "marbles" the meat with fat, but is it any wonder why it can fatten us up too? Remember, the adage, "you are what you eat"? Well, we can now update that with "you are what you eat, and what *they* eat".

Eggs have been given a bad rap because of the cholesterol content of their yolks, but it is only oxidized cholesterol that may be truly harmful to our arteries and hearts (think powdered eggs). If you like eggs, cooking them in a way that keeps the yoke "runny" rather than cooked will minimize oxidation. The egg yolk is full of nutrients that the body can easily absorb, including twice as many antioxidants than are found in an apple: Vitamins A, B, C, D, E and K in addition to iron, biotin, zinc, lecithin and choline. All of these help contribute to brain function, healthy metabolism and disease prevention. The healthiest eggs to buy are from local farmers who let their hens pasture and eat what is in their natural environment. The yolks are often brighter yellow-orange as compared to eggs found in the supermarket.

Ask your local farmer if they supplement their chickens with soy or corn feed. If they do, make sure they are the organic varieties since most soy or corn is genetically modified. Pasture-raised hens produce eggs with more healthful levels of Omega-3's than are found in the eggs from conventionally raised hens. The living conditions for conventionally raised hens are inhumane and stressful. Chickens are lined up next to hundreds if not thousands of other chickens in caged pens and don't even have room to turn around. They, like the cows, may be fed genetically modified cornmeal, and some are bred so that their breasts grown unnaturally large, so much so, that some of these chickens can't even walk because they are so top-heavy! Check out Dr. Mercola's website www.mercola.com for some great videos on the subject. Once you've seen them, you'll never want to eat regular chicken ever again!

I'm not even going to talk about what they do to conventionally-raised pigs because the last video I saw almost made me vomit. There is much controversy in some nutrition circles on whether eating pork is healthy. Many religious groups traditionally avoid pork but it is not clear why. It is possible that parasites harboring in pigs are easily transferred to humans and thus the religious guidelines were created to avoid this problem.

Recently I read an interesting study from the Weston A. Price Foundation Newsletter that used dark field blood analysis to determine whether eating unmarinated pork caused any negative effects on the blood as compared with eating marinated pork. The study authors wanted to see if there was a scientifically valid reason why traditional cultures who consumed pork only did so after it was marinated. In this study, they compared unmarinated pork with pork marinated 24 hours with apple cider vinegar, pastured prosciutto and pastured bacon from the same local farm that raise pork humanely and without antibiotics or hormones. They also used unmarinated lamb as a control.

Fascinatingly, in three healthy volunteers, their blood analysis was completely normal when eating each of the meats, with the exception of when they consumed unmarinated pork. When they ate the unmarinated pork, their blood cells started stacking up on each other, an unhealthy state called rouleaux formation. Since reading this study, I've only eaten bacon from a regional source and the one time I forgot and ate pork pot roast at someone's house over Christmas, I immediately experienced hip pain. I deduced that I was having an inflammatory reaction in my gut which resulted in the hip pain.

In addition to the Basic Level guidelines, here are the guidelines for the next level which minimizes dairy and gluten.

Intermediate Level Guidelines:

- ☐ Choose organic produce over conventionally grown produce, especially the fruits and vegetables in the Dirty Dozen (see Resources), the ones most heavily laced with pesticides and herbicides.
- ☐ Choose local or pasture-raised sources of beef, goat, lamb, poultry, and eggs over conventionally raised sources.
- ☐ Choose local and/or humanely raised pork if you eat it and remember to marinate it overnight in the fridge (apple cider vinegar for example) before you cook it.
- ☐ Choose Wild Alaskan Salmon and low mercury tuna if you like tuna. I exclusively buy my raw sushi grade salmon from Vital Choice Seafood.
- ☐ If you eat processed food, try to choose the organic versions that have been minimally processed and have few ingredients.
- ☐ Eat leafy green vegetables daily if seasonal.
- ☐ Eat two different vegetables with lunch and dinner.
- ☐ Consider adding a "greens" superfood shake as part of your breakfast. I use Amazing Grass Chocolate Superfood shake but there are other good brands.
- ☐ Go gluten-free, sticking to organic whole grains including gluten-free whole oats, brown rice, quinoa, millet and amaranth, soaking or fermenting them for maximal nutritional digestion.
- ☐ Limit grains to one meal a day.
- ☐ Minimize outside dining and bring your own food when you travel whenever possible.

☐ Replace vegetable oils with organic extra virgin coconut oil, organic grass-fed butter or organic ghee for cooking.

☐ Reduce consumption of vegetable oils with the exception of olive oil for salads.

☐ Do not eat junk food (chips, candy, candy bars, cookies, cakes etc.).

☐ If you eat dairy, stick to raw or low-temperature pasteurized cultured dairy, such as kefir and max one serving per day.

☐ If you eat nuts and seeds, it is best to buy them soon after harvesting, and store them in the fridge to prevent rancidity.

☐ Use Celtic Sea Salt or Himalayan Crystal Salt (my favorite) in your food to add flavor and minerals.

☐ If you eat soy or corn, make sure it is non-GMO.

☐ Drink ½ your body weight in ounces of pure structured or spring water daily.

☐ Make bone broths and drink one cup daily.

Pain Relief Advanced Level

At this level, you will adopt everything in the basic and intermediate levels consistently. In addition, you will consciously rotate your food so that you are not eating the same things day after day. You will also be avoiding grains and dairy entirely. This is the ideal diet for someone with a long history of intestinal issues likely related to leaky gut. Once pain and abdominal symptoms are gone for a few months, you can start introducing gluten-free grains back into the diet slowly to see how you feel. Grain, however, should never be a staple in the Advanced diet, which is similar to the Paleolithic diet (also known as the Caveman or Primal diet).

Advanced Level Eating Guidelines:

☐ Eating exclusively organic fruits and vegetables; buying local whenever possible.

☐ Avoid all dairy except organic grass-fed butter or ghee.

☐ Add pasture-raised local eggs to your diet for extra nutrients and protein.

☐ Go grain-free (no gluten, corn, oatmeal, spelt, quinoa, rice etc.).

☐ Eat pastured and/or organic land animal meats two meals a day and consider adding nutrient-dense pastured organ meat on a regular basis.

☐ Make your own bone broths and drink 1 cup per day or cook it into your food.

☐ Rotate your foods every day as much as possible so that you are not always eating the same thing, which can require some creativity. Rotation helps to prevent the development of food sensitivities and gives you a more well-rounded nutritional profile.

☐ If you eat nuts and seeds, buy organic, and soak or sprout them before eating. If this is too much work, you can buy them sprouted online. They are absolutely delicious this way.

☐ If you eat legumes, make sure they are sprouted so that the anti-nutrients are washed away in the water used to soak them. Some people do not digest the nutrients from legumes very well and do better eating meat. I find this true of people who have blood type O. If you know your blood type, this may be helpful to you. Go to www.westonprice.org for more on sprouting your food. Beyond Organic also sells sprouted grain snacks in case you don't want to sprout them yourself. See Resources for link.

☐ If you eat soy, make sure it is organic and ideally fermented such as in miso, natto and tempeh because the nutrients are more bio-available that way and there are natural probiotics used in the fermenting.

☐ Eat grass-fed organic butter, extra virgin coconut or palm oil instead of using highly processed vegetable oils with the exception of expeller pressed organic olive oil and flaxseed oil which, when raw, is very healthy according to most nutrition experts.

☐ Add fresh raw organic vegetable juices that you juice yourself on a regular basis, daily if you like, unless you suffer from diarrhea. I use the Omega 350 Vertical Masticating juicer because the juice lasts for up to 72 hours unlike juice from centrifugal juicers. The device is easy to clean and has a small footprint thereby using up less counter space.

☐ Buy most of your meat and produce from local farmers markets when available. Otherwise shop at www.USWellnessMeats.com or Beyond Organic online stores.

☐ Shop almost exclusively at your local health food store for most of your other groceries instead of at the regular supermarket.

☐ Rarely dine in restaurants unless they purchase meats and produce from local farmers.

☐ If you like sushi, eat Vital Choice wild Alaskan salmon whenever you can. If you eat tuna, get low mercury tuna from Vital Choice.

☐ Make all your own salad dressings from scratch with organic olive and organic apple cider vinegar. Personally I love Carlson's Cod Liver Oil Lemon Flavored so much, it has become my favorite salad dressing! You can get it at most health food stores or online.

If you don't like to cook, eating healthy can seem like a chore because it takes more preparation than popping a frozen dinner into the microwave. During the work week, I have found it challenging to prepare quality meals for lunch and dinner, especially when I have limited time between work and skating. If you are super-busy like me and wish you had a personal chef, then I have a great resource for you.

While researching the "Paleo" diet lifestyle, I came across a company who makes delicious gluten-free, grain-free, sugar-free, soy-free, dairy-free meals using local organic seasonal vegetables and grass-fed, hormone-free meat. These meals are made by a *real* Paleo chef (and athlete), Chef Richard Bradford.

Guess what? Chef Richard and his team freezes these flavorful cooked meals in BPA-free, gluten-free sealed plastic and can send them straight to your home! At approximately $11 per meal (5oz. meat and 7 oz. vegetables), these pre-made paleo meals actually save me time and money. Because of the quality of produce and meat I usually buy at the natural food store, I spend just as much when I cook it myself. Furthermore, the propane used to cook my meals and heat my water to wash dishes adds to the cost and inconvenience.

The pre-made paleo meals take approximately five to ten minutes to reheat on the stove, thus saving me preparation time. That means I have plenty of time to eat a relaxing dinner before I going skating. Doing the dishes takes a few minutes rather than a whole half hour. We eat Chef Richard's yummy creations for lunch and dinner five days a week. On the weekends, my partner and I enjoy cooking, since we can take our time.

Chef Richard and I got together and created a meal pack just for people who want to eat well and heal their chronic pain. We call it the Dr. Karen's Pain Relief Success Pack and you can find it at www.karenkan.com/painreliefpaleo. This is a special pack that contains grass-fed beef, turkey and chicken, and the vegetables dishes are nightshade-free (since some people with arthritis are sensitive to nightshade vegetables such as eggplant, bell peppers, tomatoes and potatoes).

Is Eating Healthy Expensive?

It may seem to the average American that eating organic is much more expensive than purchasing cheap subsidized food products made by the corporate food giants. The price tag of most organic food is indeed higher than conventional food, but making choices based solely on the sticker price is like robbing Peter to pay Paul. Eating toxic or nutrient-sparse food is going to cost you one way or another. If you could add up the true cost of poor eating, including medical bills, prescription drugs, time away from work, poor quality of life because of chronic diseases, and early death, it would be a no-brainer to eat well. Furthermore, I have found that when people truly eat quality food, they actually are less hungry and may consume less food overall because the body is getting the nourishment it needs with fewer empty calories.

Nutritional Supplements

I was taught, erroneously, in medical school that if my patients ate a healthy diet, they would never require supplements. Unfortunately, most of us have not eaten purely organic food our entire lives and our soil was deemed nutrient depleted even back in the 1930s. Can you imagine the nutrient depletion in our soils today with mono-culture agribusinesses producing most of the food in America? It's not a pretty thought. You'd have to eat a heck of a lot of food to make up for what our food system lacks. Furthermore, you need supplements to repair an unhealthy body.

In my practice, supplements are chosen individually for each patient based on their muscle testing. That being said, there are some basic supplements that are safe and beneficial that I recommend to almost everyone, especially those with chronic pain. I've listed these below. Keep in mind that the dosages that I recommend to patients can really vary based on their muscle testing, so the dose ranges I've given below fall under the most "common" recommended doses. Links to some of the brands I've listed appear in the Resources chapter.

Hydration Supplements

As I mentioned in the chapter on hydration, there are many ways to get structured water. If you haven't read that chapter yet, you might want to do that now. If you have an old natural spring nearby, this may be your best bet. You might like to use Willard Water® supplements to make the water clusters smaller so that you get more water into your cells. I've noticed an appreciable difference in how my body feels when I use the Willard Water® versus when I don't. When I use the Willard Water® consistently, my bowel movements are better, my body feels less thirsty, and my skating ability is improved. Cellular hydration is essential if you're experiencing chronic pain.

Probiotics

Probiotics play an important role in healing the gut and I think everyone should be taking them, especially if they've ever been on antibiotics or long term medications such as birth control or anti-inflammatory drugs. Taking probiotics is a must in our modern society. With the daily onslaughts of toxins and chemicals we are exposed to, our immune system needs all the help it can get. The gut, functioning as an important part of our immune and nervous systems, stays healthy when it has enough "good" bacteria or yeast supporting it.

Natural probiotics can be found in fermented foods and cultured dairy although I always recommend taking a supplement. The brands I'm currently using the most that you can purchase online include: Culturelle®,

RAW Probiotics by Garden of Life®, Prescript-Assist™, and Ethical Nutrients™ Intestinal Care DF and Florastor®. In the office, I also use Genestra™ HMF Replete and Integrative Therapeutics™ Enterogenic Intensive 100 (100 billion CFU per capsule) and Syntol AMD. Available in pharmacies only is a brand called VSL#3® which contains 112.5 CFU per capsule. A minimum of 10 billion CFU's daily is preferred, and many people require more in order to rebalance their intestinal flora.

A large number of people in my practice have an overgrowth of pathogenic yeast/fungus in their intestines, most likely from the use of antibiotics. For these folks, many do well with Syntol AMD, a probiotic/prebiotic combination product that also contains specific enzymes to digest the cell walls of dead yeast attached to the bowel wall. A prebiotic is a supplement that contains fiber "food" for the healthy bacteria probiotics. The ones in Syntol AMD tend to cause less intestinal gas than do other prebiotic formulas.

Often when one uses probiotics, the dying yeast can cause a severe "die-off" reaction as the cells burst open. Its contents ferment in our bodies before they can be removed. This detoxification reaction, also known as the Herxheimer reaction, can cause symptoms of fatigue, feverishness, chills, muscle aches, flu-like symptoms, headache and rash. Syntol AMD has the ability to digest cellular components of the dead yeast before they ferment and cause uncomfortable detoxification reactions. In my practice I use muscle testing to determine the best brand of probiotics for each patient along with the optimal dose.

Magnesium

Magnesium is highly deficient in our society yet serves a vital function in over 300 biochemical reactions in our body. Magnesium deficiency causes weak bones, muscular contraction and pain. Toxins can accumulate due to magnesium deficiency which can also cause or contribute to chronic pain. Without magnesium, your cells cannot manufacture the molecule of energy, ATP.

For people in chronic pain who do not have diarrhea, I will use a combination of oral magnesium in the form of an amino acid chelate, such as magnesium glycinate or magnesium bisglycinate, and transdermal magnesium oil or lotion. Oral dosages commonly range from 300 to 800 mg a day in divided doses, cutting back if one experiences diarrhea. If someone has fibromyalgia, I'll often use Ethical Nutrients Malic Magnesium tablets (also called Metagenics™ Fibroplex when you get it from your doctor). Transdermal magnesium doses range from 10 sprays to upwards of 48 sprays per day for Ancient Minerals magnesium oil or around three teaspoons of Ancient Minerals magnesium lotion per day. Again, in my practice, I will muscle test each patient to determine his optimal dose.

Another form of magnesium I'm using more and more is liquid ionic magnesium. The brand I use is called Nutrilink Mag Force and it is available online at www.nutrilinkenergy.com. Mag Force uses state-of-the-art technology to reduce magnesium to the smallest atomic level so that assimilation in the cells is enhanced. Unlike other ionic magnesium formulas, Mag Force is "charged" with subtle energy. In other words, it is "alive" with Qi whereas most other formulas have not been enhanced this way. I also use their Nutrilink Mineral Force formula in the morning. It is also "charged" with subtle energy. You may wish to get both. The only major disadvantage of the Nutrilink formulas is that they need to be refrigerated and they are difficult to transport when you are travelling because they are liquids.

Currently, I take upwards of nine Metagenics™ Fibroplex (Ethical Nutrients Malic Magnesium) per day in divided doses as that is what my body muscle tests for. Sounds like a huge dose, I know, but people with a history of fibromyalgia often require that much. In addition, I use about 3 teaspoons of magnesium lotion in the morning and about one ounce of Nutrilink Mag Force before bed. Often, I also take about an ounce of Mineral Force in the morning with my green superfood shake.

Fish Oil

The omega-3 fats found in fish oil act as an anti-inflammatory agent in our bodies. There are also many plant sources of omega-3, such as flax, walnuts and hemp, but many people cannot efficiently convert these short-chain omega-3 fats to the forms needed by our bodies. Fish such as wild Alaskan salmon or sardines contain healthy omega-3 oils. Interestingly, grass-fed meat has similar omega-3 profiles, but conventionally raised meat does not. If you do not eat omega-3-rich fish or grass-fed meat several times a week, you should consider taking fish oil.

When it comes to fish oil, it is important to buy a quality brand. There are many brands on the market, so it is important for you to purchase a brand that is as pure as possible and thus safer and more effective. I do not trust brands you can get over the counter in drug stores, mainly because their production standards are not ideal and they only meet the minimum American standards for purity. Furthermore, many are made by pharmaceutical companies who do not necessarily have your best interests at heart. What you are looking for are brands that process the fish within hours of catching it. This requires smaller fishing practices.

Norwegians are well known for their higher standards of fish oil, so purchasing brands like Nordic Naturals® or Carlson's® will guarantee fresher oil. Certain brands like Quell™ and Minami use a toxin-free low temperature process that supposedly maintains the healthy structure of the oil so that it doesn't get heat-damaged. Of late, I've been gravitating to minimally-processed salmon oil because the antioxidant astaxanthin is naturally part of the oil and it is helpful to those experiencing chronic pain. I've been using Biopure™ because my colleague, neurotoxin expert, Dr. Dietrich Klinghardt searched the world over to find the best fish oil which could be made available to regular consumers.

Some experts have been using krill oil instead of fish oil because it contains more concentrated omega-3's and has been shown to be more effective in lowering cholesterol than the same dose of fish oil. Since we know that cholesterol is the result of inflammation, it makes sense that krill oil may work for those in chronic pain. I haven't used it much in my practice yet because I'm waiting for more scientific data before making the switch. Keep in mind that krill oil is often twice as expensive as high quality fish oil. As long as I know krill is sustainably harvested, it might be a great new supplement to add to my practice.

Many holistic nutrition experts feel that fermented cod liver oil is the best Omega-3 oil to consume because of the fat soluble Vitamins A and D contained naturally in this oil. The only brand available in the United States is Green Pasture, available online through several distributors. Top nutritionists at the Weston A. Price Foundation feel that the nutritional combination of fermented cod liver oil and high vitamin butter oil helps us assimilate the minerals and vitamins better into our bodies as compared with taking other forms of Omega-3's. I take a teaspoon of this combination every day.

Multivitamin/Mineral

Whatever you do, please don't run out to the drug store and purchase a cheap multivitamin/mineral formula. So many drugstore brands have thick waxy coatings that your body can't digest (containing high levels of magnesium stearate), using artificial colors and dyes to make them look palatable. These vitamins are made from isolated pharmaceutical grade ingredients. For specific clinical purposes I still use the purest forms of isolated vitamin or mineral formulas when necessary, but in general, I prefer whole food vitamin/mineral supplements. As usual, I will muscle test my patients to see what their bodies are saying is best for them.

The two brands I'm currently recommending are Innate Response Formulas® and Garden of Life®. Granted whole food supplements are more expensive, but the body assimilates and absorbs whole food nutrients better than isolated nutrients. Furthermore, both products are raw as well as free of dairy, soy and gluten. Both brands have age-specific multivitamin/ mineral formulas. I recommend that you research them and see which one you want to try. Innate Response Formulas® is available through healthcare practitioners, whereas, Garden of Life® is available through health food stores and online. Although the former is available online as well, the company does not guarantee the quality of the product if sold by discount supply houses or Amazon.

Vitamin D₃

Vitamin D is a fat soluble vitamin that is clearly deficient in most of my chronic pain patients even though it is a natural vitamin that your skin produces during sun exposure. Eating quality animal meat will more likely give you better levels of Vitamin D because it is fat soluble, but adding fermented cod liver oil may be helpful to boost Vitamin D levels as well.

Vitamin D deficiency is the rule rather than the exception in the northern hemisphere. My patients often forget to take it during the summer months because they are in the sun so much but when I retest them in the fall, their levels have invariably dropped. Some experts advocate buying a tanning bed, but many people have difficulty producing Vitamin D in their skin due to age or illness. Vitamin D deficiency can increase your risk of joint and bone problems, as well as colon, prostate and possibly breast cancer. There are 600 receptor sites in the body for Vitamin D including the brain and the heart. One of the reasons I recommend it for those in chronic pain is because Vitamin D deficiency contributes to chronic muscle pain.

Vitamin D$_3$ is also called cholecalciferol and is considered the more active and bioavailable form of Vitamin D$_3$ to take. The average dose required in most adults is 5000IU daily. Most allopathic doctors will balk at how "high" that dose sounds, but if you ask for a blood test, the 25-hydroxy Vitamin D level, you want to aim for a result of 50-80ng/mL. Levels under 30ng/mL are considered deficient, whereas levels over 100ng/mL (rare without supplementation) may be toxic. Even with daily supplementation of Vitamin D$_3$ in doses of 5000 to 10,000IU daily, your levels will not rise very quickly. You may wish to recheck your levels every few months to make sure you're in the healthy range. If, however, your levels are dangerously low (below 20ng/mL), then you may want to recheck your levels within a month, just to make sure you're absorbing the brand you're taking.

By the way, if your doctor insists on giving you the prescription Vitamin D$_2$ (ergocalciferol) 50,000IU once a week, don't bother. Firstly, I had patients whose Vitamin D levels didn't improve with this dosing so I switched them back to a natural supplement at 5000IU daily. Secondly, I had a patient who told me that she started having stomach pain after starting the prescription Vitamin D$_2$ and guessed it was something to do with the "green gel" coloring they used in the pharmaceutical. We stopped it and her stomach pain disappeared. Understand that in order for a pharmaceutical company to patent and thus make money off a natural substance, they must mutate it because natural supplements aren't patentable. When drug companies have to artificially change the structure of the Vitamin in order to sell it and make money, it makes it hard for people like me to trust how safe and effective it truly is. I'd rather stick to the more natural forms.

Getting enough "healthy" fat in your diet not only helps you with your Vitamin D levels, but also helps you absorb Vitamin K (from animal fat) which improves the way calcium gets integrated into stronger bones. Vitamin K_2 is considered important to prevent calcium from being deposited in arteries and joints. Vitamin K is produced in the intestines by the "good" bacteria. One study showed that taking broad-spectrum antibiotics can severely reduce Vitamin K production in the gut by nearly 74% in people compared with those not taking these antibiotics. Diets low in animal meat can also cause low Vitamin K levels. One form of Vitamin K_2, called menaquinone-4 (MK-4), is available in animal meat. The other is menaquinone-7 (MK-7) which is made from natto (fermented soy) can be purchased as a supplement. People at risk of low Vitamin K should probably take a supplement in the form of MK-7 along with their Vitamin D_3, especially if they are vegetarian.

I use several different "doctor-only" Vitamin D brands in the office, but I suggest you start with a whole food version that is available to non-practitioners from Garden of Life® called Vitamin Code® Raw D_3. Alternatively, I'd recommend taking Green Pasture fermented cod liver oil which includes Vitamin D as well as other nutrients that help its absorption. In my office, I also use Pure Encapsulations® and Innate Response Formulas® Vitamin D_3. The latter includes Vitamin K as well as Vitamin D.

Vitamin C

Vitamin C is so important in many holistic circles that some health centers offer high dose Vitamin C by intravenous drip. Vitamin C helps with wound healing, supports healthy detoxification, and neutralizes harmful free radicals. Because I use the LifeWave Y-Age Glutathione patches every day, I know that my own Vitamin C gets regenerated to some extent. Contrary to what we were taught in medical school, large doses of Vitamin C do not seem to cause kidney stones in people.

Because it is water soluble, unlike Vitamin D, it is more beneficial to dose it several times a day rather than to take one giant dose, especially if you have a chronic illness. Because it can cause loose stools and gas at higher doses, this may be a good reason to limit each dose to 2000mg. Everyone's dose is individual and in general, most patients in my practice muscle test for between 3000 and 10,000mg a day. When someone has or is about to get a respiratory infection, we usually bump up the dose. Interestingly, the higher dose does not contribute to loose bowel movements until the patient begins feeling better from his respiratory illness. At that point, the patient knows to cut back on his Vitamin C dose.

There are many forms of Vitamin C including the cheaper ascorbic acid, mineral ascorbates and whole food Vitamin C. Brands I recommend include Metagenics™ Ultra Potent-C, Garden of Life® Vitamin Code RAW Vitamin C, and Emergen-C® and Country Life Acerola chewables with bioflavenoids for those who don't mind the 3 grams of sugar. Some are more expensive than others, but in my practice I just muscle test to see what would work best for each individual patient.

Digestive Enzymes

Many of my patients who have chronic pain do not have the ability to make adequate amounts of digestive enzymes to stay healthy. Digestive enzymes are necessary not just to digest your food in your digestive tract, but also to digest cellular debris such as decayed cells, fibrin, fatty proteins, and other unwanted materials that normally accumulate in the blood. Debris in the blood can make the blood cells stick together. Not only can this cause pain in some people, it can cause blood clots in others and is considered a primary cause of heart attacks due to blocked arteries.

If you have digestive issues, it may be beneficial for you to take digestive enzymes with your meals. I use several brands including Innate Response Formulas® Digestive Enzymes Clinical Strength, Garden of Life® RAW Enzymes, and Enzymus Medical Devigest ADS. The latter includes high levels of specific enzymes to digest dairy and gluten but isn't appropriate for people with low stomach acid conditions because it contains bicarbonate.

Often as we age, our ability to make stomach acid declines. Certain people need additional hydrochloric acid in order to digest their food and nutrients properly, especially the elderly. Holistic nutritionists often recommend taking a tablespoon of organic apple cider vinegar in a glass of water and sipping the concoction over dinner. Betaine HCL is a supplement that can also help boost stomach acid. Unbeknownst to most people, a lack of stomach acid can manifest the same type of "acid reflux" symptoms as too much stomach acid. In fact, the latter condition is fairly rare.

Long term use of acid reflux medications is harmful because they prevent the proper digestion of food. In addition there isn't enough acid to kill unwanted parasites and bacteria found sometimes in ingested food. If swallowing apple cider vinegar in water or taking Betaine HCL produces a significant burning feeling in your stomach, you probably don't need it. If it has no effect, it means that you probably could use some extra acid.

In addition, taking specific enzymes between meals in order to remove debris from your blood may be extremely helpful in relieving chronic pain symptoms. These are what we call systemic enzymes. Adequate blood flow to your muscles and joints depends on free-flowing blood. Enzyme blends have been shown to decrease inflammatory levels and improve muscle and joint stiffness. Wobenzym® PS is popular among holistic physicians treating people in chronic pain. Serracor NK and Enzymus Neprinol AFD are also helpful for patients with fibromyalgia and arthritis. Using digital blood microscopy, researchers have documented that using systemic enzymes such as these helps to reduce the debris (dead tissue and cellular components) in the blood. This may be the mechanism whereby they effectively decrease chronic joint and muscle pain.

Eating Well is Lifelong Choice

If you give your body the proper fuel so that it can function optimally, get rid of toxins and repair damaged tissue, your chronic pain may become yesterday's news. Eating well shouldn't be considered a fly-by-night pursuit, however, just to get rid of pain. When most people start making positive changes in their diet a remarkable thing happens. They start making other positive changes in their life. They start feeling happier and have more energy. They make better decisions most likely because their brains are functioning better. In a short amount of time, "bad" food choices no longer taste good to them, and in fact, they can start craving organic salads, fruits and vegetables instead of pasta, cookies, cakes and chips.

These days, even if I happen to eat a gluten-free organic chocolate chip cookie that is fresh from the oven, I definitely don't yearn for another because my body says "enough" because the cookie is too sweet. Snacks I used to be addicted to often don't appeal to me any longer because they taste unsatisfying. I don't overeat like I used to anymore, especially since I began juicing regularly and eating more "paleo". So don't worry that you're going to miss all your favorite foods. A lot of my past favorite foods no longer taste good to me because my body just simply rejects them and I'm literally no longer attracted to them. Instead I crave things like roasted organic beets, locally grown grape tomatoes, organic pea shoots or bone broth.

Unlike most of the doctors who might tell you that it is "normal" for your body to break down as you age, I'm going to tell you otherwise. Your body will function well if you treat it well and the aging process can be reversed. Nutrition is just one piece of the puzzle, but an important one. Developing lifelong healthy eating habits will not only keep you healthier and happier, you'll age gracefully and have a greater opportunity to enjoy life. It's well worth the effort. Believe me.

Chapter Summary

- Without nutrients, the body has a hard time healing itself and malnourishment is a cause of chronic pain.
- There are many nutritional myths. Understanding the truth will result in your understanding what to eat to make up a nutrient-rich diet.
- There are three pain relief nutritional guidelines outlined in this chapter. Choose the one you want to start with and make the dietary changes you resonate with most.
- Eating poorly is much more expensive in the long run than eating well.
- Supplements are almost always necessary to support the body in healing itself.
- Make eating well a lifelong habit and your body will respond by slowing or even reversing the aging process.

19

MOVE THE BODY—MOVE THE QI

Exercise is a necessary component of healing. Even if you've been inactive due to pain or lack of motivation, it is vital that you move your body. Now I'm not suggesting that you go from couch potato to marathon running, the latter not being particularly healthy for the average chronic pain patient. Some degree of body movement is highly desirable because the energy that flows in our channels can get "stuck" especially with ill-health. In Traditional Chinese Medicine, the stuck energy is called stagnant Qi. Stagnant Qi is having roadblocks every few feet on the energetic highway of the body. Not only can it cause chronic pain, it can prevent other body and organ systems from functioning optimally.

Daily body movement is ideal. If you haven't been particularly active, you'll have to take it easy at first and do what feels manageable. In this chapter I will describe a few different types of movement forms that are suited to many people with chronic pain. Some are easier than others and I'll try to be clear on what form of exercise is best for those with different types of pain conditions.

If you're already an athlete, like me, or have stayed fairly active despite having chronic pain, it will be easier for you to incorporate other healthy forms of movement. Sometimes, however, I find that my patients push past their body's limits and thus keep re-injuring themselves due to lack of awareness or just plain stubbornness. It is good to keep moving, but it isn't good to ignore your body's pain signals to the point of pain. The types of movement forms I describe in this chapter are fairly well tolerated and some will actually help balance out the body so that you will be able to return to the other types of activities you used to do and enjoy.

For example, if you're an avid downhill skier, I want you to be able to ski to your heart's content. If you've missed golfing because of chronic pain, I want you to heal in order to able to return to golfing. If you hate raking, however, I'd much rather you hire someone else to do it instead. Martyrdom and obligatory "chores" that are known to cause pain are absolutely not helpful in the healing process and set you up to feel victimized.

Instead of giving you the usual spiel about getting enough aerobic exercise, I'm going to share with you my specific suggestions for exercises that aid in healing chronic pain. It doesn't mean you shouldn't do aerobic exercise that raises the heart rate and exercises the cardiovascular system. I'm just not going to be covering that ground here where our focus is on pain relief.

Qi Gong & Tai Chi

Chinese Qi gong exercises are generally gentle and are designed to move the Qi, the energy, within the energy channels as well as boost your energy "battery". Qi gong is an ancient form of movement and there are many different teachings. I had a friend, Toni, who told me once that she went to several Qi Gong classes and got nothing out of them, but yet everyone else in the class was raving about its beneficial effects. The type of Qi Gong she was learning entailed sitting in a cross-legged position and imagining the Qi flowing up and down her channels. Even though she was a good at visualizing, she just couldn't experience the immense value others did. I told her that for her body, she may actually need to move her body in order to get the same beneficial effect.

The Qi Gong I am most familiar with is a simple set of exercises called the Eight Silken Movements. It was originally derived from a complex set of approximately 64 exercises, but eventually was distilled to just eight so that the average person could learn and master them. A few of the movements may still seem difficult if you haven't been able to bend forward, for example, because of back discomfort. If you are interested in learning Qi Gong and there are no Qi Gong practitioners nearby, I recommend that you check out Spring Forest Qi Gong. It is probably the best known home study course available and there have been some independent studies validating Spring Forest Qi Gong as an effective modality for chronic pain. There is a free video at www.SpringForestQigong.com with Master Chunyi Lin on moving the Yin and Yang energy. If you enjoy this easy exercise, like I did, then Qi Gong would be an excellent way to circulate the energy in your body and to balance your energy for self-healing.

Qi Gong movements tend to be gentle, deliberate and slow. Although it may look incredibly easy, focusing on the energy and breath as you do the exercises takes a little bit of practice. Just like anything new, it might seem a little foreign when you first begin, but like many others, you may derive intense pleasure, calmness and pain relief with practice.

Look up Qi Gong practitioners in your local area. It really helps to have a teacher with whom you enjoy working. If you can't find one, you may wish to join the Spring Forest Qi Gong community online. If chronic pain has really restricted your ability to exercise, Qi Gong may be the best movement form to try first.

Tai Chi, another Chinese movement form, is gaining popularity in the West. It is considered a slow-moving martial art and even small towns like the one I live in has several Tai Chi teachers. In Hong Kong and China, it is common to see elderly people practicing Tai Chi together every morning in the park. It keeps them supple and strong. From the very young to the very old, Qi Gong and Tai Chi exercises are simple yet beneficial. I believe that it not only helps to condition the body, but also the mind and spirit.

Tai Chi for Arthritis is a special Tai Chi program created by Dr. Paul Lam. It is easy to learn and safe even for the elderly. Studies have shown that this program relieves pain and improves quality of life. Many arthritis foundations worldwide are supporting it. With over 15,000 certified instructors worldwide, millions of people have benefitted from this simple program. For more information, go to www.TaiChiforArthritis.com.

Cellercising

I love bouncing up and down on my Cellerciser. It looks like a rebounding mini-trampoline, but has very specific features that separate it from other rebounders. In fact, I highly discourage anyone with pain to buy a cheap rebounder because it may cause jarring injury to the joints. When you lift weights, you exercise a particular muscle against the forces of gravity. When you Cellercise, every single one of your 75 trillion cells are being "exercised"-in fact over 100 times gravity! This beneficial stress to the cell walls helps strengthen them.

Even our internal organs get benefit from bouncing up and down on the Cellerciser. When our connective tissues get weak, our organs and other body parts tend to sag. By Cellercising, you can reverse this trend because all of your connective tissues are being exercised, not just your muscles. In addition to conditioning your body's cells, you may experience better sleep, less stress and improved lymphatic draining (and removal of toxins) just by Cellercising 10 minutes a day.

After enjoying my own Cellerciser, a friend brought his own rebounder to my office so we could do a head-to-head comparison. I won't name the brand, but let's just say his rebounder was one of the best-selling brands in gyms in the United States. It really looked like a replica of the Cellerciser and I couldn't tell the difference between the two until I jumped on it.

My friend's rebounder was significantly lighter than my heavy-duty Cellerciser. It was difficult to open and I could see from the side that although my friend had hardly used it, the frame was actually warped! I jumped on his a few times, then jumped on mine. Jumping on his rebounder had a hard "end feel" at the bottom of the bounce. It didn't bother me that much, but I could feel the difference. Mine, on the other hand, had a soft "end feel" and the material didn't cave in. To achieve even more objectivity, I asked my acupuncture colleague, Ann, to lightly bounce on both and give us feedback. She first bounced lightly on my Cellerciser, then on my friend's rebounder. Within a few bounces on my friend's rebounder, she stopped and said, "This one is hurting my knee" and got off. Ann didn't have major knee issues but she developed pain all the same using the cheaper rebounder.

The Cellerciser is made with the patented soft-bounce digitized triple-tiered tapered TRI-FLEX™ spring. The triple-tiered tapered spring adjusts to the weight of the user automatically. The Cellerciser is the only piece of equipment with this patented spring which is made of hi-carbon steel wire with an excellent annealing/temper-treated finish. Typical rebounders often use a canvas, nylon or plastic mats that can stretch, rot, or mildew. The inferior material, weave and stitching can cause the feet to sink or pronate toward the middle causing ankle problems, knee problems, and lower back problems. The Cellerciser mat is woven with space-age materials that do not wear out despite consistent use, and it discourages your feet from pronating (turning inwards) while you bounce. I've had mine for over five years and I've never had to replace a spring. If it squeaks a bit, you can oil the springs with some essential oil. Then it is extremely quiet.

The Cellerciser comes in two models. The Half-Fold folds in half and has a carrying case that you can sling over your shoulder. The Tri-Fold model is heavy-duty and can fold neatly into a triangular formation into a case that has wheels. I've taken it on trips with me, although it's pretty heavy to lift in and out of a car so I usually have James help me with that. The Half-Fold costs around $393 and the Tri-fold around $499 and both come with a balance bar which I highly recommend. If you purchase a Cellerciser online, add the extra 2-hr DVD "Cellercise-The Ultimate Exercise" to your cart. Then when you checkout, use coupon code *DRKAREN* so that you get the DVD free. I just bought this DVD ($40 value) and it's awesome!

When first Cellercising, use the balance bar at all times until your strength and balance increases. The bar is meant to be loose so that you learn to keep your balance with minimal gripping. You'd be amazed at how many out-of-shape people feel wobbly the first time they use the Cellerciser! Even people who exercise daily (such as walking) can have difficulty because their current exercise regimen doesn't test their balance or equilibrium.

The reason I recommend the Cellerciser is two-fold. Firstly, it is a great exercise to move the lymphatic fluid in the body. The lymphatic channels are an important part of our detoxification system. The lymph channels don't have a muscle pump like the circulatory system. Thus, lymphatic fluids only move with the help of muscle action from the arm and leg. Even lightly bouncing on the Cellerciser with two feet barely off the mat, an exercise called the Baby Bounce, can profoundly improve your lymphatic circulation, which in turn, can help you get rid of toxins and heal your body.

Unless you're already a conditioned athlete, I'd recommend starting out with just two to five minute sessions of Baby Bouncing one to three times a day. Stand with both feet on the Cellerciser about hip-width apart and just bounce lightly. Keep your knees soft and your hands lightly touching the balance bar for support. After a week of this, you may wish to try some of the other exercises shown in the book or on the DVD.

It feels so good to bounce that it can be addicting. Five minutes go by quickly especially if you're playing your favorite tunes on the stereo as you bounce. Remember how natural it was as a child to be jumping on the bed or couch? Children intuitively gravitate to jumping on beds because it is fun but also because it feels good to bounce. Cellercising is the grown-up way to getting healthier while having fun.

The second reason I recommend the Cellerciser is that *all* the cells in your body are actually flexing and stretching while you bounce! If you put your right hand over your left shoulder muscle while you bounce gently, you'll feel this muscle contracting and relaxing with each bounce. It is quite an incredible feeling. Your nervous system is also getting a tune-up. Your balance can improve almost immediately after Cellercising just for a few minutes as demonstrated in the $40 Cellercise DVD. Lastly, Cellercising may be more efficient than biking or walking as an aerobic exercise so you can save some time as well as your joints while you exercise.

The people that may not be able to tolerate bouncing are people with severe neck injuries or headache. If that's you, then you'll have to try some of the other movement forms I recommend first. I watched a demonstration by Cellerciser inventor David Hall where he actually bounced someone therapeutically. A woman with chronic unrelenting pain was instructed to lie on the Cellerciser, her head resting on a pillow and her legs propped up on a chair. David then proceeded to straddle her torso and gently bounce on the Cellerciser for several minutes. If you ever have the opportunity to have someone "bounce" you, it is a heavenly feeling, sort of like being rocked to sleep.

After the demonstration, the woman had no more pain. Even the next day, she proclaimed that her pain was completely gone and apparently it never returned. I'm not absolutely certain about the mechanism of healing in this instance but I suspect that the bouncing "reset" this woman's nervous system.

Meridian Stretching

I absolutely love meridian stretching. When done as a stretch as well as a resistance exercise, it makes me sweat very quickly! It is called Meridian Stretching because each of the main stretches work on each of your primary acupuncture meridians. By doing Meridian Stretching, the flow of energy improves in the meridians. Not only do you become more flexible, but also your pain levels go down and your overall energy goes up. Balancing your meridians via Meridian Stretching also has wonderful side benefits when it comes to your mind and spirit.

The meridians that are the most "stuck" will tend to propagate similar stuck emotions. By stretching the tight meridians, the stuck emotions tend to naturally heal themselves. According to the creator, Bob Cooley, who suffered debilitating pain after being hit by a car, when the meridians become more balanced, you will naturally gravitate to things that are for your highest and greatest good. So in other words, you'll likely find yourself reaching for an apple instead of cheesecake!

Meridian stretching is unlike anything I have tried before. The idea is that you resist the stretch the entire time using the same muscle groups you are stretching. It's hard to explain it so you should check out some of the Flexible Strength YouTube videos to get an idea of how to do these exercises. I have them on a playlist on my YouTube channel: www.YouTube.com/karenkanmd. I can only do about six or eight repetitions of each stretch (especially if I resist both directions) at a time because it is so intense.

When done correctly, you won't injure yourself, which is possible with passive stretching. Passive stretching is what we learned in grade school. In passive stretching, the muscle you are stretching is allowed to be relaxed as you are stretching it. For people who are really tight, however, I have found that passive stretching can actually tear muscle tissue and cause injuries. Meridian stretching, on the other hand, requires you to resist the force of the stretch for the entire time. Having the muscle you are stretching fully engaged in a state of contraction prevents it from being overstretched or torn by accident.

Although I am considered quite flexible compared to most people in their forties, I had lost a lot of flexibility because of my illness. I remember the first time I tried meridian stretching. I was shocked at how "warm" I got after just a few stretches. I could feel the fibrous tissue of my fascia finally stretch so that my muscles and joints could move more freely. It was a feeling I never felt before with regular passive stretching. With time you may be able to use maximal resistance when doing the stretch and that allows for old scar tissue to be broken up.

Having a certified Meridian Stretching trainer help you stretch makes it easier for people with co-ordination problems or who have difficulty understanding how to do exercises from a book or video, both of which are available on the Meridian Stretching website. For more information on Meridian Stretching, or to find a certified professional, go to www.meridianflexibility.com.

Yoga

Yoga has grown in popularity so much so that almost every town in America has a yoga class. It isn't hard to find certified yoga instructors. Even if it looks intimidating from photos you may have seen where yoginis are stretched into pretzel-like shapes, don't be scared to try it. I was using a Rodney Yee yoga videotape long before I was able to get into a real class. I really liked it and eventually got to attend a couple of live classes with Rodney himself. You can do yoga in the privacy of your home using DVDs, but finding a beginner's class with a good instructor is ideal. The problem with home-study is that it is easy to get into bad habits. It made a world of difference when I actually got professional instruction.

If you have many yoga teachers in your town, try them all out. It is important that you resonate with your teacher. Some people like teachers who have a more masculine energy. Often that masculine energy appeals to followers of Bikram Yoga (done in a heated room), Ashtanga/Power Yoga, and Kundalini Yoga. Of course, I'm generalizing, but I think most seasoned yoga practitioners would agree that certain yoga types are more Yang (masculine energy) than others. If you have significant pain, however, I would recommend that you start with Hatha or Iyengar yoga which is more Yin (feminine energy). In fact, ask the yoga studio whether they have a *restorative* class. Even though there is a lot of resting in restorative yoga, it is amazing what it can do for the body. Restorative yoga is the ultimate form of Yin energy. If you are a super-busy-achiever type of person, then Yin is really what you need, even if you naturally gravitate to more challenging exercise.

Whether you'll enjoy yoga and whether it is safe for you ultimately depends on your teacher. I've been with teachers who are very experienced, but who aren't intuitive and I've hurt myself. Other teachers, sensing my tendency towards competitiveness, have nipped my compulsive perfectionism in the bud and have gently supported my yoga in becoming softer and more forgiving.

The one thing I want you to know about yoga is that how you breathe is as equally important as how you move. Yogic breathing, which is breathing through expanding the belly, has benefits all by itself. When you learn this type of breathing, you can apply it to any movement form as well as throughout the day to relieve stress.

Walking

Walking is highly underrated, and you don't need lessons to know how to do it. Walking uses the lower leg muscles to pump the lymph back up towards the heart, thus helping your body's detoxification. By increasing circulation throughout the body, walking moves the Qi. As no special equipment is required, walking is inexpensive and simple. Any length of walking is better than none, so if you've decided that your main exercise will be walking, make it a consistent habit.

There are a few things that can make walking even more beneficial than before. One is walking in nature. Clinical studies have shown that even just viewing pictures of nature has healing effects on the body. The presence of trees, flowers, wildlife, etc. makes for a more healing environment than does a busy downtown street.

Walking barefoot provides extra health benefits because you'll be Earthing (see Chapter called Get Grounded). Walk barefoot only if you have a safe place to do so, where you won't get injured–such as a clean beach. By connecting with the earth, you will be grounding all the dirty, positively charged particles from your body into the earth. At the same time, you'll be absorbing the beneficial negatively charged anti-inflammatory particles back into your body. I have to admit that I'm a little squeamish to walk barefoot on bumpy ground, so I bought special grounding flip flops to wear when I walk around my yard to "earth" outside.

Chi (Qi) Walking is a movement form that marries the benefits of Tai Chi and applies it to walking. Unlike regular walking, Chi Walking requires you to really be in touch with your body, your center and your energy. In Chi Walking (www.chiwalking.com), five mindful steps are utilized in the program. The purpose is to reinforce the body-mind connection and improve awareness so that you are energized in this practice.

The first step involves aligning your posture and your intentions. The second step is engaging your core using your lower abdominal muscles for stability as well as engaging your willpower. The third step is creating balance between the upper and lower body and between the left and right sides of your body. Creating mental balance is also part of the third step. The fourth step involves choosing to walk with inner strength and grace as well as making small positive choices in your life. Lastly, the fifth step is about moving forward with consistency and confidence while mentally focusing on spaciousness.

A girlfriend of mine does Chi Running and she loves it. She says that she runs "from her core" and that when she is focused on doing Chi Running, her running seems almost effortless. This friend of mine, whose legs were in a cast in early childhood, is now running eight-minute miles and half marathons. Unless you are already a runner, I would not recommend running as your primary exercise. It can be hard on the joints especially if you do not have correct form. If you are already a jogger or runner, however, I'd recommend that you learn Chi Running. Once you practice this form of running, I don't think you'll ever go back to "regular" running.

Fascial Stretching

One of the best do-it-yourself resources on fascial stretching is the book by Ming Chew, Permanent Pain Cure. I first heard about it from a friend whose frozen shoulder was "cured" by doing the exercises in the book.

The fascia consists of tough connective tissue fibers that envelope and connect all the physical structures in your body including organs, muscles, bones, and nerves. If it weren't for the fascia, all your internal organs would drop down to the bottom of your pelvis in a disorganized pile whenever you stood up! If you've ever cooked a steak, you'll recognize the fascia as the tough whitish membrane that attaches the fat to the meat. The fascia is chewy and is not very easy to eat.

Healthy fascia should be flexible, but after an injury, it can become restrictive like a scar. Surgery actually creates more scar tissue and restricts the fascia even more and can often lead to chronic pain. In Ming Chew's book, you can learn the various fascial stretches to relieve tension and pain in various parts of the body. Together with the nutritional and other suggestions in this book, fascial stretching can make a huge difference in how your body feels and functions. One of my quotes is: *healthy fascia = healthy body*. Consider getting a copy of Ming Chew's book, Permanent Pain Cure, so you can stretch out your fascia.

Enjoy Yourself

Moving the body is an innate requirement for humans. We are not meant to sit still or at a computer desk for hours at a time. When we do, our breath becomes shallow and the energy in our bodies becomes slow and stagnant, affecting all areas of our health. Although I've only recommended a handful of my favorite movement forms, you are not limited to these. What's most important is that you choose something you enjoy. When you enjoy what you do, your body will automatically feel better. The neurochemicals involved in the process of enjoyment are healing to your body, mind and soul.

For example, I feel most connected to the Divine when I am figure skating. I love the feeling of gliding along the ice in a balletic pose while listening to beautiful music. My emotions connect with my spirit which connects with my physical body as I feel the blade glide along the ice. Even though figure skating is one of the hardest sports to perfect, my body enjoys it, so I keep doing it. It isn't as balanced as I would prefer, since I tend to spin and jump in only one direction, but the joy I derive from skating supersedes these considerations. Skating with my partner, James, is particularly joyful because I can feel the connection and energy exchange as we skate. At some point I may decide that repeatedly flinging my body into the air is too dangerous, but part of me wants to accomplish what others consider "impossible" for someone my age. So for now, I'm going to continue my pairs skating.

Dancing is another movement form I absolutely love. Although I don't perform any longer, I find dancing allows me to feel the music within my cells. I wish I could take you to the African dance class that I drum for.

My partner and I do live drumming for a dance class and it is incredibly fun. There is nothing quite like dancing to live drumming because the drumming vibrations penetrate into your core and ground you. Every dancer leaves the class smiling. In our class, we have an older woman who has mental and physical disabilities. Her caregivers bring her weekly to our class and even though she can't follow all the movements, she enjoys the music and continues to attend. She even participated with us in a stage performance once! The amazing thing is that with continued dancing, she has become stronger and more coordinated than when she first started.

If you like dancing but you don't feel comfortable being in a class, it doesn't matter. Just turn up the stereo in your private living room and dance to your heart's content! Just promise me you'll take it easy the first few times if you haven't been exercising for a while. My dream for you is that you will fall in love with one of the movement forms I've discussed and become a certified instructor in order help others in your community.

Chapter Summary

- Physical movement helps circulate Qi, the energy of life, throughout the body, and is a necessary component to healing chronic pain.
- Movement forms such as Qi Gong and Tai Chi specifically use breath and movement to circulate Qi consciously in the body and are pain relief modalities in their own right.
- Cellercising helps to circulate the lymph which can diminish pain due to sluggish lymphatics as well as help tone the muscles and connective tissue.
- Meridian Stretching helps to break up old fibrous scars in the fascia, thus allowing full range of motion of joints and muscles.
- Yoga is an ancient movement form that has a restorative component to it that has been shown to be helpful to those in chronic pain.
- Chi Walking elevates simple walking to a form of healing by incorporating five mindfulness steps.
- Ming Chew's fascial stretches can repair restricted and tight fascia which is causing or contributing to your chronic pain.
- It is vital that you enjoy the movement form you choose because enjoyment is part of the healing process.

20

SLEEP WELL TO HEAL WELL

Why Sleep is Important

Sleep is highly underrated. We are a society that applauds overwork and overachievement and under-appreciates the benefits of rest and rejuvenation. As an example of this attitude, the average American employee receives about two weeks paid vacation a year. With seniority, that may increase to four weeks, but not often. In Europe, workers typically receive six weeks paid vacation or more. I've had patients exclaim that they can't sleep more than six or seven hours a night, until they retire from their jobs, after which they begin sleeping at least eight hours.

Before the advent of the light bulb, people slept upwards of nine or ten hours a night. In the winter, they slept more (due to shorter days) than during the summer. Nowadays, most people are lucky to get seven hours of sleep. Easy illumination, televisions and computers keep people awake and stimulated for a greater proportion of time, and that includes me.

So why is sleep so important? It is important because sleep is *rejuvenation* time for the body. In addition, important hormones and neurotransmitters are released during different stages of sleep. If you do not get enough sleep, you may become deficient or unbalanced in some or all of these natural bio-chemicals.

I have a patient that I'll name Peter, who came to me complaining about problems sleeping. He'd wake up groggy and tired and complained of brain fog. He had suffered a head injury while skiing a few months prior, so I sent him to my massage colleague, Marie, to evaluate his cranial system. During his initial treatment Marie discovered that when Peter fell asleep on the treatment table, he actually gasped for air and even stopped breathing several times. When she alerted me to the problem, I urged Peter to undergo a sleep study. In the meantime, I also suggested that he try wearing his LifeWave Y-Age Aeon anti-stress patches behind his right ear during sleep because this acupuncture point, Triple Burner 17, is located close to his brainstem, the part of the brain controlling breathing.

I wasn't sure it was going to help, but given his head injury I thought it couldn't hurt.

To my surprise, Peter reported sleeping soundly the first night he wore the patch on this acupuncture point and hasn't had any gasping or breathing problems since. What was also interesting was that Peter lost approximately five pounds of excess body weight within the first few days of sleeping deeply. He'd been trying to lose weight to no avail, but once he was able to sleep, he was able to take off the extra pounds. I surmised after this incident that the reason Peter couldn't lose the weight was because his poor sleep prevented him from making important hormones, like growth hormone. Growth hormone promotes lean body mass, and when in low levels encourages unwanted fat storage.

When you don't get adequate deep sleep, your body can't repair itself and is in a constant state of "breakdown" also called *catabolism*. Even if all your other health habits are pristine, you can still have problems healing chronic pain if you don't sleep well. Patients with chronic fatigue and fibromyalgia have a horrible time sleeping. I should know since I used to be one of them. During my sickest months with fibromyalgia, I remember sleeping upwards of 12 to 14 hours a day, but still woke up exhausted and groggy. Every bone and muscle in my body ached. I felt like someone ran over me over with a truck. I couldn't believe that after sleeping so much, I could still feel exhausted. What I didn't realize then was that I was not getting deep, *rejuvenating* sleep.

Stages of Sleep

There are several sleep stages you're supposed to go through if you're sleeping well. Each stage of sleep has a different accompanying brainwave pattern. Each of these patterns is vital to normal functioning of our adult brains and bodies. During the lighter stages of sleep, your brainwave is in alpha, a relaxed state. Many meditative practices can also put you into an alpha brainwave state. When external, linear, beta brainwaves relax into slower, internal non-linear alpha brainwaves, heart rate, respiration, blood pressure and the body's general metabolism also slows down.

As you deepen your sleep, your brainwave switches to theta, a slower brainwave state. This state is also known as the dream state or REM (rapid eye movement) state. During this time a crucial part of the brainstem, called the Reticular Activating System (RAS) goes into a special state in which it literally closes off the muscular control signals from the brain to the body. So, during the whole period of Theta brainwave state, dreaming sleep, the entire body is essentially paralyzed and makes no movement. This is supposedly a safety mechanism that prevents us from hurting ourselves as we dream. There are certain people who suffer sleep paralysis whereby their bodies are paralyzed but they are actually fully awake. This is very frightening for someone to experience, especially the first time. The opposite is true for sleepwalkers, people who enact their dreams while they are still fast asleep.

The theta portion of sleep is where the Emotional Body recuperates, heals and "tunes" itself. There are various levels of dream material which get processed during this state. Some dreams are clearly re-experiencing the day's events to clear them out, while deeper theta dream states are associated with the clearing of deep emotional traumas-sometimes back to childhood. It is the emotional state of theta sleep that is the most important, not the content apparently.

Older children and adults with ADD (attention deficit disorder, also referred to as ADHD) tend to have predominantly theta brainwaves, even while awake. Unable to get their brainwaves into the beta, the alert and focused state, people with ADD are literally dreaming while awake. Creative as they are, without the ability to be stay in beta brainwaves, people with ADD have difficulty focusing on one thing at a time. Their brains are too busy taking in the "big picture" with all of its distracting details. My partner, James, is really good at noticing subtle mistakes the movie makers make. I hardly ever catch these mistakes. For example, he'll notice that in one scene, the car window is smashed and then in the next scene it isn't. His theta-dominant ability is not that helpful, however, in a workshop situation if the instructor is at all boring.

In the deepest stages of sleep, your brainwave switches to delta wave. This is where the body is in its most quiescent, stress-reduced, restful state. There are several levels of delta waves, each one slower than both alpha and theta. This is believed to be the state where the body does most of its self-healing and rejuvenating work. As the brainwaves sink deeper into slower and slower Delta brainwave patterns, the body goes into the lowest blood pressure, heart rate, metabolism, respiration and body temperature it experiences. This is the time at night in which the body regenerates, recuperates and heals, re-tuning itself for the next day. There are no mental or emotional processes, and interestingly, no sense of time. This is the most difficult time to try to awaken a sleeping person.

During normal sleep, your body cycles through the different stages of sleep which is why you'll often have many different dreams. If you're not dreaming well, it is less likely that you're going deeper into delta wave sleep. If you're not getting into deep delta wave sleep, then your body can't rejuvenate. That is why getting quality sleep is vitally important to heal your chronic pain.

Take the quick quiz below to assess whether you are getting adequate quality sleep. If not, I have some suggestions on how you can. Check off the statements that are true for you regarding your sleep patterns:

- ☐ I sleep eight or more hours most nights of the week.
- ☐ I sleep through the night without waking up until it is time to get out of bed in the morning.
- ☐ I usually wait no longer than 10 minutes to fall asleep.
- ☐ I don't have to go to the bathroom to urinate during sleeping hours.
- ☐ I wake up refreshed and I don't need coffee or other stimulants to wake me up.
- ☐ I am aware that I dream every night.
- ☐ My dreams are vivid, colorful, and I can recall the details when I first wake up.
- ☐ I do not snore when I sleep.
- ☐ I do not wake up due to pain.
- ☐ I go to sleep before 10:30 PM every night consistently.

If you didn't check off all or most of the above statements, then you may have a real problem with quality sleep. Lack of quality sleep not only perpetuates chronic pain, but also prevents important hormones from being released. In addition to chronic pain, likewise, fatigue, foggy-thinking, irritability and memory problems can result from chronic sleep deprivation.

Sleep Hygiene

Sleep hygiene is a term that doctors use to describe a list of sleeping "do's" and "don'ts" for their patients. Having good sleep habits can really make a huge difference in relieving and preventing chronic pain. Out of all my bad habits, I think sleeping is my worst. I'm a night owl and I love to stay up late, usually working on the computer. As you'll see from the list below, that habit is really a no-no. In addition, I'm often skating in the evenings when the ice time is available, so I end up wide awake before bedtime. Even though I don't get up early, it would serve me better to get to bed at a decent time and stop "activating" my brain and body so late at night. Here's the list you can refer to for proper sleep hygiene:

DO:

- ✓ Retire to bed at a regular time each night.
- ✓ Go to sleep no later than 10:30 PM at night, preferably earlier.
- ✓ Sleep in a completely dark room avoiding artificial light.
- ✓ Associate your bedroom with sleep, not work.
- ✓ Have a quiet relaxing bedtime routine.
- ✓ Have a regular exercise routine; vigorous exercise earlier in the day and relaxing exercise (like yoga) later in the evening.
- ✓ Make sure your bedroom and bed is comfortable, ideally having bed coverings made of natural materials like cotton or bamboo.
- ✓ If you read before bedtime, read something light and pleasant.
- ✓ Reduce or eliminate coffee if you have trouble sleeping at night.

DON'T

- ✗ Do "work" in your bedroom. Instead use an office or separate space to work.
- ✗ Watch TV or use the computer within one hour of your bedtime.
- ✗ Watch the news at all, but especially in the evenings: disturbing images will imprint into your subconscious as you sleep.

×   Eat large meals right before sleeping.

×   Take a hot bath right before bedtime. Do it earlier in the evening as the body temperature needs to drop before sleep.

×   Use caffeine or stimulants, especially twelve hours prior to bedtime.

×   Drink alcohol on a regular basis if you have trouble sleeping and especially if you wake up between 1–3AM (Liver Meridian Energy dominant time).

×   Have a television or a clock radio in your bedroom or a fluorescent light bulb by the bed. The electromagnetic radiation can disturb your sleep.

×   Keep a cell phone on in your bedroom unless it is on airplane mode.

You may wish to download a copy of the Sleep Hygiene document from the Center of Clinical Interventions. See Resources for links.

Why Drugs Don't Help

Millions of people worldwide are dependent on sleep medications. Some are available only by prescription and others are over the counter. The over the counter drugs are often older drugs that are antihistamines. The side effect of these antihistamines is somnolence which is why they will have a warning on the box not to operate heavy machinery while using the drug. These drugs make you feel groggy in the morning. Furthermore, both prescription and over the counter sleep medications do not tend to encourage the brain to go into healthy deep sleep. In other words, your brain doesn't get into delta wave sleep. In fact, if you ask most people hooked on these drugs, they will tell you that they rarely dream, revealing an inability to even attain theta wave sleep, a sleep stage lighter than delta.

Aside from the side effects, the problem with long term use of sleep medications is they only cover up the symptoms. They do not get to the root of the problem. Healthy sleep habits along with specific energy tools can help the brain and body relearn how to sleep deeply.

How to Get Quality Sleep

To get the most rejuvenating sleep possible, you need eight hours of solid sleep without interruption. You should be dreaming every night and those dreams should be vivid, colorful and easy to remember when you first wake up. Ideally when you wake up, you should feel well-rested and refreshed, not groggy and tired. For people who haven't slept this way in decades, it seems like a tall order. Even small improvements in the quality of your sleep can have profoundly beneficial effects on your chronic pain.

Below is a list of strategies I recommend to improve quality sleep besides practicing proper sleep hygiene. Try one or more of them and see what works best for you. A combination approach often works well.

Earthing

Sleeping on top of an Earthing bed sheet or mat helps to ground you and decrease the stress in your body. I find sleeping earthed simply heavenly so I recommend it to everyone. My mother calls it her "magic carpet". Why she calls it a carpet I'll never know, but as long as she's happy with how she feels sleeping on it, I'm happy. I have discovered that investing in a fitted bed sheet works even better for whole body pain than just the half sheet, so if it is affordable for you, get one for yourself.

Magnesium

Magnesium helps with relaxation. It is also required for energy production in addition to over 300 biochemical reactions in the body. Magnesium taken orally or applied on the skin (transdermal magnesium) can help your body relax into a deep sleep with consistent use. Depending on your bowel's tolerance, you can take between 300mg to 500mg orally in the evening, use magnesium oil of up to 48 sprays on your skin or 1 oz. of Nutrilink's Mag Force. If you like baths, then take a warm magnesium salt bath an hour before bedtime. Doing so can really help you sleep. Please read the chapter on magnesium for more detailed dosing information.

Silent Nights Patches

One of the most effective energy tools I've used to improve sleep in my patients is the LifeWave Silent Nights patches. These patches are drug-free and use infra-red energy to communicate to the body's energy field. The Silent Nights patches help the brain get into deeper brainwave states, such as delta wave. In the process of deepening sleep, these patches support the body's healthy production of melatonin and serotonin, two important neuro-hormones.

Melatonin is also an antioxidant that protects nuclear and mitochondrial DNA. Many people use melatonin as a supplement to help them sleep. Although this is often effective, I have a couple of concerns with regards to supplemental Melatonin. Traditionally melatonin was made from cow pineal gland extractions. In some countries, the sale of melatonin over the counter has been banned because of concerns of disease being transmitted from infected cows. In the United States, melatonin is sold over the counter and most of it is synthetic, so there is little risk of disease. What I have found, however, is that my patients who take melatonin as a supplement often complain of grogginess in the morning. This side effect does not seem to happen when someone is using the Silent Nights patches. I believe that being able to support your body's own production of melatonin is a better option than taking a supplement.

Serotonin helps us feel relaxed and happy. Serotonin is an important neurotransmitter and the one that is manipulated by anti-depressant medications. Adequate serotonin levels are believed to improve sleep and mood. The LifeWave Silent Nights patches can support healthy serotonin levels while improving quality sleep. Please note that in Europe, these patches are called Silent Nights MD and they are designated as a Class I phototherapeutic medical device. The ministries of health in Europe are much more open to alternative technologies compared with the U.S. Food and Drug Administration, so it isn't surprising that these patches are growing in popularity among European healthcare professionals.

The nice thing about these patches is that they work relatively quickly. My favorite acupuncture point to use with these patches is Governing Vessel GV24.5, which is also known as the third eye. This acupuncture point is found in the middle of your forehead just above the eyebrows. If that point doesn't work for you, there are several more you can try. I have links to videos online where I show you exactly how to find these acupuncture points and how to use the Silent Nights patches.

LifeWave Y-Age Aeon Patches

While I recommend Silent Nights patches for night time use to help you sleep, I also recommend the LifeWave Y-Age Aeon patches during the day to help you reduce stress. By balancing your cortisol (stress hormone) levels during the day, you'll have a better chance of sleeping well at night. I have many patients just using the Brain Balance protocol I taught in Chapter 6 who tell me that their sleeping and dreaming has improved even without any other sleep remedy. Read the chapter on Balancing the Brain to learn which acupuncture points I use most successfully with the Y-Age Aeon to support natural pain relief. Sometimes I use the Y-Age Aeon patches at night at the same time I use the Silent Nights patches to get really deep sleep. When I combine them, I'll often use Silent Nights on the third eye acupuncture point GV 24.5 and then use the Aeon patch over an area of inflammation or on one of the acupuncture points listed in the Y-Age brochure.

For very stubborn insomnia cases in my practice, I will recommend a combination of LifeWave Y-Age Aeon patches during the day, and Silent Nights and Y-Age Carnosine patches at night. The Carnosine patches used in conjunction with the Silent Nights can be particularly powerful. Having the Carnosine patches on board at night helps the body go into "repair" mode while you sleep and many people who have tried this combination rave at the depth of sleep they are able to achieve.

Delta Wave Sleep Music

I have a library of various delta wave sleep audio programs created by Dr. Jeffrey Thompson. There are various types available: some have music and some incorporate nature sounds. Dr. Thompson's brainwave entrainment music works by training the brain how to produce synchronized brainwaves. This process is called brain entrainment. As you listen to this music repeatedly, your brain will begin to "entrain" to the slow delta wave brain pulses created by Dr. Thompson's delta wave music. Literally, over time, your brain will learn to "sleep well" on its own. Dr. Thompson recommends listening to the entrainment music for at least twenty-one days in a row to get the greatest benefit. Some of my patients keep the music playing softly while they sleep. See Resources for links.

Breathing Exercises

Traditional yogic breathing has long been known to help with relaxation and sleep. One of the easiest breathing exercises is breathing slowly in through the left nostril while obstructing the right with your right index finger and then exhaling through the right nostril while obstructing the left nostril with your left index finger. Breathe in only through the left and out only through the right. This helps to activate the right side of the breath, causing relaxation.

Exercise

Exercising regularly helps the body normalize many processes including sleep. While you don't want to be exercising vigorously near bedtime, any form of exercise you choose will be better than none. Meditative exercises like Tai Chi, Qi Gong, and yoga can all be helpful to improve your sleep and mood. I've found that after doing Meridian Stretching, my body is so relaxed that sleep is inevitable. Cellercising using the Baby Bounce technique before bed can also help relax your body before sleep. Read the Chapter 19 Move the Body-Move the Qi for more information about these forms of exercise.

Journaling

If you're someone who tends to worry a lot, it may be helpful to write your worries down in a journal in order to "let them go" to a Higher Power. In a similar fashion, you can share your worries with Worry Dolls. Worry Dolls are small dolls handmade in Guatemala. The idea is that if you're worried about things, instead of worrying all night, you tell your worries to these dolls and put them under your pillow before you fall asleep. According to folklore, the dolls are supposed to do the worrying for you so you can release those tensions while you sleep. Although many buy them for their children, I think they are great even for adults!

Sometimes I get inspired ideas as I lie down to go to bed, so it has been helpful to have a journal by my bed to jot these ideas down. By doing so, I don't get anxious about forgetting them. Not all insomnia is a result of worry. Sometimes I get too excited about an idea and can't get grounded enough to fall asleep, so journaling is very helpful. One night, I actually wrote a whole book before I could fall back asleep!

A fantastic way to use your journal before bedtime is doing the Gratitude exercise. The purpose of this exercise is to focus on what you are grateful for. In this exercise, you list all the things that you're grateful for that day. It could be that you were grateful that it was sunny and warm and you got to "earth" barefoot outside. Or maybe you were grateful that your husband made dinner and you didn't have to. By focusing on what you're grateful for right before sleeping, you create happy, peaceful energies. Your subconscious mind is then programmed for positivity as you drift asleep. It is one of the reasons I ask my patients not to watch the television news before bedtime. Our subconscious minds are highly programmable, which is why commercials are so effective in brainwashing us. By intentionally programming the energy of gratitude right before you fall asleep, you'll be programming your subconscious mind to create more positive experiences in your life.

Another great use for your bedside journal is to write down your dreams. The more intent you are about capturing your dreams on paper, the more dreams you'll tend to remember. Dreaming is a way of processing subconscious emotions, so by journaling them, you may be able to interpret these messages for own personal growth and healing.

You may also ask for guidance or healing while you sleep. This can be very interesting. One night I decided to ask for guidance around healing my body. In my dream, I was in a large hotel with my family, ready to go to the all-you-can-eat buffet at the hotel restaurant. I was first in line, so I couldn't wait to get to the salad bar to see what was there. To my dismay, every single food item had flies on it. I was really disgusted and disappointed. When I woke up, I interpreted the dream as a message that

I really needed to take responsibility for how food is nurturing my body. I began to pay more attention to where my food came from and how it was processed. By having more control over what I was eating, I was able to appreciate how much healthier my body felt.

Progressive Relaxation

Progressive relaxation is a form of meditation whereby you alternate between contraction and relaxation of sequential parts of your body. Most people start at their toes and work their way up to their heads. My Kundalini yoga instructor likes to do this meditation at the end of our class to get us completely relaxed into the final yoga pose called Corpse pose (also known as relaxation pose). The technique is easy so I'll share with you how to do it.

As you lie face up in bed, you start with your toes. Curl your toes up vigorously for about five seconds, and then relax them. Do this several times. Remember to keep breathing. Then move up to your calves and alternate contracting and relaxing them for a few rounds. With each progressive cycle, you move up the body alternating contraction and relaxation until you get all the way up to your face. When you get to your face, you tightly squeeze your eyes, nose and mouth shut for five seconds before you fully relax. Sometimes in a big class, I don't know how my teacher keeps a straight face watching us all contort our faces for the last part of this exercise! At the end, you just relax and breathe, allowing the energy to flow throughout your muscles. This simple exercise has helped countless people to relax before falling asleep. Try it and see if it works for you.

Reduce Negative Qi

Negative Qi (Chi) is a term used to describe energy that is detrimental to your body, mind or spirit. Although we can't control all the negative energies around us, we can minimize them, especially in the place where we sleep. Negative Qi can take the form of electromagnetic smog, chemicals or even negative emotions.

Electromagnetic smog can stress the body when it is most vulnerable, which is during sleep. If your sleeping isn't ideal, you may wish to remove all electrical equipment from your bedroom with the exception of a battery operated clock. Sometimes the glow from digital clocks can interrupt the pineal gland's function to help you sleep. So a dark bedroom is better. Furthermore, investing in a Gauss meter that checks the dirty electricity emanating from your electrical outlets may be prudent. They aren't very expensive and you can lend them out to friends and family so that they can check their homes as well.

Ideally the EMF coming out from your outlets should register less than 60 G. If they register more, you may wish to purchase some filters. These filters are called Graham-Stetzer filters. The old filters I used to have were very noisy because they would click and pop as they filtered the "dirty" electricity. Recently I purchased a set from Greenwave Filters which I love because they are very quiet. I addition, I don't lose an electrical outlet because you can plug in any two or three-prong device into the bottom of it. In my office I have two filters for each of my treatment rooms, where the dirty electricity registered over 1700 G. I find that I am both calmer and more relaxed in my office and so are my patients.

Another way to clear negative energy from your sleeping space and home is using a product called Clean Sweep by Energy Tools International. This water-based energized spray is odorless and is sprayed in any space where you want to clear negative Qi, including negative emotions. If your bedroom has been a place where arguments or illness have taken place, it would be a good idea to clear these negative energies so you can heal. Spraying your bedroom nightly is a great way to improve quality sleep. You can even spray yourself before bed, from your head down to your toes to clear your own energy field. Clean Sweep is a great energy tool for super-sensitive types, who tend to be a sponge for outside energies. See Resources for links.

Essential Oils

If you like pleasant scents, then you may like using essential oils. They can be applied to various places on the body, even acupuncture points, to help you sleep. Lavender essential oil is the most widely known for improving sleep.

Other essential oils used for this purpose include Valerian, Velviter, Roman Chamomile, Lemon Balm, Sweet Marjoram, Jasmine, and Sandalwood. Many companies make essential oil blends that are specifically designed to help you to sleep more deeply. Ideally you'll want to purchase oils from a company that makes therapeutic-grade essential oils.

Acupuncture points that you can use with essential oils include temples (Triple Burner 23), inside wrists (Heart 7 or Pericardium 6), inside ankles (Kidney 3 or Spleen 6) or third eye (GV24.5).

Subtle Energy Supplements

In an earlier chapter, I mentioned the company Nutrilink. They make supplements that are subtle-energy enhanced. My patients with extremely stubborn sleep problems often get relief with a combination of taking the Nutrilink Mag Force (take at night), ANS Support, Brain Support and Sleep Aid, the descriptions of which can all be found on their website www.NutrlinkEnergy.com.

Chapter Summary

- Quality sleep is essential in order for the body to self-heal.
- Many people do not realize that they are not getting adequate sleep.
- Practicing proper sleep hygiene helps you set the stage for quality sleep.
- Sleep drugs do not help you get into the proper stages of rejuvenating sleep and thus are a poor long term solution.
- Energy medicine tools are available to support the body's getting into natural sleep rhythms without having to resort to drugs.
- Exercise, journaling and progressive relaxation are inexpensive ways to enhance your sleep experience.

SECTION D

YOUR SPIRIT: HEALING THROUGH YOUR HIGHER SELF

"If you're really spiritual, then you should be totally
independent of the good and the bad opinions of the
world . . . you should have faith in yourself."
-Deepak Chopra, MD

21

WHY RECONNECT WITH SPIRIT?

To be perfectly honest, I would not have "reconnected with spirit" if it weren't for the suffering my illness caused. And I say "reconnected" rather than "connected" because we are always connected to our spirit. It's just that most of us don't know how to access this sacred place.

In the depths of my illness, I was angry, resentful and depressed. The last thing I thought of was consciously connecting to my spirit. I just wanted to be fixed! Have you ever thought that too? Yup, I just wanted all the pain, fatigue, and sorrow to disappear . . . instantly. I didn't have an extra ounce of energy to "push" any further. I was done. I was desperate. I had given up totally.

Desperation–are you there yet? Maybe not. Maybe you won't have to get to that painful place. Or maybe you *do* have to in order to create real empowered change. I don't know. Only your Higher Self knows. If you don't like to be told what to do, then you may very well have to experience complete surrender like I did in order to heal.

I still remember the desperate moment when I re-connected with my spirit, my Higher Self. I was in bed, crying as quietly as I could, while lying next to my husband. I wanted to go to sleep and never wake up. As the tears rolled down my face, I suddenly felt a voice inside me say gently, "You have a choice, you know". It stopped me in my tracks. I countered stubbornly, "No I don't! I have to stay in this marriage even if it kills me. Divorce just isn't right! I don't want to be a bad person! I don't want to fail." The voice continued gently, "Ok, if that's your choice, then you can continue on your current path and nothing will change. It's ok if that's what you choose". At that moment, I realized that by accepting the status quo of feeling obligated to stay in my marriage no matter what, I *was* making a choice.

Do you ever feel like you don't have a choice? Many people don't, and I empathize. I know what it's like to feel obligated. It feels heavy and yucky in my body. I had no idea that that type of energy was literally clogging up my energy channels and making me sicker and sicker. All the acupuncture, herbal supplements, and counseling in the world would not have done one bit of good if I had not finally listened to my Higher Self, my intuition, and had the courage to choose a different path. Of course, these tools supported me in the process by helping me balance and increase my energy so I could take action.

For me, the path I chose was getting up the courage to stand up for myself and separate from my husband. I knew this path would be wrought with extreme emotional backlash as both my husband and parents would feel devastated by my decision. Since childhood I had always felt responsible for everyone's feelings, so it was extremely difficult for me to make a choice that might hurt another's feelings. And indeed, it was heart-wrenching to witness my father crying for the first time in my life. The pain was great, yet the pain of ignoring my spirit, my soul, was greater, so I stood firm and weathered the storm.

Fast forward ten years. I could not have guessed back then who I would be today and how happy my life is. I couldn't have guessed that my ex-husband would forgive me and go on to marry a woman who was a better match for him and father two beautiful children. I couldn't have guessed that my parents, would not only forgive me, but lovingly accept my new partner. The gifts that have come from my reconnection to spirit are countless.

If someone were to ask me the one thing that made the most difference in my healing, I would say "reconnecting to spirit". The reasons you may wish to reconnect with *your* spirit are plenty, and healing your physical pain is just one of those reasons. Here are some others:

- Living a life of joy and purpose-feeling like you are making a difference in the world
- Being able to access your intuition to help you make positive choices so you and others can reap the benefits
- Discovering your mission through self-acceptance and appreciating your unique gifts
- Enjoying your life, your relationships, regardless of any challenges life may throw at you
- Appreciating that you are an amazing, unique, fabulous soul and that the world needs you
- Having fun and experiencing the joy of conscious creation

- Serving the world by being your true authentic self

Can Being "Spiritual" Help My Pain?

Having chronic pain slows you down doesn't it? Does it prevent you from enjoying your life? Did you ever take your "health" for granted before you experienced chronic pain? The answer for many is *yes*.

Just for a moment, put aside any arguments or "buts" you may have and consider this thought: *Your chronic pain is exactly the opportunity your spirit created in order to grow you spiritually.* What if this were true? What would that mean for your life right now? Could it be that your chronic pain is not actually an obstacle in your life, but an invitation to reconnect with your Higher Self? If you are reading this chapter, it is likely that you've somehow attracted this thought into your consciousness. Whether you consider it or ignore it is up to you.

Think about this possibility: what if pursuing the relief of chronic pain became a spiritual journey? What if you discover more opportunities to develop happier relationships, joyful livelihood and prosperity in the process? How open would you be? Reconnecting with spirit can help you heal your chronic pain. It's a matter of jumping in and seeing your illness as an opportunity rather than as a burden.

In my experience, my openness (and desperation) to connecting with spirit was responsible for my relatively quick recovery from fibromyalgia. Most people do not recover from fibromyalgia. In fact, few are able to return to work and most people become permanently disabled. Although I cannot say my health is "perfect", I appreciate that my pursuit and deep desire to be healthy has brought many wonderful opportunities and I am enjoying the *process* of healing. Healing is a process, not an end point. You've probably heard the saying, "It's the journey, not the goal". Healing is like that. It is a journey of self-discovery and self-development whereby you may also experience the physical healing of symptoms.

Spiritual Healing

According to quantum physicists as well as spiritual mystics, energy comes before form. In other words, before something gets manifested in "reality" as solid matter, it has to be transformed from one energy form to another. Thought is energy and through a process of manifestation, can become a tangible thing that we can touch, taste, hear, smell or feel. Healing the spirit is synonymous with healing at the quantum level.

Out of all the processes outlined in this book on healing chronic pain, I feel that my spiritual healing was the number one most important factor in my healing. Consider this thought: *everything you are experiencing is for your highest and greatest good.* Sounds weird doesn't it? Maybe the thought even angers you? But just for a moment, imagine if you will, if this were true. Then how would that change your perspective concerning your chronic pain?

So what does the process of spiritual healing feel like anyway, you might wonder? Well, it feels different for everyone, but I can describe the process that I often witness in my patients:

1. A crisis, illness, or unpleasant situation gets our attention.
2. This situation gives us an opportunity to choose how we perceive it. If we perceive it as "bad" and resist it at every turn, we suffer. If we perceive it as an opportunity and choose to use it as a way to grow our spirit, we enjoy the process.
3. When we can perceive the situation as a calling of our spirit to grow ourselves bigger than we were before, we manifest the courage it takes to expand beyond our comfort zone.
4. When we've expanded beyond our comfort zone and integrated our new experiences, we get to know ourselves on a much deeper level and appreciate newly developed strength and skills. We learn to appreciate the opportunity our pain has brought us to allow our spirit to grow. In the process, we are less attached to the outcome and more vested in the actual experience.
5. We perceive our world differently as our spirit evolves, letting go of pre-existing beliefs and judgments at each level and we start to understand how everything we think and do affects every other being in the Universe.

6. As we spiritually evolve to higher levels, our joy increases as we experience healing on many levels: health, relationships, money, and career, to name a few.

In the next few chapters, I'll be introducing you to some "spiritual" concepts and exercises so that you can experience how accessing your spirituality can support you in healing your chronic pain. Hopefully, you'll manifest much more than just healing your physical symptoms.

Chapter Summary

- Your chronic pain may be an opportunity rather than an obstacle to experiencing a full and happy life.
- Reconnecting with spirit, your Higher Self, may be one of the quickest ways to recover your health.
- In addition to symptom relief, there are many "side" benefits from acknowledging and working with Spirit in your life.
- The process of spiritual healing may feel different for everyone, but many people find that they grow to enjoy it.

22

DOES PAIN SERVE A PURPOSE?

Pain: Friend or Foe?

You may experience body pain when something isn't balanced in your life. I tell my patients that when we live our lives unconsciously, we're not always aware of whether our decisions are for our highest and greatest good. In fact, we are often making choices that hurt us rather than heal us. When we make these kinds of choices, The Universe, or our Inner Guidance, has a way of nudging us to show us that we're not following our soul's path. The nudge starts with something small, like getting a new unsympathetic boss at work, but if we don't take the hint, it can be bigger, like a car accident. If we still don't listen to our Inner Guidance, sometimes we need what I call the "Spiritual 2x4" across the side of the head - an event so big, that we can't miss it. That's what happened to me.

I think I've always had a Type A personality, someone who is such an achiever that every waking moment is dedicated to some goal or prize. In school, if I got 98% on a math test, I'd focus on the 2% I failed to get right. When I failed my first A.R.C.T. piano exam at the Royal Conservatory of Music in Canada as a teenager, I stayed in bed and cried for almost three days straight. My motto was: *failure is not an option.* If you're a perfectionist, take heed. As you'll read in the pages to come, perfectionism is almost a guaranteed way to block your own healing. Crazy isn't it? But it's true.

When I made the commitment to build my eco-house with my husband despite the vehement objections of my family and the concern of close friends, I didn't ever once consider that maybe, just maybe, it wasn't the right decision for me. I wasn't at all concerned with what was for *my* highest and greatest good. All I was concerned about was the happiness of my husband. I thought that if I could finally make him happy, then I would be happy.

I layered more responsibility on myself to become a better person. It seemed like my goal in life was to be better, never being satisfied with who I was in the moment. There was always something better to look forward to, it seemed, and I wasn't going to be satisfied until I got *there*. Unfortunately, there is no such thing as "there". There is only *here*. And truthfully, I wasn't happy here.

So after years of pushing through the grueling schedule at medical school, the stressful jobs in underserved medical communities and finally embarking on house-building and not listening to my Inner Guidance, I finally received a "Spiritual 2x4" blow to the head. My descent into physical, mental and emotional misery was fast after that, like sinking into quicksand. My life was so busy and fast before I got sick that I wasn't even remotely aware of the subtle signals from my psyche urging me to choose a different path. My Type A personality combined with my stubbornness created such an overwhelming situation that only a major catastrophe could slow me down enough to listen to my soul.

Pain Means Pay Attention

Pain can also be a sign that you are being called to pay attention to something important in your life, be it your lifestyle, beliefs or relationships, for example. So think for a moment about your own life. I don't know *exactly* why pain has entered your life, but I do know the life patterns that are associated with it. What follows is a list of questions for you to start thinking about: what your pain is asking you to pay attention to or what purpose it may serve in your life. You might want to jot a few notes down in a journal when answering the following questions.

1. What events were happening in your life before you began experiencing pain?
2. Where and when in your life have you done things you really didn't want to do, but thought you *had* to in order to be accepted? loved?
3. Do you ever say to yourself, "I'll be happy when such-and-such happens" as if happiness depends on something happening in the future rather than being a state of mind in the present?
4. How often do you think to yourself, "Things would be great if only so-and-so would do such-and-such (to make my life easier)?"

5. How much attention have you paid to treating your body well, nurturing it with enough nutrition, exercise, sleep?

6. How much attention have you given to what your thoughts are focused on? Are they focused mainly on what's wrong with your life or what's right with your life?

7. Has life been centered on your daily activities and your to-do list with little or no attention focused on your life's purpose or spiritual growth?

8. Do you ever wonder why you're here on earth and what your purpose is supposed to be in the grand scheme of the Universe?

9. How often do you choose someone else's well-being or needs over your own?

10. How balanced is your lifestyle? Do you balance rest with activity?

11. How much energy do you spend taking care of your physical, mental, emotional and spiritual health on a regular basis?

12. What might you be gaining by being disabled or in pain (Example: people feeling sorry for you, being nicer to you, feeling more supported by loved ones)?

When we take the time to evaluate how well we are taking care of ourselves, physically, mentally, emotionally and spiritually, we can then appreciate the role that pain has in our lives. Just because our bodies are self-healing organisms doesn't mean that we can just put our lives on autopilot and assume that no matter how we treat ourselves, our bodies will bounce back.

Having pain symbolizes the opportunity to take full responsibility- maybe for the first time in your life-for your health and well-being.

Healing Others through Your Experience

Alice had a nagging pain between her shoulder blades. She had all sorts of other issues, so we didn't start addressing this pain until some of the more urgent issues were dealt with first. This nagging pain suddenly flared up. One of her energy therapists said that there was an energy "hole" in the area. Whenever I'd acupuncture that part of the spine, the skin would turn beet red, indicating a source of inflammation.

Alice, being a remarkably sensitive and empathetic person, would easily be drained by family relationships. It dawned on me one day that she was so sensitive that she could literally "take on another's pain". I was inspired one day to ask Alice if she ever thought about her role as a healer. Many of us who are healers are what intuitive physician, Judith Orloff, M.D., calls *intuitive empaths*. Alice was an intuitive empath although she never thought about "healing" other people. During this conversation, I spontaneously asked Alice whether she would be willing to endure this type of pain if she knew that in the process she was healing someone else. Unequivocally, she said "Yes".

What's most interesting to note is that after Alice and I had that conversation, her pain seemed to quickly subside. I performed acupuncture on the area one last time and there was no redness. Later, she found out that a friend had been diagnosed with cancer of the spine in that exact area where she herself was feeling pain. She remembered our conversation and wondered whether or not her own pain was connected to her friend's. Life is a mystery, so we'll never know for sure, but it didn't surprise me to find out that this friend experienced a spontaneous remission of her cancer, much to the surprise of her doctor.

So here are my questions for you: If someone you knew needed healing from a serious illness or disease, would you accept temporary pain if it meant you'd be helping him or her? If, in healing your own chronic pain, you somehow make it easier for other to heal theirs, would you sign up for this "spiritual" assignment? These are just questions for you to ponder.

Wounded Healer—Developing Compassion

I used to think that every healing professional worth his or her salt should be perfectly healthy. If not, why listen to what he/she has to teach? While it is true that we must practice what we preach, I now believe that it was presumptuous of me to "blame" healers for not being perfectly healthy themselves. Some of the best healing professionals I've known have endured significant illness. It has taken my own personal experience with illness and imperfection to realize that one of the benefits of experiencing pain firsthand is learning compassion.

Before I got sick myself, I thought of myself as being compassionate. I was popular and patients loved me. But underneath the mask of tolerance, I still judged my patients for not working hard enough to get well. I blamed them for eating poorly. I blamed them for smoking. I blamed them for staying fat. It wasn't until I got sick myself that I finally developed true compassion for my patients. When I would wake up in the middle of the night with every bone in my body aching with pain, I understood how horrible it was to suffer pain. When I was so exhausted that I couldn't even make a phone call, I understood what my patients with chronic fatigue syndrome were going through.

These days, instead of perceiving pain as the enemy, I appreciate it as a teacher. It is human nature to live life on autopilot, without consciousness, getting our "to-do" lists done every day, but pain has a way of waking us up to the present. Pain has taught me compassion. I believe that although my stressful lifestyle contributed to the development of my illness, I shouldn't blame myself for it. Instead, I am grateful for the experience so that I can learn compassion and help countless others who are in pain as well.

Many of my patients are healers, but they don't know they are. They have the "wounded healer" archetype. What this means is that part of their life purpose is to experience "wounds" as part of their spiritual journey so that they may move beyond them and teach others how to live empowered lives. It doesn't mean that everyone has to be a professional healer if he or she has the wounded healer archetype. People who heal themselves from a wounded to an empowered place radiate the kind of compassionate energy that empowers others whether they recognize it or not.

Don't Blame Yourself

Many people erroneously believe that they are in pain because of something they did wrong. Although it might be true that you could have taken care of your body better in the past, be compassionate with yourself. I've had a hard time with self-compassion because I can be extremely self-critical. The words, "could've", "should've", "would've" come up quite a bit in my thoughts, but now I know these are my defenses. Do you ever hear yourself saying these words? From this point forward, eliminate these words and focus on the present. When you catch yourself in a self-critical mode, see if you can gently recognize an old pattern and then stop your negative train of thought right away.

Taking responsibility, without blaming others or past situations is very healthy and is different from feeling guilty about being at fault. Each moment is an opportunity for you to take responsibility, i.e. to choose a healthy thought or to let go of an unsupportive unhealthy thought. Every time you choose self-compassion over self-criticism, you are feeding your spirit!

Another belief that I held that I have since let go of is the belief that if I did everything "right", I would not be in pain. It bothered me when spiritual gurus I admired manifested illness because I believed that they should be healthy if they were doing things "right". Thanks to my spiritual teacher, Pat Jones, of Healing Adventures, I now realize that this just simply isn't true. Many spiritual and holistic health gurus enjoy perfect health. But when they don't, it isn't necessarily because they didn't eat right or thought the wrong thoughts. Pat explained to me that some souls come into the world with a contract to bear the burdens of others so that the world can be healed by their actions. Jesus was such a person. He wasn't ill, but he willingly accepted death on the cross in order to teach us compassion and the immortality of spirit. Spiritual teacher Ram Dass was struck with a severe hemorrhagic stroke at the age of 65 in the middle of writing his book, Still Here: Embracing Changing, Aging and Dying. His struggle with faith and his spiritual healing have now become legendary and an inspiration to all who suffer.

Living on Autopilot versus Living Consciously

If nothing else, the experience of chronic pain, or any other illness for that matter, is an invitation from spirit to live consciously rather than on autopilot. Living on autopilot means going through our day without a thought or care as to what we truly feel or believe. It means taking action without conscious choice and letting our childhood programming direct our lives, whether or not that programming is for our highest or greatest good. Often, it is not and we need to "grow up" to make our own conscious choices in order to be truly fulfilled and healed.

Chapter Summary

- Pain is a useful sign that something is amiss or out-of-balance in your life.
- Pain may be signaling that you need to wake up and pay attention to something in your life that may not be serving you.
- Pain symbolizes an opportunity for us to take full responsibility for our health and our happiness.
- We can choose to see pain as an opportunity, rather than as an enemy.
- Some people are "wounded healers" whose purpose in life is to empower others to heal from a place of compassion.
- Pain may be an invitation to start living from our conscious selves rather than living on autopilot.

23

SELF-ACCEPTANCE

A natural progression seems to occur in the healing process that seems to be mirrored in my experience with patients seeking pain relief. Why is it that one person will read this book and overhaul her lifestyle and habits while another will just put it aside and do nothing? It is likely that if you're reading this, you don't believe in "quick fixes", but I'm sure you know people who do. In the past, I felt frustrated by my patients who didn't take my medical advice. Many doctors feel this same frustration.

Finally after years of suffering from my own illness, I've shifted to a new place of acceptance. It has greatly helped me to realize that even if my patients don't do one iota to help themselves, I can still love and accept them. By accepting them where they are in their journey, it gives them the opportunity to accept themselves. What I finally discovered is that my *relationship* with my patients is more important to the healing process than any tool or advice I can offer!

Jason, one of my patients, had an addiction. As soon as he drank one beer, he couldn't stop drinking. One day he arrived at my office drunk. He could barely look me straight in the eye. I could feel his self-loathing, his shame and his utter embarrassment. Somehow, he got himself to the appointment. Most people would have felt too vulnerable to come, yet Jason showed up and I was ever so grateful that he did. The healing work we were able to accomplish that day was amazing.

Jason trusted me enough to voice the emotional anguish he was feeling. We used two energy tools to help him: the Uhe Desensitizing Method and Tapping. It didn't take long before he felt a significant shift and he left the appointment more healed than when he came in. The entire experience was very moving and I was able to appreciate that we both received a healing that day, not just him. I was transferring this feeling of self-acceptance to Jason. He felt from me what he could not yet feel for himself. When you can get to the place where you accept yourself and all your so-called faults, you will shift into a deeper place of healing.

Although I would love to see every single one of my patients take full responsibility for his or her health and wellness, it would not be reasonable to expect that. Sometimes I don't even want to take personal responsibility for myself, so how can I expect them to? We are all human, so to be fallible and imperfect is part of our charm. In this chapter, I'd like you to consider what stage of the healing process you're at and invite you to fully accept yourself at this stage. Just for the sake of illustration, I'm going to arbitrarily label these *stages*. Since these stages are arbitrary, someone may vacillate between Stage 1 and Stage 2 or Stage 2 and Stage 3. The stages are on a continuum. If you're an achiever, see if you can refrain from making this some sort of contest about "who's best", but rather be perfectly honest with yourself. This is an exercise in self-acceptance.

Stage 1 Healing: Symptom Relief

When we first experience pain that doesn't go away on its own, we often start to get frustrated. Sometimes we wonder, what's wrong with my body? At this stage, we care little about how our pain impacts our spiritual development. We just want it gone. It inconveniences us. It makes our lives miserable. It is annoying. Sometimes we judge ourselves as having done something wrong and then feel guilty about it.

At this stage, when we seek professional help, whether it is through traditional or non-traditional means, we're really just looking for symptom relief. New patients who come for their first appointment with me who are in Stage 1 will often look a little dumbfounded when I begin talking about how their thoughts and beliefs are impacting their pain. People in Stage 1 often aren't ready to make profound life changes. They just want to get back to their lives and keep going on the path they were already going on until they were so rudely interrupted by their pain problem.

The best therapies for those in Stage 1 are likely to be those that provide quick relief (like LifeWave IceWave Pain patches) but don't require much thought or personal development work. Often, people at this stage give their power over to their doctors, therapists, acupuncturists and just want them to "fix" what is wrong. Though it is common for people at this stage to follow the instructions of their healthcare providers, they will often do the bare minimum because they really don't believe that their lifestyle, their thoughts and their habits make that much of a difference. The level of self-responsibility at this stage is low. Similarly, the level of self-empowerment is also low at this stage.

There is absolutely nothing wrong with being at this stage of healing. It is beneficial if you are at this stage to fully own where you're at and not feel guilty about it. Being fully *conscious* in your decision to take limited responsibility for your condition makes you miles ahead of those who do it unconsciously.

My patient Stella came to me with increasing stiffness and pain in her back and legs. Her golf game was severely limited and she was frustrated. I took a thorough history and noted that she was taking many medications including a cholesterol-lowering statin. Statins are a group of drugs notorious for blocking the natural healing mechanisms of the body by blocking Co-enzyme Q-10 production. When I added up the nutrient depletions she had due to her medications, it was clear why she wasn't healing. She was open to removing some gluten from her diet but not terribly convinced it was going to change her condition. She agreed to start taking a high quality co-enzyme Q-10 formula, but I found out later from my assistant that the look on her face when she saw the price (about $1 a pill) meant she wasn't going to keep taking it. No matter how long I counseled her or how many times I explained to her how her medications could be contributing to her pain, she never took the next step which was to at least take a higher quality nutritional supplement. Even though I told her from the first visit that people on statin drugs can sometimes take twice as many acupuncture treatments to see results, I wasn't surprised that she stopped coming. If I had convinced her to continue her treatments, we might have been successful, but I knew she wasn't going to invest more time and energy into her treatments. She was in Stage 1.

I had another patient in Stage 1 who was in her eighties. She responded surprisingly well to the acupuncture treatments, but had a problem list a mile long. I knew we weren't going to be able to "cure" her of everything with just acupuncture alone. After I determined she was gluten-sensitive and suggested that her condition would heal much faster if she removed it from her diet, she decided to stop coming after the third visit. Her thinking was: *"Thanks, but at my age, I'm not going gluten-free!"*

Stage 2 Healing: Curious Awareness

In Stage 2, people tend to be more inquisitive about the reasons for their experiencing chronic pain. At the beginning, the reasons may seem simplistic, such as "my injury just never healed" or "I have arthritis because my mother had it", but in this stage, people are much more open to alternative explanations. Although in Stage 2, people don't take full responsibility for their health and well-being, they often stick with the treatment plan because they have tried lots of traditional therapies without results.

At this stage, people are willing to make small or medium changes in their lifestyles and habits. Furthermore, they have bought into the belief that they have a major role to play in their healing. They realize that they are not just passively receiving care from a doctor but instead, are actively participating in their wellness. The openness of this stage makes these patients really fun to work with, especially when they suddenly gain insight into the power they have within to change their experience.

Jenna had a life-threatening condition due to a drug reaction. She came to me out of desperation. She was unable to work. When I mentioned that she should remove EMF stressors from her bedroom as well as try going gluten-free, she did it immediately. Her new-found health is now inspiring those around her. Now she is an advocate for gluten-free living and shares with me new and wonderful gluten-free resources that may help others. Jenna is well on her way to Stage 3 Healing.

Stage 3 Healing: Co-Creation

Sometimes we are fast-tracked into Stage 3 because we've reached "rock-bottom" like I did with my illness. The status quo, if painful enough, will often convince someone to do whatever it takes to feel better.

In Stage 3, there is no question that when we experience pain relief, we are overjoyed, but we are not *attached* to being pain-free all of the time. At this stage, we realize that something other than our ego is driving us. We feel that there is a link between our experience of pain and our personal transformation. At this stage, we see our pain relief as a spiritual journey rather than as an end point. We may notice that when we re-experience physical pain, we instantly go into self-blame. But as we develop higher consciousness, the self-blame melts into self-compassion. And we may re-experience this pattern many times over and yet each time, it feels new.

Some people who are in Stage 3 Healing feel an urge to share their experiences with others to lessen their burden of suffering. Many of them become teachers and healers in their own right, even if they don't do it professionally. People in Stage 3 are on a continuous journey of healing. They understand that old wounds may show up when they least expect it, so that they can be healed. They take fewer and fewer things personally yet take more and more things responsibly. In other words, they begin to realize that in every moment of every day, they can choose to feel either victimized or empowered. It matters less what choice they make. Rather, it is the acceptance and understanding that they have a choice. This is one of the most profound healing experiences in Stage 3.

In Stage 3 Healing, our experiences become fun and enjoyable. Even pain becomes a reminder to become more conscious. It is very easy to become unconscious of our spiritual process when we are comfortable so pain is sometimes a reminder for us to "wake up" again.

Remember, there is no "better" or "worse" when it comes to the healing stages. I just made them up based on my personal observations of my own experience and my experience with patients. The purpose of this chapter is for you to accept your own healing stage so you can let go of expectations that may be keeping you feeling guilty or sad. Maybe you're in Stage 2, but really do not resonate at all with anything I wrote about Stage 3. That's perfectly fine. You don't have to get to Stage 3. It isn't a destination. It isn't a goal. It is just an observation. On the other hand, you may be in Stage 1, feeling guilty that you really don't want to change your diet or sleep earthed or try brainwave music even though you think you "should". Now I invite you to let go of the guilt and just accept that in Stage 1, you really just want symptom relief!

Chapter Summary

- Part of the spiritual healing process is accepting where you are and letting go of guilt and expectation of where you think you should be.

- Self-acceptance is part of the holistic healing journey.
- The Stages of Healing are arbitrary descriptions of the level of personal responsibility one feels in the healing process.
- Learning to accept whatever Stage you are in is healing in and of itself.

24

THE GIFT OF BEING PRESENT

Countless spiritual teachers advise us to become more "fully present" and tell us of the wondrous benefits from being in this state. These teachers include Deepak Chopra, MD, Eckart Tolle, Carolyn Myss, Pema Chodron, and Neale Donald Walsch, to name a few. Frankly, at first, I didn't buy it. I didn't understand what they meant by "being present". Why couldn't I just *do* something to be present? How was I supposed to just *be* present? I began trying to meditate. Often I'd fall asleep or just start thinking about my next big project. If I did visualizations, movements or listened to Dr. Jeff Thompson's brain entrainment music, I felt great! But I couldn't just sit there with nothing to do and just "watch my thoughts" for very long. I really thought that sitting meditation was the pinnacle of what I was supposed to *achieve*. Presence, however, has nothing to do with achieving.

I'm embarrassed to admit that I used to secretly make fun of people who'd spend their vacations at Ashrams meditating all day. *Boring*, I thought. My judgment was that if these people really wanted to change the world, they should get off their butts and do something useful. Today, I think very differently. Full-time monks and "professional meditators" are accomplishing something amazing with their meditation practices. I'll share with you why what they're doing is as important as what scientists or activists are doing to help heal the world of suffering.

Before having fibromyalgia, I was like the Energizer® Bunny. No one could keep up with me. My need to achieve was so great that once I finished one project, I was on to another, barely giving myself a chance to breathe or even celebrate my accomplishments. This habitual "doing" was actually an unconscious way for me to escape what was really troubling me-low self-esteem.

Somehow I grew up with the unfortunate, common perception that I wasn't good enough. No matter how many outside awards and accolades I received, I still felt like a fraud on the inside. My outer confidence was a mask because inside I was terrified that someone might discover I wasn't perfect. My quest for perfection led me down the path where I eventually burnt myself out and became disabled.

You see, although my body looked "healthy", my mind was stuck in old repeating patterns and my spirit was all but withered away. Thanks to my illness, I had absolutely no choice but to slow down and re-evaluate everything I had believed since birth. I literally came to a point during my illness where I felt I had the choice to continue going down my habitual path of unconscious "doing", or bushwhack through a new, yet undiscovered path of presence where I could regain my health again. Many spiritual teachers call that moment of choice "the dark night of the soul". My spirit had to use my illness in order to get my attention. This may be true of you too.

What Presence has to do with Healing

Carolyn Myss said it best when she explained that healing the physical body requires most of your spirit, i.e. "energy circuits" to be functioning in present time. As I discussed in the Mind section of this book, past emotional trauma or old non-supportive beliefs siphon energy away from the present moment, leaving you with less energy to heal. The practice of being present is a way to recover these lost energy circuits and reintegrate them into present time. The hardest thing about being present is that it isn't really an action. It is, however, a state of being.

The present is also the state from which you manifest your future reality. There is a humorous saying that goes, *"If you have one foot in the past and one foot in the future, you're in a position to piss all over the present"*. Please excuse the harsh language, but I think the point is made! The more we can recognize and choose being present, the more we can live from a place of true choice. Living from a place of choice means never being a victim of circumstances. Your ability to influence the outcome of your desires stems from your moment to moment choices. These choices include the choice to perceive anything that happens to you as an opportunity or as a curse.

It takes courage, persistence and willpower to question our automatic perceptions and choose which ones we want to keep and which ones we've outgrown. These moment to moment choices require presence.

Becoming More Present

There are many spiritual teachers who can help train you to becoming more present. I'm certainly not an expert but I can offer you an exercise that has been helpful to me, so that you can practice getting the hang of it. I encourage you to do further study because you'll find that you'll resonate with some teachings more than others.

Becoming present isn't a goal per se, but a practice. Yoga teachers often call their personal yoga ritual their "practice". Many spiritual teachers refer to a meditative "practice". Being present, like riding a bike for the first time, takes practice. At first, it might feel foreign and you may even judge yourself as being inept at it. You might even negate the experience believing that it isn't worth your time. That's ok. Becoming more present can be one of the hardest things you'll ever practice. But let me tell you this: it is one of the most rewarding.

Practicing Presence—Exercise #1

Sit in a comfortable position with your spine straight. See if you can minimize distractions such as ringing phones, television, music etc. Close your eyes. Now, with your eyes closed, start paying attention to your physical body. At first, you might be feeling the clothes touching your skin, or the hardness of the chair or cushion underneath you. Maybe if you've done yoga or meditation before, you'll automatically tune into your breath. All of that is good.

Next, see if you can tune into the place inside your skin i.e. the interior of the body. There is no need to change anything. I just want you to tune in and notice what it feels like. You might scan up and down and notice how different parts of you feel inside. If any judgment or other thoughts come up, that's ok. When you notice them, just acknowledge them, "Ah, thanks for sharing", and then let them go. Continue redirecting any of these thoughts or judgments and return to tuning into your body. After about five minutes, open your eyes and go back to going about your day.

Practicing Presence—Exercise #2

For this exercise, as in exercise #1, sit in a quiet comfortable upright position and focus your attention inwards. Once you've tuned into the various sensations of your body and just "noticed" what they feel like, I want you to now tune into one specific area of discomfort. It may be easiest to focus on the one area of your body where you're experiencing the most pain. As you train your focus on this specific area, see if you can let go of any judgments that may naturally arise, such as, "ugh, this pain sucks!" or "I wish this would go away now!" etc.

Instead, whenever thoughts come into your consciousness, just say to them, "Thank you for sharing" and then move back to focusing on the sensation of the discomfort. Really feel the sensation without putting a label on it. Even if your mind thinks, "it feels hot"; "oh, it is really feeling tight!" just let these thoughts go and retrain your mind to focus back on just feeling. Immerse your senses into this focused area. Often you may start to feel it shift and change, but you're not trying to make it change. You're not trying to make it go away. Even if the pain does go away (and don't be surprised if it does), see if you can let go of any emotional attachment to the experience.

Instead of hoping the pain will disappear next time you do this exercise, just be with "what is". As spiritual teacher, GP Walsh, likes to say, this is the Art of Allowing. You can learn more about this art by checking out his free introductory course (see Resources for link).

Whenever I practice the first exercise, I am aware of a feeling of vibration throughout my body. There isn't any emotion, just the feeling state. To illustrate how this can work in everyday life, I'm going to share a story about how "being present" helped me release intense fear one night.

As a teenager, I was enraptured by suspenseful horror movies. Movies like "The Amityville Horror", "Carrie", and "Halloween" were classics that I enjoyed. After getting fibromyalgia, I found that I could not really enjoy scary movies very often because they could drain my energy. A couple of years ago, I decided that I was going to watch a scary movie called "The Ring". A friend of mine had enjoyed it, so I thought that I was strong enough to start watching scary movies again. Well, "The Ring" turned out to be one of the scariest movies I ever watched. The special effects were especially haunting and I was scared something was going to crawl out of my television when the lights went out! After watching "The Ring," I could barely fall asleep the next two nights because my mind would conjure up images from the movie over and over again.

What made things worse for me is that I knew I was draining my energy by making myself so scared by reliving the scenes in my head, yet I couldn't seem to concentrate on relaxation exercises either. The movie had a cliff-hanger ending and it bothered me that there wasn't a resolution to the movie. Over time, I finally forgot about the movie and was able to sleep normally and to walk by the television late at night without freaking out.

Guess what happened? The sequel to the movie, "The Ring 2," came out on DVD and my friend offered to lend me the movie. I couldn't resist. I just *had* to watch it! Once again, after watching it, I scared myself silly and couldn't fall asleep. This time, however, instead of trying to breathe and relax, and calm myself, I decided to dive right into the scared feeling. Scenes from the movie kept running around in my head, so I redirected my focus to my body. I became curious about what was going on in my body. In other words, I asked myself, "What does being really scared feel like in my body?" I directed my attention within and was surprised at what I found. I felt waves of huge pulsing energy throughout my entire body. This energy was so big, it was literally shooting out of my hands and feet! The sensation was so interesting, I investigated further and found that my heart was beating so vigorously that I could feel the heaving of my chest wall, up and down. Wow! I never noticed this sensation before. Everything I felt was new and curious to me. As soon as I noticed myself thinking these thoughts, I'd go back to focusing on the experience. The next thing I knew, I was sound asleep and woke up bright-eyed and bushy-tailed the next day.

So what happened to me and why was I able to fall asleep? Instead of resisting my feeling of being scared, I consciously dove into it and became curious about what that experience was like. I was so fully *present* with my experience of feeling scared, that I didn't have time to re-live the scary scenes of the movie (which would have been experiencing the past). Being fully present meant that I could no longer be scared. Instead I was just present to what *is*.

This experience has reminded me over and over again of the power of being present. Resisting our experiences rather than diving into them creates the opposite effect that we desire. However, it is natural to resist what is uncomfortable. Here's the cool part. You can be resisting what is uncomfortable and then fully acknowledge your resistance in the present and consciously *feel* your resistance! You can't really "do" presence wrong!

When we experience pain in our bodies, it is often the result of stagnant energy. There isn't enough movement of energy, whether that is related to emotional issues, nutritional issues, or spiritual issues. No matter the cause, just putting your attention on the issue without judgment or intention other than to just be present with it, often gives the area enough energy to move through the stagnation. However, being attached to that goal causes restriction and more stagnation, because in that attachment, fear comes up and that means you are no longer present to what is.

Chapter Summary

- Being present means having all of your spirit or energy circuits in present time.
- The present is the state from which you manifest your reality.
- Being in the state of presence takes practice, just like any skill.
- True holistic healing includes the practice of being present with our experiences whatever they may be.
- Bringing focused, gentle attention to a painful area through the practice of presence may help to shift your experience of it.

25

BODYWISDOM™

I'm absolutely thrilled to be able to share with you BodyWisdom, created by my friend and colleague Lion Goodman. BodyWisdom is a coaching process for dealing with uncomfortable experiences, feelings, or problems (including chronic pain). Using BodyWisdom, a coach can help clients process their experience fully, and discover its source. This enables the experience to complete its creation cycle, and thus shift or disappear. You can also use the process to coach yourself in shifting the chronic pain experience. I've been given permission by Lion to reproduce his article here:

BodyWisdom is part of *The BeliefCloset Process®*, a sophisticated healing methodology that can transform negative and limiting beliefs into positive and empowering beliefs. For more information about this, go to: www.TransformYourBeliefs.com.

BodyWisdom is a process for:

- ✓ Making direct contact with any uncomfortable experience, feeling, problem, or concern,
- ✓ Discovering its source, and
- ✓ Allowing it to complete its creation cycle, and thus change or disappear completely.

Note: This exercise is intended to serve as an exploration of human consciousness. It is not intended to treat or cure any physical, mental, or medical condition. If the condition you are exploring does not clear up after using this exercise, see a doctor or obtain medical advice from a licensed medical professional.

BodyWisdom can be used to explore any persistent or unresolved problem or issue. For example:

- I have an uncomfortable feeling and don't know what to do about it.
- I keep having the same negative experience over and over again.

- I have a persistent pain.
- There's something that won't heal.
- I can't let go of a particular experience.
- I don't know what I'm feeling.
- I have a problem but I don't know how to resolve it.

Background Theory:

Every *experience* moves through a *Creation Cycle*. It has a beginning (appearance), a middle (experience), and an end (disappearance).

When experienced fully, an experience will complete its Creation Cycle and disappear (or change).

When an experience is *resisted* (in any of the ways it can be resisted) it will persist, repeat, or become more energetic. There are many ways to resist an experience:

- ignore it, deny it, or pretend it's not important
- suppress it, shun it, forget about it, decide not to experience it
- think about it, figure it out, or any other mental process
- label it and/or talk about it
- do something about it, or do something else
- feel another feeling, or go numb and feel nothing
- remember a similar feeling or experience and compare the two
- get distracted, put your attention on something else
- dissociate (*disassociate*) by separating yourself from your body
- enter another component of consciousness (identity, voice, sub-personality)
- etc.

When a person is confronted with a situation and doesn't know what to do, he or she will do something he/she <u>does</u> know how to do (e.g., dissociate, resist, suppress, etc.).

The key to clearing an unwanted experience is to become *willing to experience* it.

When resistance turns to willingness, the experience is allowed to complete its original intent, completing its Creation Cycle.

BodyWisdom Instructions:

One person takes the role of the coach, and the other takes the role of the client.

The coach asks a series of questions, directing the client's attention to a specific body sensation in order for the client to experience the sensation fully. When a sensation is experienced fully, it will change or disappear. If it doesn't change or disappear, it either: 1) has not yet been fully experienced, and requires more attention, or 2) it has a message that has not yet been received. To deal with the latter case, a direct dialogue with the sensation enables the message to be received.

The coach's attitude should be reverent, respectful, appreciative and honoring of whatever comes up. Answers can sometimes be surprising, so accept every response as if it is perfectly normal (even if the client says "the sensation is the shape of an upside-down giraffe."). Treat every answer and sensation as if it is a report from a child you love and want to encourage. Enjoy yourself, the other person, and the exercise.

This exercise is intended to help clients get in direct touch with feelings, memories and experiences that have been set aside, forgotten, or repressed. Emotional responses to the exercise are expected and are treated as part of the exercise. In extremely rare cases, a client may have a very strong emotional reaction during the exercise (fear, trauma reaction, big upset, etc.). If this should occur, simply say: "We're ending the exercise now. Please open your eyes, and let me know what you experienced." This will bring the person back into normal consciousness.

The coach starts by asking, "What are you experiencing that you would prefer not to experience?" Allow the client to describe it in detail. If the problem, issue, or discomfort is being experienced *now,* in the present moment, the coach asks the client to place his attention on his body, and feel whatever sensations are present *right now* in his body. These sensations should be associated with the problem, issue, or discomfort the client wishes to be rid of. The client needs to describe the sensations in detail.

If the problem, issue, or discomfort is something the client experienced *in the past,* ask the client to remember what the experience felt like, and to reproduce the feeling by remembering the experience vividly, as if it were happening right now. Then ask him to describe, in as much detail as possible, what the sensations feel like that are present in the body right now. [What is being experienced in the present may be different than the person's experience in the past. Use whatever comes up in the present moment, not memories of what things felt like in the past.]

The coach listens carefully to the client as he describes the sensations, and takes notes throughout the exercise to help in remembering the details. Note that sensations are often felt or experienced outside the physical limits of the body. ["This cloudy feeling goes out ten feet past my body." "It weighs ten thousand pounds."] Accept whatever the client says about his experience.

It is important to make a distinction between terms for 1) physical sensations and 2) feelings (or emotions). In this exercise, we are working exclusively with physical sensations such as weight, size, form, temperature, color, movement, and shape. We are *not* working with feeling or emotion *labels* such as anxiety, fear, anger, sadness, grief, etc. Labels are sometimes useful, but not for this exercise.

Every emotion can be felt as a set of sensations. Sadness, for example, is usually associated with a sensation of heaviness in the upper chest and/ or constriction, often extending into the throat. Anger is often associated with heat, agitation or rapid movement upward from the belly. Both fear and excitement are terms used for agitation in the chest, throat or belly ("butterflies in the stomach"). If the client uses an emotion label, say, "Okay, that word is a label we use to describe specific sensations. Feel the sensation directly inside your body, and describe what it actually feels like."

Next, the coach will ask a series of questions to direct the client's attention toward the direct experience of sensations. When a client actually *focuses attention directly on the sensation,* he or she cannot help but experience it fully.

The coach uses his or her intuition and empathy, feeling into the client's experience as he describes it. Allow yourself to feel the sensations being described, reproducing them in your own body. You will intuitively know what to ask next. Remember to take notes, because you will be repeating the descriptions back to the client periodically.

Direct the client to identify whatever the sensation feels like right now. Keep his or her attention focused on specific answers-the more specific, the better. If the person says, "It's big," ask, "How many inches across is it?" If he reports: "It's hot," ask "How many degrees hotter than body temperature is it?" This forces the client to place more attention on his experience than he normally would, which is the key to clearing previously un-felt feelings. When you repeat any question, add the word "now," since sensations change when attention is placed on them.

The coach says: "Feel the sensation, just as it is, from the center of the sensation. With your awareness, expand outward to its edges. How far out does it extend? Add: "Some edges are sharply defined, and some are fuzzy. They may gray out or fade out. If the edges fade out, look for the place where it ends, and it doesn't exist anymore." Wait for her answer, and be sure the client provides a specific measurement. (If she says, "a couple of feet," ask, "Is it two, two and a half, or three feet? Hold a measuring tape up against it and see exactly how far it extends.")

Next, ask the following questions, or similar questions that are relevant to the sensation being described. Use your natural curiosity to inquire, as if you are interested in *exactly* what the sensation's qualities are. The questions can be asked in any order. Pause between questions, and give the client enough time to look, perceive, feel, get an impression, and report back to you.

- Look at the entire sensation's shape. As you feel the overall shape of the sensation, describe it. What shape is it, exactly?
- How big is the sensation? Specifically in inches, what is its height? Width? Depth? How far into or out of the body does it start, and how far out does it extend?
- Does it have sharp and defined edges, or are they fuzzy, less defined, or diffuse?
- Is there an energetic center that it seems to emanate *from*? Are there hot spots of more intensity, or is the sensation the same everywhere?
- If you put it on a weight scale, how much would it weigh?
- [If there is pressure] How many pounds of pressure does it have, and in what direction is it pressing?
- If it had a color, what color would it be?
- If it were made of some material, what material would it be made of?
- Is it still? Or does it have some kind of movement, pulse or vibration? Describe the movement or vibration in detail.

- What is its temperature in relationship to your body temperature? Is it colder? Warmer? If you put a thermometer next to it, what temperature would it read?
- If the sensation exists in two or more places, then look to see whether the sensations are connected in some way. If they are, describe the connection.
- (Add any other questions that are customized to the type of sensation being described.)

Notice that these questions are directed at expressions of physicality. If the client attempts to label it ("It's anxiety/fear/anger."), gently bring his attention back to the sensation: "Okay, that's a label you're applying. Set that aside and feel the sensation directly. What is its size/shape/color . . . ?"

After the person identifies a few of the sensation's characteristics, say, "Okay, just allow that *<specific sensation>* be there, and make sure you're breathing." (For example: "Just allow that *six-pound four-inch-long orange hollow metal tube* to be there, and make sure you're breathing.") *Allowing a sensation to be there* requires a conscious willingness to experience it. Acceptance, or being willing-to-experience something, is required to release anything that's been resisted.

Let the person feel it "just as it is" for a little while (a few breaths). Then ask, "Is it still there, or did it change, or is it gone?"

- If it's still there, say, "Okay, just allow it to still be there."
- If it changed, say, "Okay, just allow it to change."
- If it's gone, say, "Okay, just allow it to be gone."

When a sensation is experienced fully, it will change or disappear. If it changes, the sensation may now feel entirely different, or it might be similar, or it may be a lighter version of the same sensation. Whatever the case, ask the same series of questions about the sensation *as it is right now*—as if it's a new sensation. If the client attempts to compare the current sensation to the previous one ("It's much lighter . . ."), focus her attention on the current one. For example, ask, "How much lighter is it? And how much does this one weigh, exactly?" Ask each of the questions again (as if for the first time) with this new sensation.

301

If it disappeared, ask, "How do you feel now?" or, "How do you feel without the sensation?"

If the sensation is still there and is unchanged, it either: 1) has not yet been fully experienced, and requires more direct attention in order to experience it fully, or 2) it has a message that has not yet been received. Use your intuition here. If the client has really experienced the sensation, go on to the Dialogue step. If you suspect that the client has not yet really experienced the sensation (for example, if he's been in his head instead of in his sensing body), go through the questions again, encouraging him to actually *feel* the sensation as-it-is, rather than just observe it or describe it.

The Dialogue: Discovering the Message

This step can be done anytime, but it is best used when a sensation will not change dramatically or disappear completely.

Say to the client, "Okay, now approach the sensation as if it were a person. Extend your attention to it, and ask it, respectfully, "What message do you have for me?" Listen carefully to the answer, and let me know what the message is." The coach writes down the message as the client reports it. Accept any message that comes through as valid and reasonable, even if it doesn't make any sense to you. Sometimes the messages are surprising.

Messages are usually beliefs in some form. You can also ask the sensation, "What belief are you?" This provides more information which can be utilized in the *BeliefCloset Process*.

Dialogue Theory: Every sensation and experience is an attempt to provide a signal to the individual (to the brain, the self, or consciousness), informing him of something important. *Pain* is a sensation that sends the message "Something is wrong here. Pay attention! Do something to stop it!" Other messages are beliefs, such as "You didn't protect me!" or "That hurt me!" The Dialogue allows the sensation to complete its "mission," which is to deliver a message. The message may emanate from the incomplete experience itself, or from a part of the psyche (a body part, an Identity, Voice, or Sub-personality) that has something important to say. When the original experience was resisted instead of experienced, the message delivery was interfered with or stopped. That experience continues to attempt to deliver its message to Consciousness. It repeats its message over and over, knocking on the door louder and louder, until the message is received. This is especially true of consistent pains or persisting conditions.

When your car makes a strange noise, you can ignore it (at your peril) or get it checked out by a mechanic. When a body sensation is making a noise, you have the same options. For physical sensations, the message might be "There's something wrong here. Get help!" For emotional issues, the message is often emotional. "That hurt my feelings! Make him go away!"

[Depending on your coaching or therapeutic relationship to the client, the information can be used later to explore the problem or issue further.]

Gleaning more information. There is often more information to glean, so say to the client: "Ask the sensation, 'Do you have any other information or message for me?'" Listen to the answer, and let me know what it says." If the information or message is not clear, you can ask a clarifying question. For example: "Ask the sensation: When you referred to 'them', who exactly are you referring to?"]

After you have written down the messages received, say "Thank the sensation for delivering its message. Tell the sensation that you have received its messages, and its job is done. Tell it that it may now go." Wait a few moments, then ask, "Is the sensation still there, or is it gone?" If a sensation is still there, it is usually a different sensation. Often, it is a deeper layer of the same problem or issue rising up to the surface now that the first layer has been cleared. Most often, the sensation will be gone. This completes the BodyWisdom process on that particular sensation.

Difficult, sticky and persistent problems are often stacked in layers of experiences and sensations, which we call "belief clusters." From the perspective of *The BeliefCloset Process*, these are beliefs that are sort of glued together in a matrix. They often operate together, and they reinforce each other.

When the first layer of a sensation or experience gets lifted off, other layers are exposed and are ready to be experienced. They are often anxious to take their turn at the front of the line! They may have been waiting for years to deliver their message. Somewhere down in the stack is the *original resisted experience*. If you can get the client to fully experience that one, the whole stack often melts away, and the problem disappears along with it.

As each sensation emerges, go through the entire series of questions again, as if for the first time. Every once in a while, a sensations will continue to change and morph. This is a tricky avoidance strategy-there is some strong resistance against experiencing the resisted experience! Here's a handy fix: If you suspect that there is resistance and avoidance going on, tell the person, "Feel what it feels like to resist this experience. Really feel the resistance. Increase the intensity of the resistance. Now describe the sensations associated with that resistance." Use the same series of questions to dissolve the *experience of resistance* itself. When the resistance disappears (similar to any sensation), go back and work with the original resisted experience. It will be much more easily experienced and disappear.

If the sensation has disappeared and you wish to go deeper in the session, ask, "Is there another unwanted sensation or experience you'd prefer not to experience? (or: . . . associated with that issue?)" Repeat the process for that sensation. You may also direct the client's attention to whatever she or he is experiencing right now that is resisted, unwanted, unwelcome, or uncomfortable.

Continue the process until the person feels open, free and peaceful, or until there are no undesirable sensations remaining. To end the session, say, "Okay, we're ending the exercise now."

Clients are often in a spacious, blissful state after the exercise. Recommend that they take a walk to integrate their new state of consciousness, especially before driving their car.

Chapter Summary:

Experiences are part of a Creation Cycle. When resistance of some kind interrupts the cycle, the experience gets stuck in a loop, called an "incomplete cycle," and it creates a persisting condition.

When the person becomes willing to fully experience a resisted or unpleasant feeling or experience, the Creation Cycle can be completed. This allows the experience to disappear. Often, a deeper experience or sensation will emerge, or a series will emerge that lead to the original resisted experience. Once the whole stack is released, the usual result is relief from pain or suffering, deeper insight, a feeling of freedom, and/or excitement about new possibilities.

Please write and tell us about your experiences with BodyWisdom. Email: lion@BeliefCloset.com.

BodyWisdom is a proprietary work product and is © Copyright 2009 by Lion Goodman. All rights reserved.

This exercise is intended to serve as an exploration of human consciousness. It is not intended to treat or cure any physical, mental, emotional, or medical condition. If the condition you are exploring does not clear up after using this exercise, see a doctor or obtain medical advice from a licensed medical or mental health professional. If you choose to utilize this exercise yourself or with others, you agree to take full responsibility for its use and for any results and/or consequences. When coaching others, treat each person, sensation, and experience with love, compassion and care.

If you are a professional coach, teacher, or therapist and wish to use this process in your practice, you may obtain additional training and certification from the author.

BodyWisdom™ is a part of *The BeliefCloset® Process,* a method for permanently eliminating negative and limiting beliefs from the core of the psyche. For information, appointments, or training, contact Lion Goodman: lion@BeliefCloset.com, 415.472.6500. For a free copy of Lion's multimedia eBook, *Transform Your Beliefs,* visit www.TransformYourBeliefs.com

26

EVERYTHING HAPPENS
FOR A REASON

Have you heard that saying? Do you believe it? If you do wholeheartedly agree with the statement, then keep reading. If you wholeheartedly disagree, then this chapter might really annoy you. Either way the choice is yours. If you're just curious, then keep reading, my friend!

Belief is a curious thing so we're going to revisit it in this chapter. A belief is a thought that is so ingrained, so habitual, that it becomes a truth in our minds. You don't have to believe anything I'm saying. What you believe is actually a choice. Most of us don't question beliefs such as the earth revolves around the sun like people did in the 15th Century when Nicolaus Copernicus revealed his discovery. But when it comes to sensitive topics like health, love, money, and culture, our beliefs can create an experience of suffering or an experience of joy.

So how does one *know* what to believe in? It seems as if every time I develop a new belief based on something novel that I've learned and incorporated into my psyche, another event or situation happens that causes me to question my belief. One day, whole grains and low fat are good for your health, and the next day, they are not. Another day, you hear about how the radiation from the earthquake-damaged Fukushima reactor could cause permanent irreversible damage to humankind and then the next day read a book that insinuates that our DNA's potential may be unleashed by it.

If you ever get completely confused about what you should or should not believe, then you're not alone. In fact, if this is a common occurrence for you, be happy about it because at least you're questioning your beliefs. If you are truly open and present with what is, then you're going to really enjoy your healing journey, like I do.

The Gift of Questioning Everything

When we question our beliefs, we are in an open place where we can integrate new information. If we never question our beliefs, we can become blind to new and empowering information. There is a difference between being open and being skeptical of everything. Questioning everything does not necessarily mean being skeptical. It actually means being open to the possibility of anything.

When LifeWave first launched its acupuncture patches to the general public, there was a lot of healthy skepticism. But year after year and study upon study proved that this phototherapeutic device actually worked. Early skeptics didn't even want to try the product even though it was not harmful. They just didn't want to believe the results were real. They imagined that everyone else who believed they worked was just being scammed.

I remember presenting a pain relief demonstration to a group of people a few years ago. All eight of the participants with pain who volunteered to get "patched" were relieved of pain. There was a 100% success rate. The only person still in pain was the one person who refused to try it. When we asked for feedback from the group the next day, she said that she didn't like my presentation style because I was overly casual and she preferred a more formal lecture style. Interestingly, it was her husband, a doctor, who begged her to come to the presentation. She really didn't want to be there. She wasn't ready to change her beliefs.

What Should You Believe In?

Beliefs are powerful. They form the basis for your actions, as in the story above. So how do we know what we should believe in? Well, in my experience, the easiest way to know whether a belief is worth believing in is by answering this simple question: *How is this belief serving you right now?*

That's it! The process is really that simple. Put another way, if what you believe in is currently serving you, then keep believing it. If, however, the belief has not gotten you where you want to go and is not serving you, you may wish to change your belief. When your spirit gives you an opportunity to challenge your beliefs, it is ultimately your conscious choice that guides the outcome of that challenge. For example, when I saw a tumor disappear within minutes on a live ultrasound while Qi Gong practitioners were doing a healing, it radically changed my beliefs about healing cancer. Healing for some can seem to be an arduous, slow process, yet in this instance, it was quick and painless. Not all healing journeys take decades.

Make Up Your Story

Here's one reason for believing that everything happens for a reason. If you truly believe this, then you automatically must believe that there is a purpose to your pain and suffering. Maybe you already believe there is a higher purpose. If, on the other hand, you don't believe that everything happens for a reason, then it automatically means that everything must be happening to you by chance and thus you have no power to influence your reality. The reason I choose to believe that everything happens for a reason is that *it serves me.* If it didn't serve me, then I wouldn't believe it. Am I making some sense?

Now just because I believe that everything happens for a reason doesn't mean that I honestly know exactly *why* everything happens. I don't. But that's the cool part. If you assume that everything happens for a reason and *that the reason is there to serve you in some way*, then your entire perspective on life changes. Imagine if everything that happened to you wasn't pre-labeled good or bad? What if you chose to see everything that happened to you as "good"? What conclusion would you come to about your chronic pain? How possibly could having chronic pain be "good"?

Here's the secret to living a happy life. Well, maybe not *the* secret, but *a* secret. If you entertain the perspective that *everything that happens to you is for your highest and greatest good*, a concept I first read about in Conversations with God by Neale Donald Walsch, then you are free to explore the possibilities on how it is serving you. Literally, you can make up a story about how it might be serving you now or in the future. Why do I consider this a secret to happiness? Because if you consciously perceive everything as "good", then you live in a state of happy expectation rather than in a state of victimhood.

As humans, we often want to understand why something happens, as if everything must have a good reason that we can accept or have control over. Sometimes we're looking for someone or something to blame in order to absolve ourselves of being responsible for our experiences. On the other hand, people may start misconstruing the belief that everything happens for a reason as an excuse to begin blaming people for their own problems. It is nothing of the sort. If a child repeatedly gets raped, few would blame her for attracting this experience. There is no way she would have consciously done so. And what about a mother who loses her daughter, killed by a repeat drunk driving offender? It would be inappropriate to tell her that it is for her highest and greatest good when she's in the middle of grieving.

In the first situation, most people would agree that childhood rape is undesirable, correct? But guess what? It happens. Many people have the perspective that childhood rape "should" not happen to anyone. But if that were true, then people like Louise Hay and Crystal Andrus would not be carrying out their life missions. Crystal overcame her challenging past to become an international motivational speaker, enriching the lives of millions of women worldwide. If Louise Hay and Crystal Andrus had not endured their pain *and rose above it* (that's the key choice), we would not have the benefit of these two important spiritual leaders today. I would not wish this pain on anyone, yet the ability to heal and overcome our circumstances is a human birthright and part of our soul's development.

What about the mom who lost her daughter to a drunk driver? One such mom is Candy Lightner and she is the founder of MADD, Mothers Against Drunk Driving, a non-profit organization that advocates and educates others so that more lives will be saved. After thirty years, this organization is still going strong and probably has saved thousands of lives. Would you not agree that if Candy Lightner had not suffered the loss of her daughter that this wonderful organization would never have been created?

Now it's your turn. You don't have to be a Louise Hay, Crystal Andrus or Candy Lightner. You just have to be you. If you believe that everything happens for a reason and that the reason is for your highest and greatest good, then you can start "making up" positive stories to explain why your spirit has asked you to experience what you're experiencing.

So I invite you now to take out a pen and a journal and start jotting down some reasons why you think your chronic pain experience might be for your highest and greatest good. If you're not ready for this exercise, then just leave it. It may not resonate with everyone. If on the other hand, you want to play this "make-belief reality" game with me, here are some ideas to get you going. You can start with this sentence (or something similar) and fill in the blank.

Having chronic pain may be the best thing that ever happened to me because . . .

I am learning so much about myself that I would never have known before this happened.

I appreciate myself more.

I discovered how much my family values me.

I am better at standing up for myself.

I have more compassion for others in pain.

I could never say "no" before, and now I can.

I've learned to appreciate and take care of my body better.

I've become more conscious.

I'm happier because _____.

I am learning how to receive.

I feel more empowered than ever before.

I appreciate that life is a gift.

I am sharing what I'm learning and helping others with this knowledge.

I found a tribe of people who really support and love me.

I don't take my life or my body for granted anymore.

My kids don't take me for granted anymore.

There are hundreds of reasons you can make up to rationalize how your chronic pain may be serving you. No one can prove that you're right or wrong. It is just an exercise to open your mind and heart to the possibilities. If you feel more open and more empowered after doing this exercise, then use it anytime you are feeling down or disempowered. If, on the other hand, it isn't resonating with you, that's okay. Stick to the parts of this book that do.

There's an Albert Einstein quote that I just love which goes something like this: *We can't solve problems by using the same kind of thinking (consciousness) we used when we created them.* One of the reasons why I'm asking you to consider the possibility that everything happens for a reason (and that the reason is for your highest and greatest good) is to open your mind to a new line of thinking. Maybe you've thought this way for years. On the other hand, maybe it is brand new. Take this belief for a test drive. Try it out for a while. See if it serves you or not. If it does, keep it, if it doesn't, then throw it out.

Chapter Summary

- Believing that everything happens for a reason is a perspective we can choose to entertain or not when it comes to our chronic pain.
- If we believe that everything that happens might be for our highest and greatest good, then our perspective changes. We are then never victims of circumstance, but participants in a grander scheme.
- Because we can't really know for sure why anything happens, we can just make up the reasons why we are experiencing what we are, putting a positive spin on it if we like because it serves us.
- The spiritual journey centers on choice. You can choose your beliefs based on how they affect your life. If they serve, keep them, and if they do not, then let them go.

27

FORGIVENESS

Without a doubt, the process of forgiveness is the fastest, straightest path possible to healing. When Eldon Taylor's subliminal recordings were tested on correctional facility inmates with the message of forgiveness, it had a significant demonstrable impact. When interviewed, a majority of inmates had the belief that life had "done them wrong" and they held a lifetime belief of victimhood. When the subliminal messages of forgiveness were played over and over again, these inmates showed a remarkable improvement in their behavior.

So long as we stay in a place where we feel victimized by our circumstances, we can't fully heal both physically or spiritually. Not surprisingly, one of the steps of the Tapas Acupressure Technique (TAT) involves forgiveness of self and others. Although we can't control everything that happens to us, we can influence our lives through our moment-to-moment choices. One of those types of choices is either to accept or resist our circumstances. When we accept our circumstances, it doesn't mean that we necessarily like what is going on. Acceptance means that you surrender your need to control all aspects of your life and instead, realize that you can take action from either an empowered place or a victimized place.

When we resist what happens to us, we literally cause energy to stagnate in our bodies. This stagnation can cause real pain. The resistance is often in the form of thoughts and emotions. Here are some examples of resistance:

> *This shouldn't have happened to me.*
> *What did I do to deserve this?*
> *It figures!*
> *. . . as per "usual"!*
> *I'm a good person, aren't I? Why is this happening?*
> *He should pay for what he did to me!*
> *Life is a bitch!*

Why me?

An easy way to tell if you're in resistance is to notice how often you use the words "should" or "should have" in your everyday language (or your thoughts). Another tell-tale sign you're in resistance is if you're always asking "why" something is the way it is. I often notice that I'm "should-ing" myself and I have to remind myself that this type of thinking can be quite non-productive and even toxic. When we are in resistance, we lose a lot of energy. This energy could be used to heal our bodies instead of being burned off in resistance.

Why Forgive?

To answer this question simply: *because it makes your life work better.* Resistance to what is present in our lives leads to mental and emotional suffering and eventually to physical suffering. It isn't easy, however, to let go of our resistance. Why? Because we've taken decades to learn it from our parents and our community. Vengeance and justice are commonplace concepts that have become ingrained in our mass consciousness. Unfortunately, just because it is ingrained doesn't mean it serves us.

Imagine yourself in a kayak paddling upstream against a forceful current. It isn't much fun is it? It expends an inordinate amount of energy. It's also near-impossible to get where you want to go. On the other hand, if you turned the kayak around and paddled with the current, quickly maneuvering past any obstacles such as rocks, you'd be traveling with little resistance. It would take much less energy. Life is much like a river. You can either resist what experiences it gives you or you can go with the flow and maneuver around any obstacles you may encounter. The more practice you get at maneuvering around obstacles, the faster and more enjoyable your life.

Forgiveness helps us let go of mental and emotional obstacles that serve to block the flow of our energy. As I mentioned before, energy blockages cause real physical pain in the body. Many people have experienced that by adopting new habits of forgiveness and acceptance, they enjoy their lives more and experience less pain.

313

Who to Forgive?

Think back to everyone who ever hurt you in your past. Is there anyone who, when you think of them, still brings up painful emotions? If there is, don't feel bad about it. Instead, rejoice that you've actually discovered a pathway of lost energy. Even if the painful emotion is just 2 out of 10 on the pain scale, it is worth addressing it. You can use Tapping, TAT or any other modality you choose to neutralize the negative emotions that still bind you to that memory.

Many people erroneously think that by forgiving someone, they are automatically condoning that person's behavior. Quite the contrary. When we hang on to our grudges and hurts, we mostly hurt ourselves. We prevent ourselves from moving forward in our lives with our full energy and instead leave parts of our energetic body behind in different places and times in the past. Having more energy in your body will hasten your healing.

Even if you can't think of anyone specifically that you want to forgive, sometimes we have inadvertently taken on other people's battles. I used to do this all the time. Before I recognized that my ex-husband might have had some depressive tendencies, I used to feel extremely protective of him, taking his side in any argument. In fact, it was always someone else's fault when things went wrong and I used to feel so sorry for him. It took almost a decade of personal transformation before I realized that I was doing my ex-husband a disservice. By supporting his victim mentally, I was actually adding to his misery! Instead of seeing him empowered, I was seeing him just as he saw himself-a victim.

I've noticed that I get angry sometimes when I hear about the lying or corruption that abounds in modern society. If getting angry gets me to moving into positive action, that's one thing, but if I become stuck in anger and resentment, then it is harmful. How many times have you witnessed some sort of atrocity on the news and then absorbed that negative energy, the energy of battle, into your body or your psyche? I've done it plenty of times, and it has been an autopilot response. It takes conscious awareness to catch ourselves when we go into battle or judgment. Understanding that this battle wages war inside our physically painful bodies may help us ease up on this habit.

Forgiveness Exercise

Let's check where in your life you still have judgment and where you could use forgiveness. The purpose of this exercise is for you to become more aware of your judgments, rather than trying to change them. Chances are, you will naturally resist any attempt by me to change your mind. That's okay. This is an awareness exercise. As you read the scenarios I present to you below, I want you to honestly gauge your reaction. It is okay to feel the full gamut of emotions. Just tune into whether you have a feeling of "it's not okay" or "this shouldn't happen". Please note that some of these scenarios can be disturbing, so if you are super sensitive and wish to skip this exercise, I completely understand.

- ❖ **Scenario 1:** Your neighbor's cat defecates on your lawn regularly and your neighbor denies this is happening.
- ❖ **Scenario 2:** Your child's teacher calls her a "lazy pig" and gets away with it.
- ❖ **Scenario 3:** A car cuts you off on the freeway and you almost have an accident.
- ❖ **Scenario 4:** Your colleague takes credit for work that you did and gets promoted.
- ❖ **Scenario 5:** You find out that genetically modified foods are harmful to animals and humans yet the food corporations are still allowed to sell it without labeling.
- ❖ **Scenario 6:** You learn that the government decides to give millions of dollars to corporations to bail them out of bankruptcy only to learn that most of that money went to the CEO's and boards of directors instead of to workers who were laid off.
- ❖ **Scenario 7:** A raw milk farmer was jailed and tortured by government officials for sharing his milk with friends and neighbors.
- ❖ **Scenario 8:** A thief broke into your home and stole all your prized possessions and ruined your family photo album.
- ❖ **Scenario 9:** Your child was bullied by another child in school and came home with a black eye and severe anxiety.
- ❖ **Scenario 10:** A three year old was repeatedly sexually abused by her father.

❖ **Scenario 11:** You find out that in some countries, women are still considered property, just like cattle.

❖ **Scenario 12:** The vaccine that is heavily marketed to young women to prevent cancer is not only ineffective at preventing cancer, it might be promoting it.

I'm sure you can think of many more scenarios that might shift someone into judgment and anger. There is nothing wrong with having judgment and anger as we are only human. But when the judgment and anger festers and becomes an underlying foundational element in our lives, then we're in trouble. Instead of being able to forgive and let go, while pursuing our mission and our purpose, we can get "stuck" on seeing only what is wrong with the world rather than what is right with it. The toxicity of watching nightly television news takes advantage of our minds and emotions this way.

Forgiveness Doesn't Mean Condoning

Many people automatically equate forgiveness with condoning. These are two different things. Although I may choose to forgive someone for hurting me, it doesn't mean that I condone their actions. Condoning harmful actions means that you're okay with someone's actions. Forgiveness means that you let go of your desire for vindication or vengeance and that you understand that being human means having flaws.

You can both forgive someone while at the same time taking action to protect yourself and those you love. If someone tries to hurt you, it would be appropriate to take action to protect yourself. Doing so means that you have healthy self-esteem and courage, and is a form of self-love. Protecting yourself may mean communicating what isn't acceptable to you or it may mean taking someone to court.

For example, if I'm with my beloved niece and I see someone bullying her, I'm not going to stand there and do nothing. You better believe that I'll jump right in and protect her, even if that means physically restraining the other person or calling the police for support. Even if that happens, I can still choose to forgive that person, knowing that their actions were probably learned, and that deep down, *we are all one.* I don't have to take pleasure in that person's punishment. I can choose instead to pray for healing for that person, while at the same time, upholding the boundaries that I've decided are acceptable to me.

Loving Your Shadow

One of my abundance teachers, T. Harv Eker, likes to ask in his seminars, *"Do you want to be right or do you want to be happy?"* After I heard this the first time, it really affected me. Self-righteousness was one of my "best" traits. I was often *right*, and through the years found myself pointing out the wrongdoings of others. It wasn't until I heard T. Harv's question that I paused to think about my consistent habit of wanting always to be right. I still have a hard time letting go of winning an argument. I'm not Einstein, but I'm smart enough to be right a lot of the time. That's been a major stumbling block for my healing.

Now, I like reminding myself, "Do I want to be right or do I want to be healthy?" It's taken me a lot of work to understand that my addiction for being right stemmed from low self-esteem and low self-compassion. I really didn't accept my shadow side and instead prided myself as being extra-responsible, extra-honest, extra-hard working, extra-tolerant etc. Anything I couldn't stand in another (lying, cheating, laziness, rage), was something I couldn't accept in myself. Debbie Ford, author of The Shadow Effect, shares that our shadow carries gifts. If we do not accept our shadow and learn to integrate it into our wholeness, we will have a hard time being happy in life. Many of us have learned to shun our failings, our shadows. Apparently, that's like disowning your left arm and preferring your right arm. You wouldn't cut off your left arm would you? Of course not!

As I mentioned in the chapter on self-acceptance, the ability to accept who we are today is part of holistic healing. Part of that self-acceptance is the acceptance of your shadow. When you can accept and even love the shadow side of you, you will no longer need to be right all the time. Instead, you will be able to compassionately accept other people's shadows, which will help them heal, as well as yourself.

In case you're not clear on what is considered our shadow selves, the parts we've often disowned, here's a short list:

- Our laziness
- Our dishonesty
- Our addictions
- Our lack of integrity
- Our fearfulness
- Our rage
- Our jealousy
- Our manipulations
- Our lustfulness
- Our greediness
- Our superiority complex
- Our vengeance
- Our ignorance
- Our selfishness
- Our critic

Can you think of more? If you haven't already seen Debbie Ford's video, The Shadow Effect, I highly recommend it. Forgiving yourself, accepting your shadow, and letting go of being right, will catapult you to an exciting new place of healing. Not only will this process aid you in healing physical pain, but emotional and relationship pain as well.

So aside from the benefits to healing, why accept our shadows? The answer is that each of our shadows carries with it gifts. Now that I've been able to own more of my anger shadow, I am more able to create and uphold healthier relationship boundaries.

In one intensive workshop I participated in, the students had to bring up their angry "enforcer" energy in order to tell a potential perpetrator to "back off" from harming a loved one. Although the teachers were only pretending to be the perpetrators, the energy in the room was tense and at first, many people couldn't do the exercise. Some people just swore, some cried and some laughed nervously. But until we gave the teachers the precise energy they were looking for, they wouldn't let us end the exercise. They pushed us (compassionately of course) into bringing up our shadow until we could use it consciously for a positive goal.

So aside from anger, can you think of some benefits from being lazy? Dishonest? Ignorant? Greedy? All these shadow qualities have their gifts. Personally I have great difficulty owning my lazy shadow. If anyone criticizes me for being lazy, my defenses fire up automatically. Why? Because I have difficulty accepting my lazy side. I equate being lazy with being a bad person. Now I realize that in owning my lazy side, I can finally *rest* my body instead of pushing it to the limits like I did when I first burnt out. I can forgive myself for wanting to plop on the couch and watch movies instead of working on the computer.

In the recent past, no personal attack could be more wounding to me than someone accusing me of my unacceptable shadow qualities: selfishness, laziness, and dishonesty. When I say wounding, I really mean wounding to the core! The worst reaction I'd have is when the criticism came from my parents. The accusation, *"You're so selfish"*, would send me into a tailspin of co-dependent people-pleasing and overworking. These days, I'm learning to own my selfishness and realize that this part of me is only trying to show me that I deserve to receive the gifts of the Universe. Being selfish has now transmuted into conscious self-care. Some of us really need to be *more* selfish so that we can better take care of ourselves. I am one of them.

Welcome Your Mirrors

If you're not really clear just yet what shadows you have not integrated and accepted in yourself, it is pretty easy to figure them out. Just jot down all the things that drive you crazy about other people! Our spouses and parents are great places to start. Whatever you judge as unacceptable in others is usually a shadow part of yourself that has not healed. The people in our lives are just mirrors.

If your experience of life has attracted people who criticize you, judge you or otherwise demean you, then you've really got some empowerment work to do in your life. Those mirrors in your life are there to give you the opportunity to step up and find your inner strength. Although most people are not going to easily love someone who abused or hurt them, at some point when they can rise above the experience to heal, they may realize that their new place of empowerment could only have come from the *entirety* of their past experiences, including their traumas.

Sometimes my mirror is someone who is currently at a spiritual developmental level that I've already worked through myself. By seeing where this person is at and how far I've travelled in my journey, it gives me the opportunity to pause and appreciate myself. A good friend of mine is a consummate people-pleaser. By watching him people-please and say "yes" when he really wants to say "no", it reminds me of what I used to do and how much happier I am now. In addition, I can be completely compassionate towards him instead of judging him. There is nothing greater in friendship than unconditional acceptance of another.

One of the greatest gifts of forgiveness and owning your own shadow is compassion. By accepting our own shadow sides and integrating them into our wholeness, we can choose compassion for others who are stuck in their shadow. The energy of compassion is extremely powerful. When it runs through your physical body, you receive healing, as well as well as the person you're in relationship with.

Compassion-Forgiveness Exercise

Here's a quick compassion and forgiveness exercise for you. The next time you choose to watch the television news and witness disasters or murders, see if you can catch yourself going into judgment, and immediately shift this into becoming compassionate. If there are victims in the story, send them the energy of compassion. Feel free to cry in the moment to share their pain, then consciously disengage your energy from the situation and go about the rest of your day.

If you're an extremely sensitive person, I wouldn't recommend that you do this exercise just yet because you may not have enough practice disengaging your energy from another's. The purpose of this exercise is to be able to dive in, feel someone's pain, then dive out moments later and (this is the important part) still enjoy your life. Remember how young children are when they fall down and hurt themselves? They may cry for a few minutes, but then something else interests them and within moments, they're back to playing. They don't wallow in the past for very long, unless they are old enough to have learned this habit from an adult or older sibling.

In the above exercise, see if you can also practice the energy of forgiveness for the perpetrators, if there are any. See if you can connect with their shadow via your own. As I often like to say, every one of us is a potential Hitler or a potential Mother Theresa. It all just depends on your circumstances and your choices. Even though this exercise seems simple, it isn't necessarily easy. Yet, in its simplicity, it is extremely powerful. It is similar to a Buddhist meditation called Tonglen whereby you consciously breathe in the pains of the world and breathe out compassion and love. See Resources for helpful links.

Chapter Summary

- Forgiveness and compassion are two of the most powerful healing energies on the planet.
- Learning to forgive yourself and others prevents resistance and energy loss which contributes to all sorts of pain.
- Learning to accept and integrate your shadows helps you heal at a very deep level.
- Accepting our shadows means accepting the gifts they bring to our lives.
- Others are just mirrors to us. If someone really annoys us, it often means we have a shadow quality we have disowned.

28

INTUITION IN HEALING

Every one of us has intuitive abilities. Brain researchers feel that the right side of the brain is the intuitive side and the left side of the brain is the logical side. The right side of the brain focuses on holistic thought, whereas the left side of the brain focuses on linear thought. During stress, the natural energetic connections between the two hemispheres of the brain can be disrupted. This is the brain imbalance that I described in detail in previous chapters. In order to access your intuition and act appropriately on it, you need to be brain balanced with both hemispheres communicating to each other.

I have noticed that a few weeks after my patients have been brain balancing using LifeWave Y-Age Aeon patches on a daily basis, they begin to listen to their intuition better. Not only that, they begin acting on it. Synchronicities seem to come more often and they become almost "luckier". The choices they make in everyday life seem to be more in alignment with their Higher Selves and they don't seem to be struggling as much.

My patient, Joanne, was dreading the trip back to her deceased mother's home to do the final clean up. She couldn't even think about the trip without bursting into tears. As she put it, "I was a basket-case!" She knew she couldn't put off the project much longer. She came to me to help her emotional instability. Her brain balance test was markedly abnormal. Within two weeks of patching her head with the LifeWave Y-Age Aeon patches, she reported that she had successfully made the trip to her mother's home, cleaned up the place and hardly experienced any stress. Her friends and family were dumbfounded at the shift in Joan's attitude. In my experience, when the brain hemispheres are balanced and the stress handling system is in "quiet" mode, we are more receptive to our intuitive messages.

Intuition can help you make healthy decisions when you are clear of attachments. When you are attached to a certain outcome, you can cloud your own intuition and make decisions that may not be for your highest and greatest good. Your intuition can help you, for example, with the following:

- ✓ What foods your body wants to be nourished with
- ✓ What healthcare providers/doctors would be a good fit for you
- ✓ What supplements may be helpful
- ✓ What foods you should avoid
- ✓ What relationships you need to either heal or avoid
- ✓ What healing modality is best suited to your needs and personality
- ✓ Attracting supportive people into your life

All of us are born intuitive. Unfortunately, as children, we are literally conditioned to ignore our intuition. We are forced to conform to family or society rules of behavior and conduct. I'll give you a concrete example. Have you ever seen a child refuse to hug or kiss a family member? From the parent's point of view this refusal can be emotionally devastating especially when there is no logical reason for it. Basically the child is energetically "turned off" and the refusal is based on an intuitive feeling. Very few children are consciously encouraged by their parents to follow their intuitive gut feelings. Why? Because it makes them unpopular with other family members. So great is this systematic deadening of our intuitive nature, that by the time we reach adulthood, we've all but forgotten how to access it.

When we do not remember how to listen to our intuition, we can get into a lot of trouble. Often, chronic pain is a result of not listening to our intuitive guidance. We may have refused to listen to our intuitive hits to take better care of ourselves. We may have said "yes" when we really wanted to say "no" when someone asked us for a favor. Our pain then *becomes* the intuitive message in order to get us to pay attention to what really serves us and what doesn't.

Not listening to our intuition can be really costly. It was for me. Long ago, I was interviewed by a colleague for a job. My husband and I desperately needed an income source because we were building our dream house and both of us had quit high paying jobs to do it. The doctor was extremely charismatic and to my logical mind, it sounded like a dream job. There was, however, a part of me that felt very uneasy. I didn't trust

323

this doctor, but I didn't know why. I consulted with a medical practice consultant and she had some concerns as well.

My husband, on the other hand, was also charismatic and convinced me to accept the job because he felt that nothing better was going to come along. I was convinced by my husband instead of following my gut, and I signed the contract and began working for this doctor. Within a year, I knew I had made the wrong decision. He had lied to me about how much money he could get from the insurance companies, so I never got paid for some of the work I did. Finally, we parted ways, but I was really mad at myself for not trusting my intuition. Not only did I lose money, I lost self-respect which in turn, affected my health. This is just an example of how ignoring one's intuition can be very costly.

When we're out of practice with listening and then following through on intuitive information, we become less proficient at it. We become just like a musician who never practices her art. At one time, I was able to play a perfectly executed Chopin Waltz on the piano because I practiced hours every day. But today, I can't play it well because my fingers won't play as fast as they used to and I don't remember the piece. However, if I practiced it again for a few days in a row, my muscle memory would kick in and I'd rapidly improve my playing. It is the same situation with intuition. If you practice listening to and following through on your intuition, your skills will improve.

A whole book could be written on intuition, so this chapter will provide just an introduction. One of the best workbooks on developing your intuition is The Intuitive Way by Penney Peirce. See Resources for helpful links.

Intuition Basics

In order to access your intuition, you actually have to be present in your body. You have to be able to feel your body's signals. It is the easiest and fastest way to access your intuition. People who live in their thoughts and not in their bodies are often either stressed-out or tend to daydream a lot. One clear sign that you're not in your body is if you're clumsy. I used to be incredibly clumsy. Just ask my ex-husband. I used to have bruises all over my body from bumping into walls or tripping over things. My ex-husband was afraid that one day, someone was going to accuse him of abusing me! Come to think of it, it is rare for me to accidentally bump into things these days, so I'm delighted that I'm more present than I've ever been in the past.

Your body is your most convenient and accurate intuition tool. Doing the mindfulness exercises in Mindfulness and Meditation chapter will help you to get in touch with your body at a deeper level. In this chapter, we're actually going to practice feeling our bodies when we're in different mind states. Often the earliest intuitive decisions we can make boil down to a "yes" or a "no". Although not a perfect system, if you get to know what feels like a "yes" in your body versus what feels like a "no", you'll be way ahead of most folks who don't even recognize an intuitive self.

What Intuition is *Not*

Honing your own intuitive skills takes time and patience and certainly this chapter is only a tiny introduction. So many people get confused when it comes to understanding intuition that I feel it is important to share my perspective of what intuition is not. Intuitive messages can come in many different forms. Sometimes they come as emotions, but at times this can be confusing because you might not know whether what you're feeling is intuitive guidance or just patterned responses based on your childhood programming.

Mitch, a young patient of mine, had a lifelong history of recurrent relationship betrayals. This pattern started in childhood but he was unaware of the connection until I pointed it out to him. When I first began encouraging Mitch to use his "senses" to guide his actions, he immediately began questioning whether he should follow his usual reaction of being suspicious of his sexual partner's potential infidelity. His pattern had been to date a woman, only to find out months later that she was cheating on him. He developed a habit of looking for signs of lying and betrayal in every text message, email or face-to-face conversation with any new girlfriend.

Unfortunately that behavior usually drove his partners away and indeed they would end up betraying him, just as he had feared. I explained to Mitch that his *reaction* was not his intuition per se, but rather a programmed protective response from childhood. I cautioned Mitch that his propensity to look for betrayal was not an accurate and beneficial use of his intuition but a habit that was personally damaging and unproductive.

Intuition is not often a feeling of intense fear or anxiety as many people seem to think. Real intuitive data comes through one's consciousness as a subtle "knowing" often devoid of emotional overlay. When Mona Lisa Schulz, MD, PhD, author of Awakening Intuition and Your Intuitive Advisor, was walking across the street and got hit by a truck, her mother, who was at a dinner in another part of the country, suddenly stood up and told Mona Lisa's father that Mona Lisa was in trouble. She didn't have any basis for her "knowing" and it didn't come as an anxiety attack either. She just knew.

My intuition teacher, Laura Day, author of The Circle and Practical Intuition, told me in class that sometime during the early part of 2001, she decided that it was prudent to prepare for possible earthquakes. Being an intuitive, she just followed her intuition to start stockpiling extra water, gas masks etc. in her New York City apartment. She wasn't fearful nor was she anxious about potential earthquakes. She just felt the intuitive pull to take constructive action. Unbeknownst to Laura at the time, September 11th, 2001 was going to be one of the most catastrophic events ever to happen to the United States. When the tragedy occurred in New York City, just blocks from Laura Day's home, she opened her doors to people who needed emergency supplies. Her intuition prepared her perfectly to help others in need-her ultimate mission in life.

My mother is incredibly intuitive. She often refers to herself as "psychic". The only problem is that she can also be extremely anxious. Even though her intuition is spot on with many things, her anxiety can make her intuition inaccurate as well. It sometimes frustrates my father when my mother focuses her intuitive sense on what might go wrong rather than on what might go right in any given situation. When I grew up and spiritual transformation became a passion of mine, it became obvious to me that it was my mother's childhood experiences that honed her intuitive skills to focus solely on survival and safety. I give my mother a lot of credit, however, because she is open to change. She now catches herself when she is spiraling down into negative thoughts and often is able to change her self-talk to a more positive tone.

Have you ever heard of psychics who only seem to give negative predictions? They are great at predicting deaths, cancer, job loss, divorce, but rarely give positive predictions? These types of psychics have the same problem my mother had. They probably grew up in an atmosphere where they felt unsafe and have thus honed their intuitive skills for survival only. Unfortunately, they may be unable to intuitively read anything positive. These types of psychics are dangerous and I believe should be avoided because they are not balanced in their own spiritual development and could potentially harm a client.

A good intuitive, someone who professionally reads another person's energy field, should not only be able to sense what is true for his or her client, but also be able to communicate this knowledge with compassion and a sense for what is for the client's highest and greatest good. Not all psychics are good intuitives, so I like to differentiate the two terms although many people do not. There are talented psychics who are excellent and precise in their readings, but do not have the communication skills or the compassion necessary to deliver the information that will most benefit their client. To state it bluntly, they love showing off and being regarded as talented psychics. A well-trained professional intuitive, however, is someone who reads energy accurately, but also knows how to communicate the information appropriately to best serve the client's highest interest.

As you develop your intuitive skills you will be increasingly accurate as long as you consciously continue working on shifting your negative childhood programming. That's not to say that your intuition won't ever evoke feelings of anger, fear or anxiety, but it is safe to say that if you are only relying on these emotions to give you information, you'll be missing a large portion of useful intuitive guidance. We are all human which means that our experiences will color, or filter, our intuitive guidance. Sometimes following one's intuition may lead to uncomfortable circumstances and yet, these circumstances may be for our own highest and greatest good.

A good beginner's guide to using your own intuition is to keep a private journal and write your experiences down so that you can understand yourself better. Just being open to intuitive guidance makes you much more likely to receive it than if you weren't. Keep in mind that few young musicians can play the violin like Yo Yo Ma, but with decades of dedicated practice and focus, they may be able to. Be patient with yourself and understand that sometimes you'll be "wrong", but know that every experience helps you become a better intuitive.

Intuitive Exercise #1

In a quiet place, sit comfortably, close your eyes and tune into your bodily sensations. Become aware of the feeling in your chest, your stomach, your jaw, your neck and shoulders, your muscles. Scan your body so you get a baseline of how you feel before we proceed to the next step.

After you've done a quick body scan, which should take no more than a minute or two, I want you to bring up a situation in your mind that really bothers you. It could be a recent stress or a situation in the past. If you had or have a conflict with someone close to you, use this situation. If you have stress at work, you can use that situation. The more intense the level of stress, the easier it is to work with in this exercise.

Once you have the situation in your mind, go over the details until the experience is feeling real and vivid. If anger pops up, just let it. Now, once you feel it become as real as its going to be for this exercise, scan your body again. Tune into different parts of your body and see how your body feels compared with your baseline. How does your breath feel now? Your jaw? Your stomach? Your neck and shoulders? Your muscles? What else do you notice? As you notice these sensations, don't judge them. Just notice them.

Usually the body's reaction to something the mind considers negative will be one of contraction. When I've done this at group seminars, many of the participants responded similarly: *"my jaw is tight"*, *"my stomach feels queasy"*, *"my neck and shoulders feel tight"*, *"my muscles are tight"*, *"my breath is really shallow"*, *"and I'm tired"*. It's a lot of fun to witness people noticing their body signals for the first time. They almost seem surprised and most don't realize that these are part of their intuitive feedback system.

Intuitive Exercise #2

Clear your mind from the first exercise, and keep your eyes closed so that you're not distracted by your surroundings. Your body should return to a neutral state. Now shift your mind and think of a very positive situation in your life. It could be a past event that was very positive or a current situation that you are enjoying. You could imagine playing joyfully with your children for example. You could also recall the time when you received a promotion or award. Once you've decided on the situation you wish your mind to focus on, start imagining it as if it were happening right now in the present. When it feels real to you, tune into your body and notice what it feels like. Scan your various body parts to get intuitive feedback.

When people perform this exercise, they often remark how "full" their body feels. Some feel expansive energy in their body. Others remark how deeply they are breathing and still others notice how relaxed their midsection feels compared to how it felt in the first exercise. I don't know how you will feel exactly, but if you've done both exercises correctly, your body should feel different now.

Interpreting Your Body

When the body is in a contracted state, it is also in a low Qi (energy) flowing state. It is a way in which the body says *"no"*. When the body is in an expanded or relaxed state, it is also in a higher Qi flowing state. It is a way in which the body says *"yes"*. When you learn how your body feels when it is saying "yes" versus when it is saying "no", you can use this to help you make healthy decisions in your life. The more you follow through on your body's signals, the more accurate the feedback will be with time.

If you are presented with a situation where you have to make a choice but don't know how to make it, you can try tuning into your body signals for inner guidance. For example, if you are given choice A or choice B, you can imagine yourself in each situation ("futurizing", I call it) and then tune into your body to see if you get a *"yes"* (relaxed) or *"no"* (contracted) reaction. Let's take a real-life example so you can see how this can play out.

Imagine that your doctor has given you the choice to pursue surgery versus conservative care. Now, imagine yourself pursuing the surgical route. How does the body react to the idea of preparing for and going through surgery? Contrast that with imagining yourself pursuing the conservative route. Which feels more relaxed in the body? Although you may feel that everyone would choose the non-surgical route, it is not necessarily the case.

When my father told me he was going to have to undergo cataract surgery, I diligently looked up non-surgical approaches to reverse the cataracts. Although the non-surgical approach seemed low risk and simple, my father chose the surgical route. I clearly felt in my body his increased level of comfort when he chose the surgical route. Would I have chosen that for myself? No, probably not. I would have preferred less invasive and more natural options long before considering surgery. As for my father, I felt he made the right choice for himself. The stress of having cataract surgery was probably less than trying an alternative therapy his doctor didn't approve of.

Dreams as Intuitive Guidance

A very easy way to learn to connect with your intuition is to have a dream journal. Dreaming is a way in which your subconscious can work through issues without the interference from the logical mind. Of course, sometimes we dream about what happened during our waking hours, but more often, dreams reveal a deeper message.

There are books dedicated to dream interpretation. Occasionally, I'll look things up in the book just to see if it resonates with me. For example, I was having lots of dreams about food, which could be interpreted as issues revolving around feeling nourished. Recently I began having dreams about bees. In my dream, bees were flying around me. I was afraid they would sting me, but they never did. Because of these dreams I decided to rent a movie on bees and I loved it. In the movie, Vanishing Bees, I found out that the bees were disappearing most likely due to the toxic effects of Round-up® ready genetically modified plants they were pollinating.

The movie gave me great respect for the role of bees in our lives. In addition, the dreams inspired me to try organic raw honey (unheated) for the first time. My previous attempts at eating honey left me hypoglycemic (low blood sugar) and tired. To my delight, the raw honey was well tolerated in my body. Clearly, the biochemical response of my body to unpasteurized, raw organic honey was completely different from regularly processed organic honey. Once I began eating the raw honey, I stopped having dreams with bees.

I highly suggest that you purchase a beautiful journal just to write your dreams in. Don't use it for anything else like your grocery list or your to-do list. Keep it sacred, just for your dreams. Pick a nice pen as well and maybe have a few different colors available. Each morning, when you first wake up, write down everything you can remember about your dream. Draw pictures if you can. Use whatever color pens you feel drawn to. Most importantly, write down the emotional tone of the dream. How did you feel? Sad? Excited? Angry?

Once you've written down the content of your dream, then you can start interpreting it. Sometimes having a dream book helps, sometimes it doesn't. Having a dream-journaling buddy is loads of fun, so if you have a close friend you can trust, you can do this together. Don't fret if you've never done this before and can't make heads or tails of your dreams. With time and practice, you'll begin to notice patterns and themes that stand out. Those repetitive patterns often represent very significant life themes that need attention. Bringing them into consciousness will hasten their resolution and healing.

So, will writing down all your dreams miraculously heal your chronic pain? Maybe. Maybe not. Healing by accessing your intuition, your subconscious, may mean healing other parts of your life as well, not just your body. Let me give you a personal story about a repetitive dream I was having when I was still married to my first husband.

In the dream, I was kissing him, but yet, it seemed that my mouth was always full of food. The food got "in the way" of the kissing. It was only after we chose to divorce that I realized that my intuition was trying to tell me that I wasn't speaking the truth of my soul. This inability to speak my truth was the real cause of my unhappiness and prevented me from experiencing an authentic relationship with my husband. Since that time, I've been more aware of my dreams. Listening to your intuition may save you years of heartache and pain (even physical pain!).

Dream Requests

One way of consciously using your dreams once you've gotten used to remembering them and journaling them, is to make a dream request. There are two types of requests you can make according to intuitive healer, Judith Orloff, MD. One is to request guidance around a certain situation. You could ask for guidance regarding your health, your finances, your relationships or your career for example. It is important to already be in the habit of journaling your dreams so that you remember most of them.

The other request you can make is requesting a healing. Now, here's a word of caution when requesting a healing through your dreams. Sometimes the healing can take a form that we do not expect. For example, Dr. Orloff notes that if you ask for a healing and you wake up with a panic attack, you should accept this as a sign of your healing and work with it. Healing doesn't always come in the form we expect. See if you can trust in the Universe to bring you the type of healing you need.

Muscle Testing as an Intuitive Tool

Another way to use your body as an intuitive tool is something called muscle testing. Chiropractors use the professional term, Applied Kinesiology, and use this technique to uncover all sort of information including environmental sensitivities, organ dysfunction, functional imbalances and even nutritional deficiencies. Although it takes some practice to do it on yourself, it is very easy to learn how to do muscle testing on someone else.

You can test whether something is for your highest and greatest good by determining whether your energy flow is affected by whatever you are testing. Most commonly, we use the shoulder muscle for testing. If your energy flow remains clear, then your shoulder muscle will "lock" or test strong when the tester is pressing down on your outstretched arm. If your energy flow becomes blocked because whatever you are testing is affecting you negatively, your muscle will "unlock" or temporarily weaken instead.

Say you wish to test whether or not a supplement is good for your teenage daughter. By having her hold the supplement to her chest, you can muscle test her response to having that frequency inside her energy field. If her test muscle (shoulder) remains locked, it means that the supplement supports the natural flow of energy in her body and will likely be helpful. If, however, the test muscle unlocks, i.e. weakens, it means that the supplement caused a stoppage of energy flow and is thus harmful to her.

Before you start muscle testing another person or teach another person to muscle test you, you need to understand a few precautions. First you and the person you are testing must be adequately hydrated. If either of you are not, you can get inaccurate results. Second I have found it very helpful that both parties are brain balanced. It may be helpful to first learn how to test someone's brain balance first and vice versa in order to get the most accurate results. You can watch my video on YouTube which shows how to do the testing. If either or neither party is brain balanced, you can either place a LifeWave Y-Age Aeon patch behind the right ear before muscle testing or say Dr. John Diamond's affirmations several times before muscle testing. There are other methods to ensure more accurate results available from the Touch4Health organization. These methods are referred to as the Zip Up, Switch On, and Tune In, and are available for free on at www.Touch4Health.com.

I often find that it is important to clear any overt biases you may have when testing another person. Strong preferences from either party can override the results when one or the other person has a vested interest in the outcome. Many mainstream doctors consider Applied Kinesiology and muscle testing too "woo woo" to be taken seriously, so it doesn't help when an unethical practitioner abuses it just to sell more supplements. Luckily these practitioners are rare. In my experience, muscle testing is a valuable method to obtain intuitive information when done correctly and with the subject's highest and greatest good in mind. Obviously common sense should prevail. No one can guarantee 100% accuracy with any intuitive tool, so keep that in mind as I teach you how to do muscle testing. Furthermore, you shouldn't make diagnoses with muscle testing.

Muscle Testing Technique

Please note that this technique was already taught in an earlier chapter, but I am repeating it here just in case you didn't read that chapter.

1. Ensure that both you and the person you are testing are hydrated and ideally, brain balanced. Optional: You may wish to place a LifeWave Y-Age Aeon patch behind the right ear before you begin (see Chapter 6).

2. Choose a test muscle. Often the shoulder muscles are used because they are easily accessible and easy to test. If you are muscle testing another person, you need to ask if she has a shoulder injury. If she does, you avoid using the injured shoulder for testing. Using other muscles other than the shoulders is more difficult and beyond what we can cover in this book.

3. Stand to the side of the person you are testing and have her stretch her arm in front, hands in a fist with the thumb facing the skyward.

4. Gently rest your fingertips (usually I use my left hand if the person's left arm is extended) just above the wrist bone in an adult. In a child or small adult, you may wish to move your fingertips further up towards the elbow to avoid pressing down too hard.

5. Instruct the person you are testing that when you say the word, *"resist"* or *"match my pressure"*, you will begin to direct force downwards on the wrist while her job is to resist upwards with equal pressure. Do press down *gradually*, over a count of three, as any person will not be able to resist if you press down on her wrist too suddenly.

6. Begin by practicing a few muscle tests "in the clear" meaning you'll be muscle testing that person without her holding any object next to her energy field for testing. The muscle you are testing should stay locked. If you feel a bounce or she weakens, you are either pressing down too hard, too quickly, or the muscle is an inadequate test muscle. If the latter is the case, change sides and see if the other shoulder tests better. If she does not "lock" when you do the muscle test in the clear, try to have her say her name, such as *"My name is Mary"* and then repeat the test. She should be strong (locked). If not, she may not be a testable.

7. Once both you and the person you are testing get a sense of how much pressure is necessary to feel a "lock", you can test what an "unlock" feels like by repeating the muscle test while the person is holding a cell phone (turned on) to her stomach or chest.

Alternatively, you can ask the person to say a false name, such as *"My name is Bob"*. Most people will immediately "unlock" in the presence of cell phone radiation even if they are not talking on the phone. Same goes for saying a false name.

8. Once you have practiced what an unlock feels like you'll want to get that person's energy field back to its baseline by removing the cell phone and turning it off. For some people, it can take a few minutes to return to a strong state, so I often quicken the process by having her say her name again. This usually strengthens her energy field immediately, and causes the test muscle to "lock" once more.

9. Once you've established a normal muscle "lock" in the clear, introduce the object or frequency you'd like to test. For example, if you're wondering whether cheese is harmful, you can either have them hold a small piece of cheese in their hand close to their chest or have them write the words "cheese" on a piece of paper and hold it up to their chest. If they are sensitive to cheese or if cheese will negatively affect them, their muscle will "unlock" on subsequent testing. The effect is immediate.

10. On the other hand, if you are testing to see if a course of action would be beneficial, you can have your test subjects write down what it is they propose to do and then muscle test it. If they muscle test strong, then it may mean that this particular course of action may be beneficial. If they muscle test weak, it may mean that it might not be. Remember to try to consciously let go of any biases you may have during the testing.

Keep in mind that muscle testing is not a magic crystal ball. You can't use it to win the lottery, and you shouldn't use it to make important life decisions or to diagnose medical conditions (like cancer). You can, however, use it to test for food sensitivities as well as for beneficial supplements. If someone tests weak for a particular environmental stressor, such as a food allergy, it is possible to retrain the body to accept this frequency as neutral rather than harmful by re-wiring the nervous system, which is an integral part of the energy field. I have found that the combination of muscle testing and the Uhe Desensitizing Method has greatly enhanced my patient's ability to heal from chronic pain by neutralizing environmental sensitivity symptoms.

Muscle testing can be useful to confirm intuitive hits versus non-intuitive programming. My patient Tate admitted to being disturbed by issues of erectile failure during sexual intercourse with his girlfriend. I asked him if he were to guess (i.e. use his intuition) whether the problem was physical or emotional, which one would it be. He quickly answered, "Emotional". Given what I already knew about him, I asked him to write down a couple of statements on separate cards:

- Frequencies related to childhood betrayal
- Frequencies related to romantic betrayal

Tate found this exercise very interesting so he wanted to add his own statements:

- Frequencies related to childhood sexual abuse (he thought of this one because others had asked him about it but he couldn't remember any happening in his childhood)
- Frequencies related to religious beliefs about sex (because he grew up in a religious household and thought maybe this programming might be affecting his sexual performance)

We shuffled the cards face down and muscle tested him with each statement. He went weak on the first two but not the latter two. The benefit of this testing was to make Tate aware of the subconscious frequencies that may be negatively impacting his health and happiness.

Self-muscle Testing

Self-muscle testing is a little trickier because it requires a well-practiced ability to sense your body. People who do not energetically inhabit their bodies on a regular basis may have a difficult time learning self-muscle testing. Body awareness is the key to being successful at self-muscle testing techniques. If you don't have a willing person at home to perform muscle testing with, you may wish to learn self-muscle testing as a way to access your intuitive self.

Aside from the technical difficulty in doing it well, a major downfall in testing yourself is that you can get inaccurate results if you can't remove your bias. In other words, you can change the outcome of the test if you have a vested interest in a particular test result. For example, if you're allergic to gluten but you absolutely love bread and cannot fathom a happy life without it, you may muscle test yourself as being able to tolerate bread.

Another pitfall of self-muscle testing is testing separate things, such as supplements, not knowing whether the combination will produce different results. For example, say you muscle test strong with supplement A, supplement B and supplement C. It is possible that with the combination of A, B and C, you may muscle test weak because there might be some overlap or negative interaction.

It is a good idea for you to practice self-muscle testing until you are confident that your results are consistent. When you ask your body, *"Show me a Yes"*, you should self-muscle test strong. When you ask your body, *"Show me a No"*, you should self-muscle test weak. You can also use your name and a false name, respectively, to get used to what a locked and unlocked self-muscle test feels like.

Teaching muscle testing, especially self-muscle testing is a little challenging in a book. As one of my friends likes to say, it's sort of like trying to give a haircut over the phone. For an example of how I do self-muscle testing, check out my YouTube channel. Dr. Bradley Nelson teaches six different ways of self-muscle testing in his Emotion Code workshop which is available on DVD. See Resources for links.

Chapter Summary

- Intuition is a natural in-born ability that we can learn to tap into to help ourselves heal and live happier lives.
- Your body is one of the most accurate intuitive devices. Feeling your body's responses to different situations may help you take appropriate action for your highest and greatest good.

- Intuitive hits differ from anxiety attacks and pre–programmed responses from childhood.
- You can learn muscle testing and teach it to others as a tool to help you access your body's intuition.
- Muscle testing can help you determine whether a course of action or a supplement may be beneficial for your health.
- Muscle testing should not be used to try to win the lottery, to make major life decisions, or to diagnose medical conditions.
- Self–muscle testing is more challenging than muscle testing another person, but with practice, can be an extremely valuable self-healing tool.

Section E

Getting Support

"One of the reasons that our lives are imperfect is that we are meant
to seek and experience healing relationships with one another."
-Karen Kan, MD

29

ASSEMBLE YOUR SUPPORT TEAM

Look Beyond Family and Friends

Healing is a team effort, even if the relationship is only with you and the Divine. I encourage you, however, to begin assembling a support team to help you through your journey. Even the wisest of us can't see past our own biases, so having people you can trust to support you is vital. It would seem intuitive to lean on family and friends for support, but often they are not the right people to get you to where you want to go.

By the time you've been suffering with pain for a while, your close family and friends may have already supported you in the best way they know how. Sometimes, however, they can sabotage you. Why would they do that? Well, it's not that they mean to, but if they are comfortable with who you are, they might not be comfortable with the *new* you as you embark on this healing journey.

More often than not, family members are supportive of you when you're in pain . . . to a point. After a while, though, it starts to get old when you're not getting any better. It isn't that they are bad people; it's just that they want to see some improvement. If supporting you has been stressful on them, they'll hope for a reprieve at some point. If that reprieve doesn't look as if it's coming, then they can develop resentment for having to take care of you for so long.

Your close friends and family have a vested interest in your condition. This can be a double-edge sword. On the one hand, they really want you to get better and will certainly try to help you. But on the other hand, they can easily get *attached* to a particular outcome and prevent you from making a choice that does not mesh with their preferences. I'll give you a painful example of how this can happen from my colleague's holistic practice.

A man consulted my colleague, Dr. Joan, because of a growth on his shoulder. The growth was thought to be malignant and the surgeon advised the patient to undergo radical surgery to have most of his shoulder removed. His family obviously didn't want him to die so they urged him to get the surgery. He, on the other hand, really wanted to try other options so he consulted with Dr. Joan and asked her to do laser therapy. In addition to using laser therapy, she was intuitively guided to use a new energy tool to treat the tumor. Much to her surprise, the tumor regressed. At that point the treatments stopped and my colleague felt that this man had experienced a miraculous healing.

She didn't hear from him for quite a while, but he returned months later because of shoulder pain. When he took off his jacket, she realized with dismay that the man had undergone radical surgery despite having no visible tumor. When she asked him why he had undergone the surgery which left him scarred and in chronic pain, he told her that his family had put a lot of pressure on him to do it and so he finally acquiesced. Regret is too mild a word to describe what this man was feeling when he realized he did this only to placate his anxious family.

Secondary Gain: Why We Hang onto Pain

Sometimes our family members unknowingly perpetuate our chronic pain and disability. If we are suffering, it would seem unsympathetic for our family members to expect too much of us, right? They might even treat us with greater patience or kindness. This reaction from our loved ones can promote an *unconscious* desire in us to stay disabled. Among medical professionals, this is what we call secondary gain. It's not a pretty scenario to admit to, but all of us have practiced some form of secondary gain, even as children, just to get what we want. And what we all want most is to feel happy and loved.

I experienced this secondary gain personally when I was on a family vacation at Disney World. My parents and I had been arguing early in the trip. I felt criticized for my career and relationship choices and felt their intense worry projected onto me. Half way through the vacation, I suddenly experienced terrible leg pains which then developed into fever, nausea, and vomiting.

As soon as I became visibly ill, all the criticism stopped. Both parents shifted into caregiver-mode and took extra effort to be nice to me. As I knelt next to the toilet waiting for the next wave of nausea to clear, it dawned on me that I got sick in order to stop the criticism! Because I had felt attacked on an emotional level and could not stand up for myself, my subconscious mind had to create an illness in order to stop the perceived attack. When I realized what had happened, I vowed to take better care of my emotional boundaries so that I would not have to develop illness in order to generate loving behavior from my family.

Close family and friends are comfortable with the "you" they already know. If you begin to change for your own good, sometimes they are receptive and sometimes they are not. You could be crowned the greatest chef on earth, but still be criticized by the people closest to you because they still see you as the inept teenager who burnt the toast.

When you change, don't expect your close family to applaud the change, especially when that change directly affects them. For example, if part of your healing is learning to set better boundaries and to say no to things that don't resonate with you, don't be surprised if you encounter resistance. If you've always been a people pleaser, the people around you have enjoyed this part of you and have no vested interest in your developing healthier boundaries.

A perfect illustration of the concepts I've presented here is the movie, Heidi. Heidi is a classic film (remade in 1993) about an orphan from the Austrian Alps whose natural zest for life gets sucked out of her when she is forced to live in the city to be a companion to a rich, spoiled city girl named Klara. Klara is confined to a wheelchair. When you watch this movie, pay close attention to the reaction of Klara's loved ones when she attempts to free herself from her wheelchair-bound existence after she becomes healed in the Alps. As her companion, Heidi likewise struggles through darkness while living with energy vampires. Fortunately she is able to reclaim her power so that her inner light shines again. Heidi *is* you.

Attracting Healthy Support

In order to create a healthy support team, you'll want to have people on that team who do not have a vested interest in your success (or lack of success). At least one member of your support team should be a trusted healthcare professional. This person should be someone who respects your choices, even if he or she doesn't agree with you one hundred percent.

There is no sense in going to your doctor if she is going to belittle your ideas or get angry at you for not following her advice.

If you have a doctor who is very open to alternative therapies, however, you may wish to keep this person on your support team. Most importantly, the health care professional you choose needs to have faith that you can heal. Remember, what he believes is at least as important as what you believe (see Mind section). One of the things I think I do best for my patients is that I can visualize them healthy and happy, even if they can't do that for themselves. I believe in them, even when they don't believe in themselves. I have faith in them. You want someone like that on your team.

If you don't have a holistic physician whom you can count on as one of your support team members, you can still enlist the support of other types of healers such as Reiki healers, acupuncturists, holistic chiropractors, holistic nutritionists, massage therapists, psychologists, etc. When choosing health care professionals, a really great way to tell whether you should include them on your team is by observing the following:

- ☐ Do they walk their talk?
- ☐ Do they take their own advice?
- ☐ Do they demonstrate a habit of life-long learning?
- ☐ Are they committed to their own personal transformation/ journey?
- ☐ Can they accept your choices without criticism or judgment?
- ☐ Do they accept you for who you are?
- ☐ Are they open?
- ☐ Are they vulnerable? Soft? Compassionate?

In addition to having team members who have dedicated their lives to supporting health and healing, I highly suggest that you hire a coach. This can be a life coach, a success coach or a health coach. Coaches, unlike friends, are supposed to hold you accountable to your own goals. They encourage and inspire you without dictating or controlling. Coaches help you feel that you can solve your own problems, giving you the tools to help yourself. Most great coaches have their own coaches! That is one way to tell that a coach is committed to her own growth. All the attributes of a good healing professional also apply to a coach. You may have to interview a number of coaches until you "gel" or resonate with one. Sometimes your health care professional can also act like your coach. The difference is one of accountability. A coach holds you accountable to what you say you want. A healing professional doesn't necessarily do that unless you ask him to.

Developing a Tribe

Often we grow out of our original "tribe" that we grew up in. That tribe consists of our parents, siblings, school friends etc. As we develop and mature, our needs change and we need the support of people who think like us, who believe in the same things we do, and who believe in us. We thrive much better when we realize we're not alone and that there are others who like us for who we are. Members of our new tribe encourage us to grow and change. When you can give up expecting your friends and family to give you the support you need, you will have taken a great step toward empowerment. You can attract a new tribe of people who will support your goals and your growth. It doesn't mean that you no longer love your family and friends. Instead, it means that you accept them for who they are without trying to change them into who you want them to be.

In order to attract a tribe of people who resonate with you, you need to know yourself and what you need. I highly recommend taking some quiet time to determine what the qualities are of the tribe that you wish to attract. Maybe you already have a few friends and colleagues who are already in your new tribe. Rarely is your new tribe made up of family members, but it isn't impossible. Take out a journal and jot down your wish list for your tribe. I'll give you an example of mine so you can get some ideas for your own list. My tribe consists of people who:

- ✓ are dedicated to personal growth and higher consciousness
- ✓ consciously work the law of attraction in their lives
- ✓ are compassionate and loving
- ✓ are into natural health and wellness
- ✓ are interested in the field of energy medicine
- ✓ see value in intuition in health and healing

✓ want to change the world by enhancing other people's lives
✓ believe in empowerment
✓ enact great change through love and tolerance rather than through anger and violence
✓ believe we are connected; we are all One
✓ are connected to the Divine in their thoughts and actions
✓ are healing the world through expanding their consciousness
✓ love to learn new things
✓ are willing to go out of their comfort zone
✓ will support me without judgment
✓ give me honest compassionate feedback
✓ believe in me and in what I wish to accomplish
✓ accept and respect who I am
✓ dream big, just like me
✓ are willing to do what no one else has done before
✓ can be vulnerable and authentic
✓ don't let fear get in the way of their dreams
✓ support healthy boundaries

Now it's your turn. Who do you want to have on your support team? What do you need from them? What can you give them in return? My mom once said that she disagreed with the term "fair-weather friends", i.e. people who stick around you only when you're successful. In contrast she believes that it is easier for friends to support you when you're down and out ("misery loves company"). False friends, she says, tend to get envious or jealous of you when you're too successful. She believes that true friends will be happy for you even if you are more successful than they are.

So your tribe members should consist of people who will be thrilled with your success rather than feeling competitive with it. Inspiration is good. Competition isn't. You'll want to choose a few team members who have already been where you want to go. If someone has naturally healed from the same condition you currently have, you may wish to seek his support.

Where to Find Your Team

Thanks to the internet, finding your new tribe is easier than ever. Solid, deep relationships have been forged over the "net" through social media such as Facebook, LinkedIn, Pinterest and Twitter. You'd be amazed at how many groups and pages on Facebook are holistic health related. You can even use the search engines to find groups who resonate with you. For example, you can go to www.meetup.com and search for groups in your area that are interested in similar things such as "natural health". If there isn't one in your area, maybe you can spearhead one. You can LIKE my Facebook page, for example, and interact with me and other "fans": www.Facebook.com/drkarenkan.

Learn from other holistic-minded teachers by going to their websites and social media pages to connect with their fans. Most teachers have free webinars or teleseminars that you can attend. If you get on their mailing list, you'll receive valuable information including invitations to these events where you'll "meet" other like-minded individuals. Knowing that you're not alone and that there are others like you can be wonderful and empowering. By assembling your support team, even if you haven't yet met some of them in person, you'll enjoy greater success in your healing journey.

Chapter Summary:

- Having the right kind of support is vital and part of your healing process.
- Friends and family may not be able to give appropriate support because they are too attached to the outcome.
- Be aware of secondary gain whereby you unconsciously continue manifesting chronic pain just to get attention or to get treated well.
- Choose a healthcare provider who believes you can heal.
- Being open to attracting your new "tribe" to support you is an important step in your healing.
- Actively searching for your tribe either in your community or online helps you appreciate that you're not alone in your journey.

30

OTHER HEALING MODALITIES

In this chapter, I'll briefly outline healing modalities that I haven't written about elsewhere in this book. The majority of the content in this book is aimed at teaching you self-healing tools that you can use on your own. There is, however, a profound benefit from receiving healing services from another person. We are meant to have relationships with each other and to help each other grow. To give and receive is just part of the cycle of energetic exchange during our human lives.

It is important that you open yourself up to receiving as part of your healing journey. For some people, receiving isn't an issue, but giving is. If your life has been "all about you", it may be time to actively seek out a way to give your gifts more to others who need them. On the other hand, if you're a perpetual giver and a poor receiver, you may need to actively exercise your receiving muscles.

What follows is a brief list of other healing modalities that may be helpful in your healing. Note that this list is not comprehensive and mostly includes therapies I'm more familiar with. I'm sure there are plenty of other wonderful healing modalities that I have not included. If you find one that works for you that isn't on this list, please feel free to share your experiences via my Facebook page.

When finding a healer to work with, the most important thing is the relationship between you and your healer. You could consult with the most famous healer in the world, but if you don't resonate with him, you won't benefit from what he offers. It is the healer, not the modality, who channels the healing. Finding a compassionate healer is as important as finding a competent one. You and your healer's intention, in combination with the rest of the Universe, co-create your reality. Take your time to choose who you want to work with and let your intuition guide you.

Many energy healing modalities are effective and yet few studies are available that prove their effectiveness. Out of all of them, acupuncture may be the best researched. Just because a modality hasn't been researched doesn't mean it doesn't work. Acupuncture is thousands of years old. If it wasn't effective, it wouldn't still be the primary means of health care for one billion people worldwide.

Healing is a personalized experience. It is challenging to even conduct scientific studies on healing because we now know that *intention* can change the results of a study. Furthermore, the placebo-controlled double blinded studies (that Western doctors consider to be the gold standard when it comes to drug therapies) are impossible to conduct with practitioner-based energy healing modalities. Although I always prefer scientific data to support my therapeutic recommendations, sometimes it just isn't available. The best "science" comes from trying things yourself and deciding whether a therapy works for *your* body and particular situation. As you read through the following descriptions, check in with your intuition. You'll probably be able to feel what modalities attract you. Let your intuition and experience become your best guide.

Acupuncture

Acupuncture is the ancient Chinese healing method of inserting thin, sterile needles into acupuncture points on the body and thus increasing the flow of energy along channels called acupuncture meridians. Acupuncture is probably one of the oldest natural healing methods used to treat chronic pain and has enjoyed thousands of years of success. Acupuncture can be performed by licensed acupuncturists, qualified physicians and other healing professionals (depending on a country's licensing laws).

Although I use many other modalities including acupuncture without needles for pain relief, I still enjoy the feeling I get from receiving a treatment from someone else. Acupuncture can be used not only for pain relief but for rebalancing other issues in the body, be it hormonal, emotional or energetic.

As an acupuncturist myself, I have noticed that people have more blockages these days than ever before. These blockages prevent them from healing and may include toxins and energetic pollution to name a few. As with all the healing modalities I'll present in this chapter, brain balancing (Chapter 6) before or during your treatments should speed healing. Weekly treatments are often prescribed for chronic conditions until symptoms abate.

To find an acupuncturist near you, you can go to www.medical acupuncture.org, an association of physician acupuncturists, or www.acufinder.com to find a licensed acupuncturist through national and international associations.

Alexander Technique

The Alexander technique aims to undo bad, ingrained habits of movement by reversing them back to the correct, natural movements of early childhood. Adults have often misused their bodies to the extent that they now have habitual body misalignments. F.M. Alexander, the developer of this technique, felt that the relationship of the head to the neck and back governs the way the rest of the body functions and he called this relationship *primary control.*

Teachers of the Alexander technique aim to restore the length, flexibility and coordination of the spine and head, and to re-establish the correct relative position of the two, at rest and in motion. By "unlearning" poor posture bad habits, you should gain more freedom of movement without associated aches and pains. You should also benefit from improved co-ordination and balance and improved relaxation. For more information, go to www.amsatonline.org.

The Body Code

The Body Code was created by holistic chiropractor Bradley Nelson, who also created the Emotion Code mentioned earlier in this book. According to Nelson, there are only six major areas of imbalance that cause practically 100% of all illnesses and disease in our bodies. Using his Body Code computer database along with muscle testing you can assess and treat these imbalances quickly and easily. The technique unlocks the hidden healing power of the subconscious mind. It is one of the most sophisticated, yet simple, self-healing systems ever created for non-practitioners. I've begun using this system in my practice and I absolutely love it! To learn more, go to www.bodycodehealingsystem.com.

Bowen Technique

The Bowen technique, pioneered by Thomas A. Bowen, helps to restore and harmonize the innate energy in the human body so that self-healing can occur. Another form of energy work, Bowen technique can be applied through light clothing or directly onto bare skin. The practitioner uses her fingers and thumbs to roll your muscles and other connective tissues with light pressure at specific points that may be trigger points or acupuncture points. Very few movements are used to achieve the desired results and the intent is to harmonize the body's vibration. For more information go to www.bowtech.com

Craniosacral Therapy

Pioneered by Dr. John E. Upledger, craniosacral therapy involves the cranium and spinal cord soft tissues which may become inflexible because of trauma or exposure to stress. Craniosacral therapists believe that there is a flow of energy or healthy cranial rhythm which can restore the healing capabilities of the body. It is a very gentle therapy that focuses on the psychological as well as the physical. The touch is so slight that you hardly feel anything. Whenever I receive this type of therapy, I invariably get sleepy, which is a sign of detoxification (healing). Most people find this therapy incredibly relaxing. It is particularly wonderful for children. For more information, go to www.upledger.com.

Chiropractic & Applied Kinesiology

Chiropractors use manipulation of the spine to restore the energy flow of the body. It is felt that subluxations or misalignments of joints can put pressure on spinal nerves and thus affect parts of the body supplied by these nerves. Some chiropractors focus solely on the spine whereas others also treat misalignments of peripheral joints such as knees, hips, and ankles. Some chiropractors practice applied kinesiology and can determine whether internal organs are referring pain to parts of the skeleton. By treating the true source of the pain, applied kinesiology chiropractors can get results where traditional chiropractors may not. For more information, go to: www.icak.com.

Dynamic Neural Retraining Program

Annie Hopper, founder of the Dynamic Neural Retraining System, is a Limbic System Retraining and Rehabilitation Specialist who is an expert in the field of acquired limbic system brain injuries and neuroplasticity. People with diagnoses of fibromyalgia, chronic pain, chronic fatigue and multiple chemical sensitivity syndromes often have limbic system brain dysfunction.

The Limbic System is a complex set of brain structures that are largely responsible for how we code, interpret, and remember sensory input. The limbic system includes the hypothalamus, hippocampus, amygdala, and cingulate cortex. This system is also thought to be responsible for emotional reactions and desires. People with severe chronic pain, such as those with fibromyalgia, almost always have limbic system imbalance. You can be relatively brain balanced (see Chapter 6) but still have limbic system dysfunction.

The Dynamic Neural Retraining Program consists of a combination of various Mind-Body re-programming therapies and exercises. You can learn it through a self-study course or at a live seminar. As with all exercise-based programs, consistent daily practice for at least six consecutive months is important to get the best results. For more information, go to: www.dnrsystem.com.

Feldenkrais Method

The Feldenkrais Method is a form of therapy that teaches body awareness and control and can benefit people suffering from neurological or musculoskeletal problems. Movement skills, posture, self-awareness and balance are all part of the training. The emphasis is on re-educating the neuromuscular pathways. This method can be a valuable tool in maintaining freedom from pain, especially in combination with the other methods in this book. With a Feldenkrais therapist, you will learn how to replace inefficient movement with movements that cause neither tension nor strain in your muscles and joints. For more information, go to: www.feldenkraisinstitute.com

Healing Codes

The Healing Codes are a simple yet powerful self-healing system that utilizes energy medicine. Discovered in 2001 by Dr. Alexander Loyd, a psychologist and naturopath, the Healing Codes activate powerful healing centers that can allow the body to self-heal. The Codes do this by removing the stress from the body, thus allowing the neuro-immune system to take over its job of healing whatever is wrong in the body. You can learn how to use the Healing Codes yourself by reading Dr. Loyd's #1 Bestselling book, The Healing Codes, or you can get a consultation with a Healing Codes practitioner. For more information, go to www.thehealingcodes.com.

Healing Touch

Healing touch is an energy therapy whereby practitioners use their hands in delivering intention and healing from a heart-centered place though your biofield (magnetic field around your body). Healing touch can help support physical, emotional, and mental health. The goal is to restore and harmonize the body's energy field so that the client can return to a self-healing state.

The treatment is typically administered while the client lies on a massage table with her clothes on. The practitioner then uses her hands to assess the biofield and proceeds to clear and balance it, as needed, using either gentle (still) touch over various areas of the body or off-body touch (near body but no direct contact). Most people feel a sense of deep calm and relaxation during a treatment. For more information or to find a practitioner near you, go to www.healingtouchprogram.com.

Integrative Manual Therapy (IMT)

IMT was developed by Sharon Giammatteo, Ph.D., L.M.T.C within the last thirty years. It uses a comprehensive and holistic approach to identify and address the underlying causes of dysfunction causing pain. IMT is based on the premise that the body has the ability to heal itself. IMT treatment techniques are hands-on and generally involve gentle tissue manipulative techniques that promote tissue repair, restore function and normalize structure.

IMT is unique in that it integrates manual therapy techniques for all systems in the body including bone, nerve, muscle fascia, organ, lymph and circulatory. It was an IMT practitioner who revealed that my right hip pain was due to leaky gut affecting the joint capsule. By identifying the true cause of the pain, I was able to heal internally to prevent further damage to my hip joint. For more information, go to www.instituteofimt.com.

Matrix Energetics®

Matrix Energetics® was pioneered by chiropractor and naturopath, Richard Bartlett, who discovered a way to used focused intent and light physical touch to manifest dramatic, sometimes startling changes to someone's body. At times, bones would even realign themselves. Dr. Bartlett found that he could teach his system to both healing practitioners as well as lay people during a weekend seminar, so he's been doing just that since 1992.

Matrix Energetics is a new paradigm of healing that utilizes the principles and science of quantum physics and subtle energy coupled with the power of focused intent in order to produce real physical changes. Often these changes defy rational explanation; so many people using this system call it "miraculous". Although I have not experienced this system for myself, my good friend, Dr. Dennis Lobstein, shared this with me: "*I just had a client today who was repressed emotionally and in pain with stiffness in her raised shoulders. Her husband had shoulder pain, and a friend who came with her had a sore neck with limited range of motion. Matrix turbo-charged the Qi Gong and Huna (ancient Hawaiian healing art) that shattered the repression and allowed the Qi and light (positive energy) to flow freely; then everybody in the room became pain-free immediately.*"

For more information go to www.matrixenergetics.com

Therapeutic Massage

There are many different massage techniques. Some massage therapists work in a spa and prefer to see clients who are just looking for a relaxing massage. Other therapists perform therapeutic massage where their focus is on releasing tension causing chronic pain in various areas of the body. Massage can help to release stuck fascial tissue as well as increase circulation in the skin and muscles.

Bodywork that is given by a knowledgeable and experienced therapist specializing in chronic pain is likely going to be beneficial. Some work deeply in the tissues and this can be uncomfortable but very therapeutic. On the other hand, not everyone can tolerate deep tissue work and for some people, a lighter touch is better. For example, I have found that my patients with fibromyalgia feel worse after a deep tissue massage. This could be because toxins are released during the massage, leaving them feeling as if they have the flu.

For people with fibromyalgia pain, I have found that they do much better with light pressure massage such as lymphatic massage or craniosacral therapy. Nevertheless, I encourage you to try massage to determine whether it is helpful. I believe that receiving human touch is extremely beneficial for everyone. If you do not regularly get touched because you're single, don't have children or pets, massage may be an opportunity to receive those benefits. For more information, go to: www.amta.org

Osteopathy

Pioneered by Taylor Still, an American doctor, osteopathy has been popular in North America for quite some time. Osteopathy can mend the musculoskeletal system by manipulations and pressure in order to restore proper functioning of the body. Originally osteopathy was an alternative to drugs, but in the United States, osteopaths can function as medical doctors, treating all medical problems and prescribing drugs. There are some osteopaths that do visceral (internal organ) manipulations, as well as musculoskeletal manipulations. These osteopaths are thought by some to be more "holistic" in their approach to the body because pain may be referred from a dysfunctional organ. For more information: www.academyofosteopathy.org.

Quantum Neurology® Nervous System Rehabilitation

Dr. George Gonzalez, a chiropractor, felt the need to study neurology when his wife suffered a moderate spinal cord injury. Her doctors offered no real answers for her injury or recovery. No one could tell them what was wrong, how long she would be damaged or how to support her healing. Through necessity, Dr. Gonzalez discovered a novel way of helping his wife heal from her nerve damage. The techniques and healing strategies that he developed are now called Quantum Neurology® Nervous System Rehabilitation. It is a systematic approach to evaluating and correcting every nerve in the body. Once a specific nerve is found to be dysfunctional a combination of hands-on tissue mobilization and light therapy stimulation are used as a correction.

In his book, Holographic Healing®, Dr. Gonzalez' teaches that strengthening the nervous system provides the opportunity for the body to heal itself. Although Quantum Neurology does not claim to treat or cure specific diagnoses, it re-establishes proper neurological communication within the body. Proper nervous system communication means less pain, more range of motion, more function and more life. There is hope even for severe cases. In one case, a man in a wheelchair for over two decades is rehabilitating himself out of his chair using Quantum Neurology. Most patients report positive improvements from their first session. The same techniques and strategies used on disabled patients are used on elite athletes that have gone on to win gold medals and break world records.

I had the pleasure of interviewing Dr. Gonzales on my radio show. Go to Resources to find the link to listen to the recording. To learn more about or to find a practitioner near you, go to: www.quantumneurology.com.

Reconnective Healing

Reconnective Healing is a unique form of energy healing that is taught by chiropractor Eric Pearl, D.C., who discovered years ago that he had somehow been "downloaded" with unique healing frequencies different from all other known forms of energy healing. He was able to attune other healers to this frequency and now has an international network of healers doing Reconnective Healing.

Dr. Pearl's healing powers have been studied by top doctors and medical researchers at hospitals, colleges and universities worldwide. These include Jackson Memorial Hospital, UCLA, Cedars-Sinai Medical Center, the VA Hospital, Tel HaShomer (Tel Aviv), Suburban Hospital, University of Miami Medical School, Kent College of Osteopathy (UK), RMIT University (Melbourne), the University of Oslo, and the University of Arizona to name a few. Reconnective Healing can help you heal your life, not just your body, and many seek it for its spiritual nature. To learn more about Reconnective Healing, go to: www.thereconnection.com.

Reflexology

Reflexology is a form of foot massage that was formalized in the West but has its basis in ancient healing practices in many civilizations. Various parts of each foot represent different zones of the body and different organs. By stimulating these zones, you can treat other parts of the body, including painful ones. Common contraindications to getting reflexology include early pregnancy, circulation problems, acute infections or foot infections. Reflexology can be relaxing or painful depending on which points are massaged and what areas are in need of attention. For more information, go to: www.reflexology-usa.org in the United States or www.reflexology-uk.net/site internationally.

Reiki

Reiki is a form of energy healing whereby a practitioner places her hands on various areas of the body to rebalance the body's energy field in order to support self-healing. Thought to have originally been created in 1922 by Japanese Buddhist Mikao Usu, Reiki has now been adapted into various forms by modern teachers. Often, Reiki healers will "read" the energy centers of the body, the chakras, in order to determine whether they are excessive, deficient or blocked. They then can rebalance the chakras by channeling energy through their hands.

During my own personal healing journey, I found that being trained in Reiki opened up my energetic senses. When I first learned it, I was terrified to use it because I was afraid of doing something wrong. But through the gentle and compassionate tutelage of my Reiki healer and spiritual counselor, Patricia Lee Jones of Healing Adventures, the process of learning this healing modality catalyzed a fantastic journey of self-discovery.

Reiki practitioners may be first degree, second degree and Master levels. At the Master level, the best Reiki practitioners I've known are ones that do energy healing on a regular basis and who are also dedicated to their own ongoing personal transformation. For more information on Reiki, go to: www.reiki.org.

Rolfing

A form of bodywork, Rolfing involves releasing the myofascial system-the system that includes both muscles and connective tissue called fascia. Pioneered by Ida Rolf, Rolfing is a technique that stretches and loosens the fascia so that the muscles beneath can fully relax. Doing so not only helps the physical body, but the emotional and mental bodies as well–according to Rolfing practitioners.

Ida Rolf felt that the connective tissue stored memories of traumas which can be released during a Rolfing session. The Rolfer will knead, massage and pummel your flesh using his or her hands, knuckles, fingers and elbows. It can be incredibly deep and any tender spots or knots can be eased. Compared with other forms of body work, Rolfing may be the most painful, but many people "enjoy" the feeling of having their knots released. The idea is that at the end of your Rolfing sessions, your myofascial system becomes balanced and your posture is corrected. For more information on Rolfing, go to: www.rolf.org.

Somatics™

The Clinical Somatics™ process consists of two parts: hands-on guided movement and self-care exercises that correct inefficient movement patterns as well as lengthen shortened muscles back to their natural, relaxed state. When muscles become chronically shortened from injury and stress, the entire body becomes unbalanced. Once the problematic muscles are relaxed and balanced through Clinical Somatics™, your posture should improve and it should be much easier to perform other movement activities such as walking and dancing.

Clinical Somatics™ involves actively engaging and training your brain to become aware of abnormal muscle movements patterns and contractions using specific, yet comfortable exercises. Sessions may be taught in private or group. For more information, go to www.somatics.org.

Trager Work

Trager Work was devised by Milton Trager, who was an acrobat and boxer who suffered chronic back problems and eventually became a physical therapist and then a medical doctor. His somatic re-education program stems from the belief that Trager Workers can link up the energy force that surrounds us all and reprogram the subconscious in order to release muscular tension. Small movements are taught to replace harmful learned habits.

Trager work is a system of re-wiring the body's musculoskeletal responses, not a treatment method, per se, so don't expect to receive a diagnosis. There are two parts to Trager Work. The first one is table-work and involves small gentle rocking, vibrating and kneading motions that are not painful (as opposed to Rolfing). Once the table work has been completed, your practitioner will move on to teaching you Mentastics which are simple exercises that you can do at home. These exercises will reinforce the work done during the office visit. For more information, go to: www.trager.com.

Zero Balancing

Zero balancing is an energy healing technique developed by Fritz Smith, MD in the early 1970s. It is a powerful body-mind therapy that uses skilled touch to address the relationship between energy and structures of the body. During the 30 to 45 minute protocol, the certified Zero Balancing practitioner uses finger pressure and gentle traction on areas of tension in the bones, joints and soft tissue to create fulcrums, or points of balance, around which the body can relax and reorganize.

Energy blockages can be cleared, thus amplifying vital energy in the body, by addressing the deepest and densest tissues of the body along with soft tissue and energy fields. Zero Balancing can help relieve physical pain, release movement restrictions and provide relief from emotional distress. A Zero Balancing session leaves you with a wonderful feeling of inner harmony and balance. I have really enjoyed receiving Zero Balancing because it is very relaxing. For more information, go to www.zerobalancing.com.

FINAL WORDS

Congratulations for having the courage to believe that you can heal your chronic pain. If you didn't have the courage you wouldn't have read this book. Healing is a journey and everyone's is different. I encourage you to continue learning and growing. Thanks for allowing me to be part of your healing journey!

Remember, all of us need support, so let's stay connected with each other via the web:

www.KarenKan.com
www.Facebook.com/drkarenkan
www.Twitter.com/karenkan
www.YouTube.com/karenkanmd
www.Pinterest.com/drkarenkan

31

RESOURCES

Scan the code below with your Tablet device or Smartphone using a free QR Code App and you'll be taken to the website where I'll be regularly updating the Resource list.

Section A: Understanding Your Pain

Chapter 2: How to Experience Pain

- "Traditional Chinese Medicine" National Center for Complementary & Alternative Medicine: http://nccam.nih.gov/health/whatiscam/chinesemed.htm
- Janet Travell, MD: www.janettravellmd.com
- "The Magnesium Miracle" by Dr. Carolyn Dean, MD: www.drcarolyndean.com/natural-health-books-by-dr-dean
- Reconnective Healing: www.thereconnection.com

Chapter 4: Causes of Pain—Western Perspective

- "The Magnesium Miracle" by Carolyn Dean, MD: www.drcarolyndean.com/natural-health-books-by-dr-dean
- Carolyn Dean, MD: www.drcarolyndean.com
- Elimination Diet: www.en.wikipedia.org/wiki/Elimination_diet
- ALCAT Test: www.ALCAT.com

- Heart Disease: www.digitaljournal.com/article/334943
- "The Great Cholesterol Myth" by Jonny Bowden and Stephen Sinatra, MD: http://astore.amazon.com/imacupuncture-20/detail/1592335217
- "Supplement Your Prescription" by Dr. Hyla: www.cassmd.com/books
- "The Science of Miracles" by Gregg Braden: www.hayhouse.com/details.php?ref=99&id=4022
- Gregg Braden: www.greggbraden.com
- Healing Cancer Summit: www.healingcancersummit.com
- Liver Damage from Medications: http://en.wikipedia.org/wiki/Hepatotoxicity
- Kidney Damage from Medications: www.lef.org/protocols/appendix/otc_toxicity_01.html
- Medication and Heart Attack Risk: www.health.harvard.edu/blog/common-painkillers-boost-risk-of-repeat-heart-attack-201209135305
- Medication and Stroke Risk: www.health.harvard.edu/blog/common-painkillers-boost-risk-of-repeat-heart-attack-201209135305
- Narcotics and Repeat Heart Attacks: www.health.harvard.edu/blog/common-painkillers-boost-risk-of-repeat-heart-attack-201209135305

Chapter 5: Causes of Pain-Spiritual Perspective

- Rupert Sheldrake: www.sheldrake.org/homepage.html
- Morphic Fields: www.youtube.com/watch?v=2Dm8-OpO9oQ&feature=youtu.be

Section B: Your Mind—Harness Your Internal Healer

Chapter 6: Balance Your Brain

- John Diamond, MD: www.drjohndiamond.com

- "Your Body Doesn't Lie" by John Diamond, MD: www.lifeenergyarts.com/your-body-doesnt-lie
- "How To Check Your Brain Balance" by Karen Kan, MD: www.youtube.com/karenkanmd
- "Wireless Technology and Your Health" by Stephen Sinatra, MD: www.youtube.com/watch?v=Xs2nF1LLt0Y
- Stephen Sinatra. MD: www.drsinatra.com
- HeartMD Institute www.heartmdinstitute.com
- Monosodium Glutamate (MSG), "Dr. Russell Blaylock reveals secrets of MSG toxicity": www.naturalnews.com/035243_Russell_Blaylock_MSG_interview.html
- Mercury Fillings "Smoking Teeth": www.youtube.com/watch?v=9ylnQ-T7oiA&feature=youtu.be
- International Academy of Oral Medicine & Toxicology: www.iaomt.org
- To find a Holistic Dentist: www.iaomt.org
- Symptoms from MSG: www.saynotomsg.com/basics_list.php
- Electropollution: http://electromagnetichealth.org
- Is Wi-Fi Safe for Children?: www.safeinschool.org/2011/01/wi-fi-is-removed-from-schools-and.html
- LifeWave Y-Age Aeon: www.lifewave.com/yage-aeon.asp
- LifeWave IceWave: www.lifewave.com/icewave.asp
- "LifeWave History" by David Schmidt: www.youtube.com/watch?v=isJWf2GtSDc&feature=share&list=PLB6E602431BB0CAAF
- LifeWave Energy Enhancer Patches: www.lifewave.com/energyenhancer.asp
- Dr. Karen's LifeWave Team website: www.patchtrainingteam.com
- John Diamond, MD: www.drjohndiamond.com
- How to test Brain Balance using Muscle Testing by Karen Kan, MD: www.youtube.com/watch?v=mGfPntF-7d8&feature=youtu.be
- Applied Kinesiology: www.appliedkinesiology.com
- Dr. Jeffrey Thompson: www.neuroacoustic.com
- Brain Entrainment Sound Therapy: http://neuroacoustic.com/newmil.html

- Dr. Jeff Thompson's Sound Table: http://neuroacoustic.com/sounddeliveryequipment.html
- Brainwave Massage 2.0 Audio for Beta Wave Enhancement http://astore.amazon.com/imacupuncture-20
- "Epsilon, Gamma, HyperGamma, Lambda Brainwave Activity and Ecstatic States of Consciousness" by Jeffrey D. Thompson, DC, BFA: http://neuroacoustic.com/epsilon.html
- "Healing with Love" by Leonard Laskow, MD: www.laskow.net/articles/Healing-With-Love-excerpt.shtml
- Energy Tools International Vital Force Technology: www.energytoolsint.com
- Nutrilink Energy: www.nutrilinkenergy.com
- EarthCalm: www.karenkan.com/EMF
- Radiation Protective Device for Your Cell Phone-LifeWave Matrix: www.lifewave.com/matrix.asp

Chapter 7: Change Your Mind

- "The Biology of Belief" by Bruce Lipton, MD: www.brucelipton.com/flipbook/biology-belief#/page/1
- Bruce Lipton, MD: www.brucelipton.com
- "The Genie in your Genes" by Dawson Church: www.dawsonchurch.com/books
- Dawson Church: www.dawsonchurch.com
- "The Intention Experiment" by Lynne McTaggart: www.lynnemctaggart.com/the-books
- Lynne McTaggart: www.lynnemctaggart.com
- "The pH Miracle" by Robert O. Young, MD: www.phmiracleliving.com/p-552-the-ph-miracle-revised-and-updated.aspx
- Robert O. Young, MD: www.phmiracleliving.com
- "What If? The Movie": www.infinite-manifesting.org/OwningTheImpossible.html
- The man whose teeth always grew back: www.infinite-manifesting.org/OwningTheImpossible.html

- Sun Gazers:
  http://home.iae.nl/users/lightnet/health/lightresearch.htm
- Sun Gazer Interviews: http://eatthesunmovie.com/synopsis.html
- LifeWave Y-Age Aeon: www.lifewave.com/yage-aeon.asp
- "The Mind Power into the 21st Century" by John Kehoe:
  http://shop.learnmindpower.com/book-s/1821.htm
- John Kehoe: www.learnmindpower.com
- "Choices and Illusions" by Eldon Taylor, MD:www.eldontaylor.
  com/choices-and-illusions/choices-and-illusions.html
- Eldon Taylor, MD: www.eldontaylor.com
- "Mind Programming" by Eldon Taylor, MD:
  www.eldontaylor.com/mindprogramming
- Subliminal Inner Talk Audios:
  www.karenkan.com/products/subliminal-innertalk-audio-cds
- Cancer Remission CD: www.innertalk.com/cgi-bin/
  store/agora.cgi?cart_id=4879314.5077*PH2iU1&p_
  id=CD5500&xm=on&ppinc=search2
- "Self-Hypnosis and Subliminal Technology: A How-to Guide
  for Personal-Empowerment Tools You Can Use Anywhere!"
  by Eldon Taylor: www.eldontaylor.com/self-hypnosis-
  and-subliminal-technology/self-hypnosis-and-subliminal-
  technology.html
- Lion Goodman: www.beliefcloset.com/about/about/
- BeliefCloset Practitioners: www.BeliefCloset.com/Practitioners
- Free multimedia eBook on BeliefCloset Process:
  www.TransformYourBeliefs.com

Chapter 8: Harness the Law of Attraction

- "The Intention Experiment" by Lynne McTaggart:
  http://theintentionexperiment.com
- T. Harv Eker: www.harveker.com
- The Secret: www.thesecret.tv
- The Cure Is: www.thecureismovie.com
- "What the Bleep Do We Know" movie: www.whatthebleep.com

- "The Field" by Lynne McTaggart's: www.lynnemctaggart.com/the-books
- LifeWave Y-Age Aeon Patches: www.lifewave.com/yage-aeon.asp
- Bob Proctor: www.bobproctor.com
- The Law of Attraction in Love: www.LawofAttractioninLove.com
- "The Circle" by Laura Day: www.howtoruletheworldfromyourcouch.com/?cat=6
- Laura Day: www.practicalintuition.com
- We won 3 Gold Medals! www.lawofattractioninlove.com/2010/04/we-did-it-james-and-i-won-three-gold-medals-thanks-to-you

Chapter 9: Clear Emotional Baggage

- Louise Hay: www.louisehay.com
- "Heal Your Body" by Louise Hay: www.hayhouse.com/details.php?id=263
- EFT (Emotional Freedom Technique): www.eftuniverse.com
- The Tapping Solution: www.karenkan.com/tappingsolution
- TAT (Tapas Acupressure Technique): www.karenkan.com/TAT
- Emotion Code: www.karenkan.com/emotion
- TFT (Thought Field Therapy): www.thoughtfieldtherapy.net
- Sedona Method:: www.sedona.com
- PSTEC: www.pstec.org
- LifeWave Y-Age Aeon: http://lifewave.com/yage-aeon.asp
- Free How to do TAT Booklet: www.karenkan.com/TAT
- How to do TAT Video: www.youtu.be/-rDF_qUntDg
- "The Emotion Code" by Bradley Nelson, MD: www.karenkan.com/emotion
- Bradley Nelson, MD: www.drbradleynelson.com

Chapter 10: Meditation and Mindfulness

- "The Mindfulness Based Stress Reduction program" by Jon Kabat-Zinn: www.umassmed.edu/cfm/stress/index.aspx

- Jon Kabat-Zinn: www.umassmed.edu/Content.aspx?id=43102
- "Freedom from Pain: Discover Your Body's Power to Overcome Physical Pain" by Dr. Peter A. Levine, and Dr. Maggie Phillips: www.maggiephillipsphd.com/products.html
- Peter Levine, PhD: www.somaticexperiencing.com
- Maggie Phillips, PhD: www.maggiephillipsphd.com
- Meditation: www.en.wikipedia.org/wiki/Meditation
- "Conversations with God" by Neale Donald Walsch: www.cwg.org/index.php?page=store&items=text
- Neale Donald Walsch: www.nealedonaldwalsch.com

Section C: Your Body—Supporting Your Body's Self-Healing Mechanism

Chapter 11: Acupuncture without Needles

- LifeWave Y-Age Aeon: www.lifewave.com/yage-aeon.asp
- Brain Balancing Protocol: www.patchtrainingteam.com
- LifeWave IceWave Patches: www.lifewave.com/icewave.asp
- LifeWave Research: www.lifewave.com/research.asp
- Clock Protocol: www.lifewavetraining.com/products-icewave.asp
- Whole Body Pain Protocol: www.lifewavetraining.com/products-icewave.asp
- "How to Patch" Videos: www.youtube.com/playlist?list=PL6666144788828AB0
- Himalayan Crystal Salt: www.himalayancrystalsalt.com
- LifeWave Patching Videos: www.youtube.com/karenkanmd
- LifeWave Y-Age Glutathione Patches: www.lifewave.com/yage-glutathione.asp
- LifeWave Y-Age Carnosine Patch: www.lifewave.com/yage-carnosine.asp
- Athletes that Use LifeWave: www.lifewave.com/inthenews.asp
- LifeWave Customer Service: www.lifewave.com/customerservice.asp
- LifeWave Energy Enhancer: www.lifewave.com/energyenhancer.asp

- LifeWave Silent Nights Patches: www.lifewave.com/silentnights.asp
- Dr. Karen's Patch Training Team: www.patchtrainingteam.com

Chapter 12: Get Grounded!

- Earthing: www.earthing.com
- Electrosmog or Electropollution: http://electromagnetichealth.org
- "Earthing" by Clint Ober, Stephen T. Sinatra, M.D. and Martin Zucker: www.earthing.com/category_s/1856.htm
- The Earthing Company Products: www.earthing.com/Shop_s/1824.htm
- Recovery Bags: www.earthing.com/product_p/rb.htm
- Half Sheet: www.earthing.com/category_s/1856.htm
- Earthing Premium Starter Kit: www.earthing.com/product_p/esk.htm
- Earthing Universal Mat: www.earthing.com/product_p/umck.htm
- Cortisol Levels before and after Earthing: www.KarenKan.com/earthsleep
- LifeWave Y-Age Aeon: www.lifewave.com/yage-aeon.asp
- VibesUP Divine Soles: www.karenkan.com/vibesup

Chapter 13: Magnesium Miracles

- "Interactions of Magnesium and Potassium in the Pathogenesis of Cardiovascular Disease" by Mildred Seelig: www.mgwater.com/seelig_interactions_of_magnesium_and_potassium.pdf
- Guy D. Abraham, MD: www.nutritionalmagnesium.org/research/muscle-health/337-fibromyalgia-relief-with-magnesium-study-gives-hope-to-fibromyalgia-sufferers.html
- 10 Signs You Need to Watch For Magnesium Deficiency: www.ancient-minerals.com/magnesium-deficiency/need-more
- Methods for Testing Magnesium Deficiency: www.energyfanatics.com/2009/11/07/methods-testing-magnesium-deficiency

- "Calcium and Magnesium in the Drinking Water" by World Health Organization: apps.who.int/iris/bitstream/10665/43836/1/9789241563550_eng.pdf
- USDA Chart of Magnesium Rich Foods: www.ancient-minerals.com/magnesium-sources/dietary/#dv-chart)
- "Transdermal Magnesium" by Mark Sircus, OMD: www.drsircus.com/books
- Mark Sircus, OMD: www.drsircus.com
- "Magnesium Miracle" by Carolyn Dean, MD, ND: www.drcarolyndean.com/natural-health-books-by-dr-dean
- Carolyn Dean, MD, ND: www.drcarolyndean.com
- Ancient Minerals Magnesium Oil: www.ancient-minerals.com

Chapter 14: Food Sensitivities and Pain

- "Wheat Belly" by William Davies, MD: www.wheatbellybook.com/wheatbellybook/bps/index?keycode=222188
- William Davies, MD: www.wheatbellyblog.com/about-the-author
- Stool Testing: www.enterolab.com/default.aspx
- Saliva Testing: www.biohealthlab.com/test-menu/immunology/gluten-intoleranc
- ALCAT blood testing labs: www.ALCAT.com
- "The Gluten Connection" by Shari Lieberman: http://glutenconnection.com/uof/glutenconnection
- Shari Lieberman: www.drshari.net
- Applied Kinesiology: www.appliedkinesiology.com
- "Seeds of Deception" by Jeffrey Smith: www.seedsofdeception.com
- Jeffrey Smith: www.seedsofdeception.com/about
- NAET (Nambudripad's Allergy Elimination Technique): www.naet.com
- Uhe Method: www.UheMethod.com
- Emotion Code: www.karenkan.com/emotion

- Bioimpedance Monitoring: www.cnm.es/~mtrans/PDFs/ Bioimpedance_for_physicians_rev1.pdf
- "Water & Salt" by Barbara Hendel, MD: http://www.himalayancrystalsalt.com/specialties.html
- Barbara Hendel, MD: www.dr-barbara-hendel.com
- Toxins Leaching From Plastic: www.organicconnectmag. com/wp/plastic-planet-uncovers-the-truth-about-plastics/#. UQRpPfIZ-Sp
- Xenoestrogens: www.en.wikipedia.org/wiki/Bisphenol_A
- David Wolfe: www.davidwolfe.com
- Masaru Emoto, MD: www.en.wikipedia.org/wiki/Masaru_Emoto
- Water Distillers Guide: www.youtube.com/watch?v=- 8uk64iG4zc&feature=youtu.be
- Jeff Green on Fluoride Toxins: http://articles.mercola.com/sites/ articles/archive/2012/02/04/jeff-green-on-fluoride-toxins- part-2.aspx
- Dr. Mercola Interviews Jeff Green on Fluoride: www.youtube. com/watch?v=5Y8JcOnZJJI&feature=youtu.be
- Healed Salt Water Hastens Plant Growth: www.transitiontoparenthood.com/janelle/energy/support.htm
- Quantum Age StirWand: www.americanbluegreen.com/stirwand.html
- Fenestra Research Laboratory Evaluation of the StirWand: www.himalayancrystalsalt.com/pdf/FinalReport.pdf
- Willard Catalyst Water: www.drwillard.com
- Study Outlines Benefits of Willard Water: www.drwillard.com/blog/2012/11/exciting-new-study- further-outlines-the-benefits-of-drinking-willard-water
- Crystal Energy: www.wetterwater.net
- Water Vitalization Crystals: www.americanbluegreen.com/vitalization_crystals.html
- Vortex Water Revitalizer: www.alivewater.com
- Research about Vortex Water Revitalizer: www.alivewater.com/research

- VibesUP: www.karenkan.com/vibesup
- Radio show with VibesUP creator Kaitlyn Keyt: www.karenkan.com/radiovibesup
- SourxeII: www.karenkan.com/water
- Radio show with Peter Schenk-Super Charge Your Water With Your Intentions: www.karenkan.com/radiothesourxe1 and www.karenkan.com/radiothesourxe
- Himalayan Crystal: www.himalayancrystalsalt.com
- Research Results on Himalayan Crystal: www.himalayancrystalsalt.com/clinical-research.html
- "Salt Your Way to Health" by David Brownstein, MD: www.drbrownstein.com/bookstore_Salt.php
- David Brownstein, MD: www.drbrownstein.com/about.php

Chapter 16: Heal the Gut

- LifeWave Y-Age Aeon Patch: www.lifewave.com/yage-aeon.asp
- LifeWave IceWave Pain Patches: www.lifewave.com/icewave.asp
- Gut–Brain Connection: www.cyrexlabs.com/HomeVideo1/tabid/174/Default.aspx
- Healing Leaky Gut Syndrome: www.karenkan.com/radioleakygut
- Leaky Gut Cure: http://www.karenkan.com/leakygutprogram
- "Digestive Wellness" by Elizabeth Lipski PhD: www.innovativehealing.com/shop/bookstore/digestive-wellness
- Elizabeth Lipski PhD: www.lizlipski.com
- Leaky Gut Symptoms: www.leakygut.co.uk/symptoms.htm
- Intestinal Permeability Test: www.genovadiagnostics.com
- Intestinal Barrier Function Test: www.intestinalbarriertest.com
- Loren Cordain, PhD: www.hes.cahs.colostate.edu/faculty_staff/cordain.aspx?m=a
- Paleolithic Diet: www.thepaleodiet.com
- Pasteurized Milk Under a Microscope: www.westonaprice.org/modern-foods/microphotography-of-raw-and-processed-milk
- Soy Dangers Summarized: www.westonaprice.org/soy-alert

- 10 Reasons to Avoid GMOs: www.responsibletechnology.org/10-Reasons-to-Avoid-GMOs
- Weston A. Price: www.westonaprice.org
- Vital Choice Seafood (Low-Mercury Fish): www.karenkan.com/vitalchoice
- "Seeds of Deception" by Jeffrey Smith: www.seedsofdeception.com/books
- "Genetic Roulette" Film by Jeffrey Smith: www.seedsofdeception.com/books
- Jeffrey Smith: www.seedsofdeception.com/about
- Culturelle ™: www.culturelle.com
- RAW Probiotics by Garden of Life ™: www.gardenoflife.com/Products-for-Life/RAW-Digestion.aspx
- Prescript-Assist ™: www.prescript-assist.com
- Ethical Nutrients ™ Intestinal Care DF (Dairy Free): www.ethicalnutrients.mymetagenics.com/store/view/product/633
- Genestra ™ HMF Replete: www.emersonecologics.com/Products/EmersonMain/PID-SE419.aspx
- Integrative Therapeutics ™ Enterogenic Intensive 100: www.integrativeinc.com/Products/Products-by-Type/Probiotics/70667-Enterogenic-Intensive-100.aspx
- Bristol University's Stool Scale: www.en.wikipedia.org/wiki/Bristol_stool_scale
- Doctors Data Laboratory: www.doctorsdata.com
- Hakala Labs: www.hakalalabs.com
- NAET (Nambudripad's Allergy Elimination Techniques): www.naet.com
- Uhe Desensitizing Method: www.uhemethod.com
- LifeWave Y-Age Glutathione: www.lifewave.com/yage-glutathione.asp
- LifeWave Y-Age Carnosine Patches: www.lifewave.com/yage-carnosine.asp
- Kidney 27 Acupuncture Points: www.imacupuncture.com/2011/07/21/chronic-pain-relief-part-1
- LifeWave Energy Enhancer: www.lifewave.com/energyenhancer.asp

- Interview with Leaky Gut Expert Karen Brimeyer: www.karenkan.com/radioleakygut
- Karen Brimeyer's Step-by-Step Guide to Cure Leaky Gut: www.karenkan.com/leakygutprogram

Chapter 17: Reduce EMF Stress

- Electropollution: www.electromagnetichealth.org
- France's Ban on Advertising Cell Phones to Children: www.thepeoplesinitiative.org/index.php/cell-phones
- "How Taking Vitamins May be Harmful to Your Health" comment by Dr. Mercola: http://articles.mercola.com/sites/articles/archive/2008/05/06/can-vitamins-shorten-your-life.aspx
- "Public Health SOS: The Shadow Side of the Wireless Revolution" by Camilla Rees and Magda Havas, PhD: www.electromagnetichealth.org/public-health-sos-book
- Camilla Rees: www.electromagnetichealth.org/emf-remediation-interviews
- Magda Havas, PhD: www.magdahavas.com
- Electromagnetic Health: www.electromagnetichealth.org
- Earthing: www.earthing.com
- EarthCalm Quantum Cell: www.karenkan.com/EMF
- LifeWave Matrix: www.lifewave.com/matrix.asp
- Greenwave Filters: www.karenkan.com/products/greenwave-emf-filters
- Energy Tools International: www.energytoolsint.com
- Clean Sweep: http://store.energytoolsint.com/e_commerce/show_category/15
- How Sage is used by Native Americans: www.en.wikipedia.org/wiki/Smudge_stick
- EarthCalm Products: www.karenkan.com/EMF
- LifeWave Y-Age Aeon Patches for Stress Relief: www.lifewave.com/yage-aeon.asp
- LifeWave Energy Enhancer: www.lifewave.com/energyenhancer.asp

- Compact LED Bulbs-"Lighting and EMFs": www.powerwatch. org.uk/library/downloads/lighting-emfs-2011-12.pdf
- Radiation Free Headsets: www.lifebluetube.com/headsets.html
- Smart Meter Dangers: www.smartmeterdangers.org

Chapter 18: Eat Well. Feel Great.

- Olympic Figure Skating Gold Medalists Oleg & Ludmila Protopopov: www.en.wikipedia.org/wiki/Oleg_Protopopov
- Sun Gazers: http://home.iae.nl/users/lightnet/health/lightresearch.htm
- "Fat Head" Movie: www.kellythekitchenkop.com/2009/09/big-fat-lies-fat-head-movie-review-real-food-wednesday.html
- Sweetener Consumption: www.ers.usda.gov/publications/sssm-sugar-and-sweeteners-outlook/sssm273.aspx
- Weston A. Price: www.westonaprice.org/abcs-of-nutrition/health-topics
- "Red Meat Consumption and Mortality" http://archinte.jamanetwork.com/article.aspx?articleid=1134845
- "Will Eating Red Meat Kill You?" www.marksdailyapple.com/will-eating-red-meat-kill-you/#ixzz1rZygv9PM
- "In Search of the Perfect Human Diet" film by C.J. Hunt www.perfecthumandiet.com
- Vital Choice Fish: www.karenkan.com/vitalchoice
- "Wheat Belly" by William Davis, MD: www.losethewheatlosetheweight.com/losethewheatlosetheweight/index
- Glycemic Index: www.mendosa.com/gilists.htm
- LifeWave Y-Age Aeon Patches: www.lifewave.com/yage-aeon.asp
- "Nourishing Traditions: The Cookbook that Challenges Politically Correct Nutrition and the Diet Dictocrats" by Sally Fallon: www.newtrendspublishing.com/SallyFallon/index.html
- Sally Fallon: www.newtrendspublishing.com/SallyFallon/aboutSallyFallon.html
- How to Ferment Grains to remove anti-nutrients: www.naturalnews.com/024508.html

- Wulzen Factor: www.en.wikipedia.org/wiki/Wulzen_anti-stiffness_factor
- Jordan Rubin: www.jordanrubin.com
- Garden of Life: www.gardenoflife.com
- Beyond Organic: www.karenkan.com/beyondorganic
- Microscopic Photos of Raw Milk: www.westonaprice.org/modern-foods/microphotography-of-raw-and-processed-milk
- Dr. Bradley Nelson: www.drbradleynelson.com
- Body Code Healing System: www.drbradleynelson.com/body-code-more-info
- "The Truth About Eggs: What Commercial Farmers Don't Want You to Know": www. articles.mercola.com/sites/articles/archive/2012/11/21/truth-about-commercial-egg-farming.aspx#_methods=onPlusOne%2C_ready%2C_close%2C_open%2C_resizeMe%2C_renderstart%2Concircled&id=I0_1360889320822&parent=http%3A%2F%2Farticles.mercola.com&rpctoken=53576433
- Unmarinated Pork Affects the Blood: www.westonaprice.org/food-features/how-does-pork-prepared-in-various-ways-affect-the-blood
- The "Dirty Dozen" Fruits and Vegetables with the Most Pesticides and Herbicides: www.ewg.org/foodnews
- Vital Choice Seafood: www.karenkan.com/vitalchoice
- Pre-Made Paleo Meals: www.karenkan.com/paleo
- Pre-Made Paleo Dr. Karen's Pain Relief Success Pack: www.karenkan.com/painreliefpaleo
- Willard Water Supplements: www.drwillard.com
- Culturelle ™: www.culturelle.com
- RAW Probiotics by Garden of Life ™: www.gardenoflife.com/Products-for-Life/RAW-Digestion.aspx
- Prescript-Assist ™: www.prescript-assist.com
- Ethical Nutrients ™ Intestinal Care DF (Dairy Free): www.ethicalnutrients.mymetagenics.com/store/view/product/633
- Genestra ™ HMF Replete: www.emersonecologics.com/Products/EmersonMain/PID-SE419.aspx

- Integrative Therapeutics ™ Enterogenic Intensive 100: www.integrativeinc.com/Products/Products-by-Type/ Probiotics/70667-Enterogenic-Intensive-100.aspx
- Syntol AMD: www.enzymus.com/syntol
- VSL#3 ™: www.vsl3.com
- Herxheimer Reactions: www.en.wikipedia.org/wiki/Herxheimer_reaction
- Transdermal Magnesium Oil: www.ancient-minerals.com
- Ethical Nutrients Malic Magnesium Tablets: www.ethicalnutrients.mymetagenics.com/store/view/product/620
- Ancient Minerals Magnesium Oil: www.ancient-minerals.com
- Nordic Naturals ™ Fish Oil: www.nordicnaturals.com
- Carlson's ™ Fish Oil: www.carlsonlabs.com/s-12-fish-oils.aspx
- Quell ™ Fish Oil: www.quellfishoil.com/index.html
- Minami Fish Oil: www.minami-nutrition.com/langselection/index.php
- Biopure ™ Salmon Oil: www.retailbiopure.com
- Dr. Dietrich Klinghardt: www.klinghardtacademy.com/ BioData/Dr-Dietrich-Klinghardt.html
- Green Pasture: www.greenpasture.org/public/Products/ ButterCodLiverBlend/index.cfm
- Innate Response Formulas ™: www.innateresponse.com/category-s/52.htm
- Garden of Life ™: www.gardenoflife.com/Products-for-Life/ Vitamin-Code.aspx
- Broad-Spectrum Antibiotics can Reduce Vitamin K: www.ncbi.nlm.nih.gov/pubmed/7895417
- LifeWave Y-Age Glutathione Patches: www.lifewave.com/yage-glutathione.asp
- Metagenics ™ Ultra Potent-C: www.metagenics.com/products/search-products-a-z
- Garden of Life ™ Vitamin Code RAW Vitamin C: www.gardenoflife.com/ProductsforLife/ THEVITAMINCODEsupsup/TargetedNutrientFormulas/ RAWVitaminC/tabid/1646/Default.aspx
- Emergen-C ™: www.emergenc.com

- Country Life Acerola: www.countrylifevitamins.com/productdetails.php?product_id=420
- Innate Response Formulas ™: Digestive Enzymes Clinical Strength: www.innateresponse.com/category-s/53.htm
- Garden Life ™ RAW Enzymes: www.gardenoflife.com/Products-for-Life/RAW-Digestion.aspx
- Enzymus Medical Devigest ADS: www.enzymus.com/devigest
- Wobenzym ™PS: www.douglaslabs.com/wobenzymps
- Serracor NK: www.astenzymes.com/systemic-enzymes-therapy
- Enzymus Neprinol AFD: www.enzymus.com/neprinol
- Digital Blood Microscopy: www.astenzymes.com/sites/default/files/Serracor-NK_SEBkinase_Study.pdf

Chapter 19: Move the Body—Move the Qi

- Spring Forest Qi Gong: www.springforestqigong.com
- Tai Chi for Arthritis: www.taichiforarthritis.com
- Cellerciser: www.cellercise.com
- Interview with David Hall, creator of Cellercise: www.karenkan.com/radiocellercise
- Meridian Stretching: www.thegeniusofflexibility.com
- Bob Cooley: www.thegeniusofflexibility.com/bob-cooley
- Videos on Meridian Stretching: www.youtube.com/playlist?list=PL9C50ED4CA71D2A05
- Certified Meridian Stretching Trainer: https://www.thegeniusofflexibility.com/trainer-locator/
- Yoga: www.yogajournal.com
- Bikram Yoga: www.bikramyoga.com
- Ashtanga/Power Yoga: www.ashtanga.com
- Kundalini Yoga: www.3ho.org
- Hatha Yoga: www.en.wikipedia.org/wiki/Hatha_Yoga
- Iyengar Yoga: www.bksiyengar.com
- Restorative Yoga: www.yogajournal.com/basics/991
- Chi (Qi) Walking: www.chiwalking.com
- Chi Running: www.chirunning.com

- Permanent Pain Cure:http://astore.amazon.com/ imacupuncture-20/detail/0071627138

Chapter 20: Sleep Well to Heal Well

- LifeWave Y-Age Aeon Anti-Stress Patch: www.lifewave.com/yage-aeon.asp
- "ADD & Understanding Brainwaves": www.centerforadd-az. com/resources/understanding-brainwaves.html
- Sleep Hygiene Document by Center of Clinical Interventions: www.cci.health.wa.gov.au/docs/Info-sleep%20hygiene.pdf
- Sleep Medications: www.talkaboutsleep.com/sleep-disorders/ archives/insomnia_drjacobs_benzodiazepine.htm
- Earthing: www.earthing.com
- Magnesium Miracles That Can Help You Sleep: www. drcarolyndean.com/2012/12/magnesium-makes-me-sleep
- LifeWave Silent Nights Patches: www.lifewave.com/silentnights.asp
- LifeWave Silent Nights MD Video: www.youtube.com/watch?v =ehpD79KQvi0&feature=youtu.be
- How to Use the Silent Night Patches Video: www.youtube. com/watch?v=NhIeZqoqYBg&feature=youtu.be
- LifeWave Y-Age Carnosine Patches: www.lifewave.com/yage-carnosine.asp
- Delta Wave Music: www.neuroacoustic.com/sleepenhancement.html
- Traditional Yogic Breathing: www.spiritvoyage.com/blog/index. php/right-and-left-nostril-breathing-easy-and-effective-pranayama
- Baby Bounce Technique on Cellerciser: www.youtube.com/watch? v=OaFGZoGG7J4&feature=share&list=PLAD7F44BCA1C30087
- "Corpse" Yoga Pose: www.yogajournal.com/poses/482
- Electromagnetic Smog: www.electromagnetichealth.org
- Greenwave Filters: www.karenkan.com/products/greenwave-emf-filters
- Clean Sweep: http://store.energytoolsint.com/e_commerce/show_category/15
- Energy Tools International: http://energytoolsint.com

Section D: Your Spirit: Healing Through Your Higher Self

Chapter 22: Does Pain Serve a Purpose?

- Judith Orloff, MD: www.drjudithorloff.com
- "Wounded Healer" Archetype: www.myss.com/library/contracts/three_archs.asp
- Healing Adventures: www.healingadventures.com
- Pat Jones: www.healingadventures.com/healing-practitioners/pat
- 'Still Here: Embracing Changing, Aging and Dying" by Ram Dass: http://ramdass.hostedbywebstore.com
- Ram Dass: http://ramdass.org

Chapter 23: Self-Acceptance

- Uhe Desensitizing Method: www.uhemethod.com
- Tapping: www.karenkan.com/tappingsolution

Chapter 24: The Gift of Being Present

- Deepak Chopra, MD: www.chopra.com/aboutdeepak
- Eckart Tolle: www.eckharttolle.com
- Carolyn Myss: www.myss.com
- Pema Chodron: www.pemachodron.org
- Neale Donald Walsh: www.nealedonaldwalsch.com
- GP Walsh: www.conversationswithg.com
- GP Walsh's Complimentary Introductory Course: www.karenkan.com/justallowit

Chapter 25: BodyWisdom™

- Lion Goodman: www.beliefcloset.com/about/about
- BodyWisdom™: www.TransformYourBeliefs.com

Chapter 26: Everything Happens for a Reason

- Bladder Tumor Disappears Within Minutes During Healing;
  Science of Miracles Movie:
  http://www.hayhouse.com/details.php?ref=99&id=4022
- Neale Donald Walsch: www.nealedonaldwalsch.com
- MADD (Mothers Against Drunk Driving): www.madd.org
- Louise Hay: www.louisehay.com
- Crystal Andrus: www.crystalandrus.com

Chapter 27: Forgiveness

- Eldon Taylor: www.eldontaylor.com
- TAT (Tapas Acupressure Technique): www.karenkan.com/TAT
- T. Harv Eker: www.harveker.com
- "The Shadow Effect" by Debbie Ford: www.theshadoweffect.com
- Debbie Ford: www.debbieford.com
- Tonglen Buddhist Meditation:
  www.shambhala.org/teachers/pema/tonglen1.php

Chapter 28: Intuition in Healing

- LifeWave Y-Age Aeon Patches: www.lifewave.com/yage-aeon.asp
- Synchronicities: www.en.wikipedia.org/wiki/Synchronicity
- "Awakening Intuition" by Mona Lisa Schulz, MD, PhD:
  www.drmonalisa.com/products
- "Your Intuitive Advisor" by Mona Lisa Schulz, MD, PhD:
  www.drmonalisa.com/products
- "The Intuitive Way" by Penney Peirce: www.penneypeirce.com
- Mona Lisa Schulz, MD, PhD: www.drmonalisa.com
- "The Circle" by Laura Day:
  www.howtoruletheworldfromyourcouch.com/?cat=6
- "Practical Intuition" by Laura Day:
  www.howtoruletheworldfromyourcouch.com/?cat=6
- Laura Day: www.practicalintuition.com

- September 11th, 2001: www.en.wikipedia.org/wiki/September_11_attacks
- "Vanishing Bees" Movie: www.vanishingbees.com
- Judith Orloff, MD: www.drjudithorloff.com/about-judith-orloff.htm
- Applied Kinesiology: www.appliedkinesiology.com
- "How to Test Brain Balance Using Muscle Testing" Video: www.youtube.com/watch?v=mGfPntF-7d8&feature=youtu.be
- Touch4Health: www.touch4health.com/techniques.html
- Uhe Method: www.uhemethod.com
- Tapping: www.karenkan.com/tappingsolution
- Tapas Acupressure Technique : www.karenkan.com/TAT
- Self-Muscle Testing: www.youtube.com/watch?v=cMfOC7YW_qE&feature=share&list=PLA45770859227C218

Section E: Getting Support

Chapter 29: Assemble Your Support Team

- "Heidi" Film: www.en.wikipedia.org/wiki/Heidi
- Facebook: www.Facebook.com
- LinkedIn: www.LinkedIn.com
- Pinterest: www.Pinterest.com
- Twitter: www.Twitter.com
- MeetUp: www.MeetUp.com
- Dr. Karen Kan Facebook Page: www.facebook.com/DrKarenKan

Chapter 30: Other Healing Modalities

- Find a Practitioner Near You: www.MedicalAcupunture.org
- Association of Physician Acupuncturist: www.acufinder.com
- Alexander Technique: www.amsatonline.org
- The Body Code: www.bodycodehealingsystem.com

- Bowen Technique: www.BowTech.com
- Craniosacral Therapy: www.Upledger.com
- Chiropractic & Applied Kinesiology: www.icak.com
- Dynamic Neural Retraining Program: www.DNRsystem.com
- Feldenkrais Method: www.feldenkraisinstitute.com
- The Healing Codes: www.thehealingcodes.com
- Healing Touch: www.HealingTouchProgram.com
- Integrative Manual Therapy (IMT): www.instituteofimt.com
- Matrix Energetics: www.matrixenergetics.com
- Therapeutic Massage: www.AMTA.org
- Osteopathy: www.academyofosteopathy.org
- Quantum Neurology radio interview: www.karenkan.com/radioquantumneurology
- Quantum Neurology Rehabilitation System: www.quantumneurology.com
- Reconnective Healing: www.thereconnection.com
- Reflexology: www.reflexology-usa.org or www.reflexology-uk.net/site
- Reiki: www.reiki.org
- Healing Adventures: www.healingadventures.com
- Rolfing: www.Rolf.org
- SomaticsTM: www.somatics.org
- Trager Work: www.Trager.com
- Zero Balancing: www.ZeroBalancing.com